Neurotransmitter Release

The Neuromuscular Junction

Neurotransmitter Release: The Neuromuscular Junction

This publication has been reprinted from a special issue of the *Cell Biology International Reports*, Volume **13**, Number 12, December 1989
and from
Volume **14**, Number 1, January 1990

Neurotransmitter Release

The Neuromuscular Junction

edited by

Francesco Clementi
Department of Pharmacology,
University of Milan,
Milano, Italy

and

Jacopo Meldolesi
Department of Pharmacology,
University of Milan, and
Scientific Institute S. Raffaele,
Milano, Italy

ACADEMIC PRESS
Harcourt Brace Jovanovich, Publishers
London San Diego New York
Boston Sydney Tokyo Toronto

ACADEMIC PRESS LIMITED
24/28 Oval Road
LONDON NW1 7DX

United States Edition published by
ACADEMIC PRESS INC.
San Diego, CA 92101

This book is printed on acid-free paper

British Library Cataloguing in Publication Data

Neurotransmitter release.
1. Man. Physiology
I. Clementi, F.
612.82
ISBN 0-12-176460-5

Printed in Great Britain by W. & G. Baird Ltd., Antrim

ORDER NUMBER

PO NYAATP08

BOOK NUMBER

9639468

BAY NUMBER

380-5

AUTHOR	Clementi, F.
TITLE	Neurotransmitter Release: The Neuromuscular Junction

DESCRIPTION

This is an ex-library book and may have the usual library/used-book markings inside.This book has soft covers. In good all round condition.

Contributors

C. R. Bader *Division de Neurophysiologie Clinque, Hôpital Cantonal, Genève, Switzerland*

M. Bähler *Laboratory of Molecular and Cellular Neuroscience, The Rockefeller University, New York, USA*

A. Becchetti *Department of General Physiology and Biochemistry, University of Milan, 20133 Milano, Italy*

F. Benfenati *Institute of Human Physiology, University of Modena, Modena Italy*

L. Bertollini *Department of General Physiology and Biochemistry, University of Milan, 20133 Milano, Italy*

G. Bonanno *Istituto di Farmacologia e Farmacognosia, Università degli Studi di Genova, Viale Cembrano 4, 16148 Genova, Italy*

F. Bonzelius *AK Neurochemie, Zoologisches Institut der J. W. Goethe-Universität, Siesmayerstr. 70, D-6000 Frankfurt am Main, Federal Republic of Germany*

G. Brooker *Department of Biochemistry, 3900 Reservoir Road, N.W., Washington, D.C. 20007, U.S.A.*

P. L. Cameron *Department of Cell Biology, School of Medicine, Yale University, New Haven, CT 06510, U.S.A.*

P. De Camilli *Section of Molecular Neurobiology, School of Medicine, Yale University, New Haven, CT 065120, U.S.A.*

L. Campanati *"Bruno Ceccarelli" Center for the Study of Peripheral Neuropathies and Neuromuscular Diseases, CNR Center of Cytopharmacology, Department of Pharmacology, University of Milano Medical School, Italy*

E. Carbone *Department of Anatomy and Human Physiology, I-10125 Torino, Italy*

S. Cereser *Department of Peripheral Nervous System Research, Fidia Research Laboratories, Abano Terme (PD), Italy*

G. Ceresoli *"E. Trabucchi" Department of Pharmacology, University of Milano, Italy*

F. Clementi *Department of Medical Pharmacology, Ctr. Cytopharmacology CNR, I-20129 Milano, Italy*

S. Consolo *"Mario Negri" Institute, Milano, Italy*

E. Costa *FIDIA-Georgetown Institute for the Neurosciences, 3900 Reservoir Road, N.W., Washington, D.C. 20007, U.S.A.*

G. de Erausquin *FIDIA-Georgetown Institute for the Neurosciences, 3900 Reservoir Road, N.W., Washington, D.C. 20007, U.S.A.*

G. Favaro *Department of Peripheral Nervous System Research, Fidia Research Laboratories, Abano Terme (PD), Italy*

M. Favaron *FIDIA-Georgetown Institute for the Neurosciences, 3900 Reservoir Road, N.W., Washington, D.C. 20007, U.S.A.*

A. Ferroni *Department of General Physiology and Biochemistry, University of Milan, 20133 Milano, Italy*

R. Fesce *CNR Center of Cytopharmacology and "Bruno Ceccarelli" Center, Department of Pharmacology, University of Milano, Italy*

M. G. Fiori *Department of Peripheral Nervous System Research, Fidia Research Laboratories, Abano Terme (PD), Italy*

A. Formenti *II Institute of Human Physiology, I-20152 Milano, Italy*

H. M. Gerschenfeld *Laboratoire de Neurobiologie, Ecole Normale Supérieure, 46, rue d'Ulm, 75230 Paris Cedex 05, France*

P. Greengard *Laboratory of Molecular and Cellular Neuroscience, The Rockefeller University, New York, U.S.A.*

F. Di Gregorio *Department of Peripheral Nervous System Research, Fidia Research Laboratories, Abano Terme (PD), Italy*

G. Grohovaz *CNR Center of Cytopharmacology and "Bruno Ceccarelli" Center, Department of Pharmacology, University of Milano, Italy*

A. Groppetti *"E. Trabucchi" Department of Pharmacology, University of Milano, Italy*

A. Guidotti *FIDIA-Georgetown Institute for the Neurosciences, 3900 Reservoir Road, N.W., Washington, D.C. 20007, U.S.A.*

C. Haimann *CNR Center of Cytopharmacology and "Bruno Ceccarelli" Center, Department of Pharmacology, University of Milano, Italy*

C. Hammond *Section of Neurobiology and Behavior, Seeley Mudd Hall, Cornell University, Ithaca, N.Y. 14583, U.S.A.*

R. Harris-Warrick *Section of Neurobiology and Behavior, Seeley Mudd Hall, Cornell University, Ithaca, N.Y. 14583, U.S.A.*

A. Henkel *AK Neurochemie, Zoologisches Institut der J. W. Goethe-Universität, Siesmayerstr. 70, D-6000 Frankfurt am Main, Federal Republic of Germany*

J. Heuser *Department of Cell Biology and Physiology, Washington University School of Medicine, St. Louis, Missouri 63110, U.S.A.*

W. P. Hurlbut *Rockefeller University 1230 York Ave., New York, N.Y. 10021, U.S.A.*

M. Israel *Laboratoire de Neurobiologie Cellulaire et Moléculaire, CNRS, 91198 Gif sur Yvette Cedex, France*

A. Janetzko *AK Neurochemie, Zoologisches Institut der J. W. Goethe-Universität, Siesmayerstr. 70, D-6000 Frankfurt am Main, Federal Republic of Germany*

T. Kanaseki *Tokyo Metropolitan Institute for Neurosciences, 2–6 Musashidai, Fuchu City, Tokyo, Japan*

B. Lesbats *Laboratoire de Neurobiologie Cellulaire et Moléculaire, CNRS, 91198 Gif sur Yvette Cedex, France*

A. Mallart *Unité de Physiologie Neuromusculaire, Laboratoire de Neurobiologie Cellulaire et Moléculaire, CNRS, 91198 Gif sur Yvette, France*

H. Manev *FIDIA-Georgetown Institute for the Neurosciences, 3900 Reservoir Road, N.W., Washington, D.C. 20007, U.S.A.*

M. Marchi *Istituto di Farmacologia e Farmacognosia, Università degli Studi di Genova, Viale Cembrano 4, 16148 Genova, Italy*

M. Matteoli *Department of Cell Biology, School of Medicine, Yale University, New Haven, CT 06510, U.S.A.*

G. Maura *Istituto di Farmacologia e Farmacognosia, Università degli Studi di Genova, Viale Cembrano 4, 16148 Genova, Italy*

P. C. Molenaar *Department of Pharmacology, Sylvius Laboratory, Wassenaarseweg 72, 2333 Al Leiden, The Netherlands*

F. Navone *CNR Center of Cytopharmac. and Dept. Medical Pharmac., University of Milano, Italy*

M. Parenti *"E. Trabucchi" Department of Pharmacology, University of Milano, Italy*

D. Paupardin-Tritsch *Laboratoire de Neurobiologie, Ecole Normale Supérieure, 46, rue d'Ulm, 75230 Paris Cedex 5, France*

A. Pollo *Department of Anatomy and Human Physiology, I-10125 Torino, Italy*

M. Raiteri *Istituto di Farmacologia e Farmacognosia, Università degli Studi di Genova, Viale Cembrano 4, 16148 Genova, Italy*

E. Sher *Department of Medical Pharmacology, Ctr. Cytopyharmacoplogy CNR, I-20129 Milano, Italy*

M. Solimena *Department of Cell Biology, School of Medicine, Yale University, New Haven, CT 06510, U.S.A.*

A. Suzuki *Laboratoire du Métabolisme de la Nutrition des Plantes, CNRA, 78026 Versailles Cedex, France*

F. T. Tarelli *"Bruno Ceccarelli" Center for the Study of Peripheral Neuropathies and Neuromuscular Diseases, CNR Center of Cytopharmacology, Department of Pharmacology, University of Milano Medical School, Italy*

F. Valtorta *Laboratory of Molecular and Cellular Neuroscience, The Rockefeller University, New York, U.S.A.*

A. Villa *"Bruno Ceccarelli" Center for the Study of Peripheral Neuropathies and Neuromuscular Diseases, CNR Center of Cytopharmacology, Department of Pharmacology, University of Milano Medical School, Italy*

W. Volknandt *AK Neurochemie, Zoologisches Institut der J. W. Goethe-Universität, Siesmayerstr. 70, D-6000 Frankfurt am Main, Federal Republic of Germany*

A. Volterra *Department of Pharmacology, Center for Neurobiology and Behaviour, Howard Hughes Medical Institute, Columbia University, New York, N.Y. 10032, U.S.A.*

E. Wanke *Department of General Physiology and Biochemistry, University of Milan, 20133 Milan, Italy*

V. P. Whittaker *Arbeitsgruppe Neurochemie, Max-Planck-Institut für biophysikalische Chemie, Postfach 2841, D-3400 Göttingen, Federal Republic of Germany*

H. Zimmermann *AK Neurochemie, Zoologisches Institut der J. W. Goethe-Universität, Siesmayerstr. 70, D-6000 Frankfurt am Main, Federal Republic of Germany*

Preface

This book comprises the contributions presented at a small meeting organized in the University of Milan to honour Bruno Ceccarelli*. Bruno was born in Torino in 1938. His scientific adventure started as a young medical student when in 1961 he joined the laboratory of Cell Pharmacology (at that time Electron Microscopy) at the Institute of Pharmacology of the University of Milano. After his MD graduation in 1963 he tried first to combine basic research and surgery; practising with considerable success in a suburban hospital. Then he decided on research and was named Assistant Professor in 1968. In 1970 he moved to New York to join the laboratory of Electrophysiology at the Rockefeller University headed by Alex Mauro. He spent two years there, also interacting with the Cell Biology laboratory of George Palade. He established a most fruitful collaboration with Alex's colleague W. Paul Hurlbut which continued up to the day Bruno died; every year Bruno spent time in New York and Paul in Milano. After returning to Milano Bruno was first named acting Professor of General Physiology and then full Professor of Pharmacology. In 1983 he became the Director of the Center for the Experimental Study of Peripheral Neuropathies and Neuromuscular Diseases, a University venture supported in part by the FIDIA Research Foundation, which is now named after him. During the night of July 7/8, 1988 Bruno died suddenly after a standard working day in which he interacted – as usual – with a number of colleagues, including both of us.

Bruno's research interests were precisely focused on basic neurobiology. After pioneer studies on the plasticity of neuronal differentiation he became interested in the structure and functioning of the neuromuscular junction, and spent the rest of his career characterizing the process of neurotransmitter release. Taken as a whole, the results obtained by Bruno and his colleagues represent the strongest available support for the widely accepted "vesicle hypothesis" of neurotransmitter release, i.e. the interpretation of presynaptic physiology that identifies the electrophysiological unitary event; the miniature endplate potential as the result of the discharge of an individual synaptic vesicle. In this area Bruno's paper with Paul Hurlbut and Alex Mauro in 1973 first demonstrated (together with another paper by John Heuser and Tom Reese, appearing in the same issue of JCB) that vesicles fuse and recycle at the neuromuscular junction. We have chosen one of those early micrograph composites for the front cover of this volume. A few years later he shed light on the relationship between fusing vesicles and the sites of the plasma membrane specifically equipped for fusion, the active zones, and finally (in 1985) demonstrated by the use of quick freezing the temporal coincidence (within 1 ms) of vesicle fusions and the development of the endplate potential following a single nerve stimulus. In the last years Bruno focused part of the work of his group on the kinetics and mechanisms of the vesicle membrane recycling and obtained important results on the specificity of the

* Bruno Ceccarelli Memorial Symposium on NEUROTRANSMITTER RELEASE: THE NEUROMUSCULAR JUNCTION, a satellite of the 12th European Neuroscience Meeting organized by the Department of Pharmacology, University of Milano, the CNR Center of Cytopharmacology, the Bruno Ceccarelli Association for Scientific Research and the FIDIA Research Foundation. Milano September 2–3, 1989.

membrane interactions involved (see also the contributions of Grohovaz *et al.* and Valtorta *et al.*, this volume). Finally, he greatly contributed to the understanding of the action of various presynaptically active compounds, such as α-latrotoxin, the black widow spider toxin that irreversibly stimulates transmitter release.

As always happens with gifted and dedicated scientists, Bruno's work was profoundly influenced by his personality and ideas. In our opinion his contribution to the laboratory was outstanding, due essentially to his three main human and scientific qualities. Firstly, Bruno was a high class experimentalist; his initial experience as a surgeon certainly helped him to carry out demanding experiments. Much more important, however, was his enthusiasm for completeness and technical perfection. We know that most of the people who had the chance to collaborate with Bruno were impressed and surprised by the large number of high quality results he always had available to support his ideas, and by his profound understanding of the technological aspects of laboratory work. Many times Bruno's interest in detail proved to be essential for solving scientific problems, as he was usually able to consider their importance within the general framework of his work. Secondly, Bruno was an excellent teacher of both medical students and colleagues in the laboratory. For many years we collaborated with Bruno in teaching at the medical school; we know how dedicated he was to this work, and how much the students (and we too) learned from him. At least as important was Bruno's interaction with the rest of his laboratory. The high quality work of Bruno's younger colleagues, which was presented at the memorial meeting (and is therefore reported in this volume), clearly demonstrates that his "school" was stimulating, comprehensive and fruitful. Last, but not least, Bruno was a gentleman. Those who over the years had the chance to interact with him, either in collaboration or in scientific competition, including two participants of this meeting, his "archrival" John Heuser (see Heuser's contribution in this volume), and Maurice Israel, who support ideas on neuromuscular junction physiology at least partially incompatible with Bruno's, were happy to acknowledge his personal and intellectual fairness. Being Bruno's closest scientific friends we can only confirm these independent judgements.

This is what we wanted to say about Bruno. The meeting was intended to gather together as many scientists who had been directly in touch with Bruno as possible, and to discuss together problems of Bruno's interest. Unfortunately, a number of Bruno's friends were unable to come including Alex Mauro, who was severely ill (he died last October). Alex however did participate in absentia. His letter, which is published in part on p. xv, was in fact read at the beginning of the meeting. Other friends who couldn't come, but we would like to thank for their interest, are Bernard Katz, Paul Greengard, Rodolfo Llinas and Ricardo Miledi. The others came, and did a superb job, which the reader can now judge from the published contributions. We, the organizers and Bruno's closest friends, can only thank them all for having beautifully honoured his memory, both from the human and the intellectual point of view.

Thanks again.

Francesco Clementi and Jacopo Meldolesi

CONTENTS

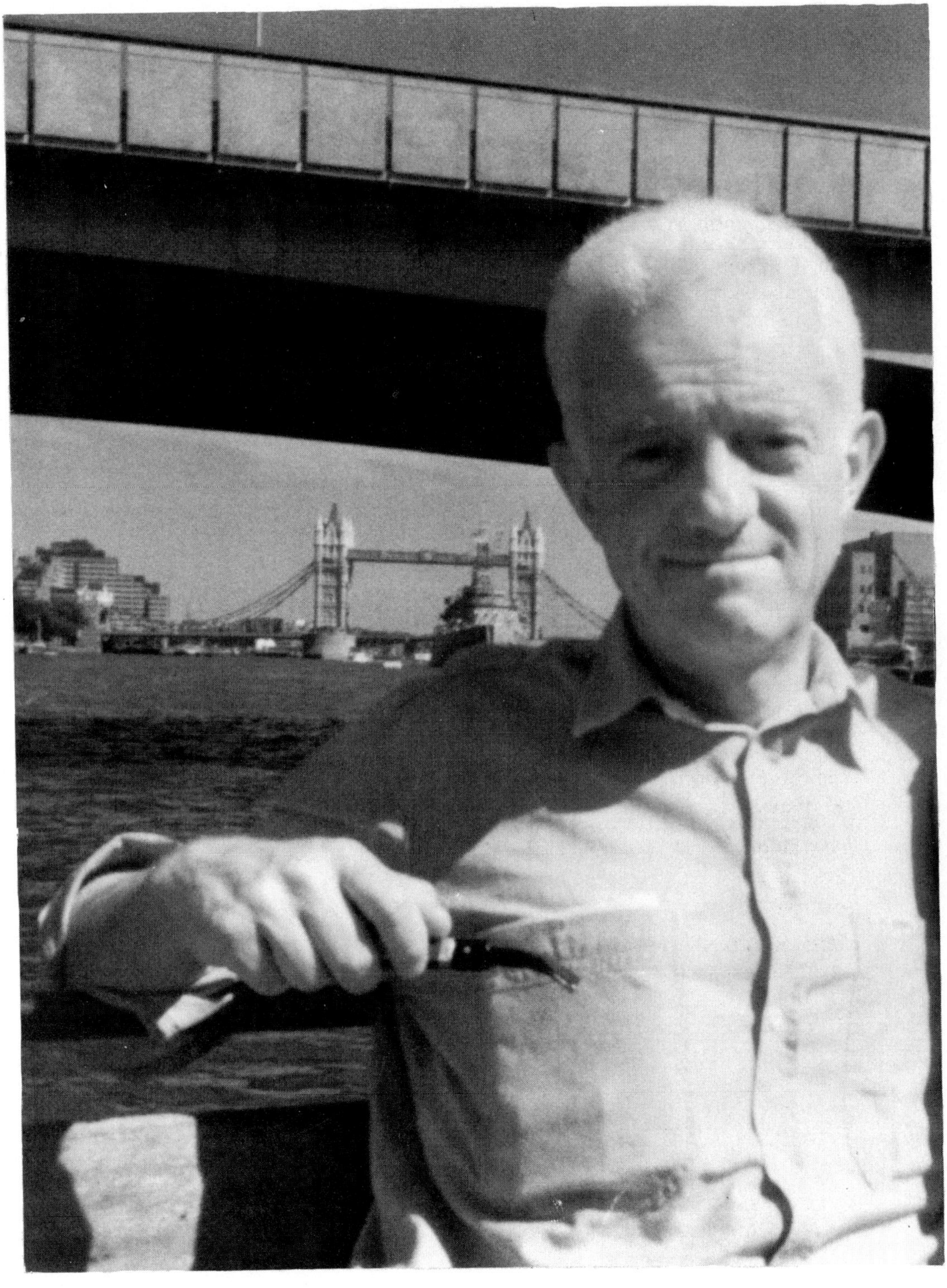

Bruno Ceccarelli
1938–1988

from the letter of Alex Mauro

Dear Friends:

I am deeply honoured and very moved to be with you, at least in spirit, to pay tribute to our dear friend and colleague, Bruno.

It seems, in some strange way, as if our memorable meeting in the summer of 1969, Bruno, Serenella and myself, at the Stazione Zoologica in Naples occurred only recently. This was our first meeting, which opened the way to a long association of friendship and scientific collaboration. (Alex then summarized the work carried out in his laboratory, in particular the two papers with Allen Clark on the release-depletion effect of the black widow spider venom at the frog neuromuscular junction). The papers captured Bruno's imagination and thus set the stage for his long-range interest in the cell biology of vesicle dynamics. This was the topic that would challenge his talents as an electron microscopist of the highest standards and drive him on to become an outstanding neurobiologist.

The wonderful collaboration with my colleague, Dr. Paul Hurlbut, is well known to experts in this field of research and has given rise to a series of exemplary papers reporting on the details of vesicle release at the nerve terminal by a variety of agents including the spider venom. Bruno's expertise as an electron microscopist and cell biologist and Paul's expertise as a biophysicist have yielded new and fundamental data on a basic mechanism in cell biology, namely, vesicle dynamics.

I wish the Bruno Ceccarelli Memorial Meeting every success with its awesome and provocative collection of papers. It is a fitting tribute to Bruno's commitment to basic science. And, of course, I send my best wishes to Bruno's colleagues for their continued success in their new laboratory which was built as a result of Bruno's tireless efforts.

Bruno personified the totally devoted scientist balanced by unfailing generosity and kindness. We shall remember him always.

Alexander Mauro
Professor of Biophysics
Rockefeller University

Secretory Organelles of Neurons and their Relationship to Organelles of Other Cells

M. Matteoli*[1], F. Navone+, C. Haimann+, P.L. Cameron*, M. Solimena*+ and P. De Camilli*#[2]

*Department of Cell Biology and #Section of Molecular Neurobiology, Yale Univ. School of Medicine, New Haven, CT 06510, USA; +CNR Center of Cytopharmac. and Dept. of Medical Pharmac., Univ. of Milano, Italy;

Neurons are highly specialized secretory cells that deliver signal molecules (neurotransmitters) to the extracellular space by regulated exocytosis. This idea was first established in the 1950's when electrophysiologists discovered the quantal nature of neurotransmitter release (Del Castilio and Katz, 1956) and electron microscopists the presence of a homogeneous population of microvesicles (small synaptic vesicles [SSVs]) about 50 nm in diameter in nerve endings (De Robertis and Bennett, 1955; Robertson, 1956; Palay, 1956). Studies carried out over the following 20 years have provided compelling evidence supporting the hypothesis that SSVs are the storage sites for quanta of neurotransmitters (Ceccarelli and Hurlbut, 1980; Torri-Tarelli et al. 1985).

Until 15 years ago or so, only a very short list of neurotransmitter molecules were known, and nearly all of them were non-peptide molecules (the so-called "classical neurotransmitters") (Hökfelt et al. 1980). These molecules can be synthesized and/or loaded into vesicles in nerve terminals and this is consistent with the property of synaptic vesicles to undergo local exo-endocytotic recycling at the axonal ending (Ceccarelli et al. 1973; Heuser and Reese, 1973). A few neurons, such as the hypothalamic neurons projecting to the neurohypophysis, were known to secrete peptides via secretory granules reminiscent of secretory granules in endocrine cells. These neurons release their products into the blood like endocrine cells, and were thought to represent a very special type of neurons (Scharrer and Scharrer, 1954).

This simplified view has now been replaced by one in which individual neurons are seen as cells capable of secreting a cocktail of peptide and non-peptide neurotransmitters via at least two distinct types of secretory organelles. SSVs are thought to contain classical neurotranmsitters only. Peptide neurotransmitters are packaged in a separate population of vesicles, which have a larger diameter (> 60nm) and an electron-dense core (large dense core vesicles [LDCVs]) (Hökfelt et al. 1984; Coulter, 1988; Matteoli et al. 1988). LDCVs may also contain amine neurotransmitters (Klein et al. 1982). In contrast to SSVs that can be reloaded with content in nerve terminals, LDCVs can only be assembled and loaded with secretory peptides in the perikaryal-dendritic region of neurons where the rough endoplasmic reticulum and the Golgi complex are localized (Russel, 1987). The relative proportion of LDCVs to SSVs varies from terminal to terminal. For example, LDCVs are relatively

---

[1] Dr. Matteoli's permanent address is: Istituto Fisiologia Centri Nervosi del CNR, Milano, Italy

[2] To whom correspondence should be addressed

abundant in nerve terminals of the hypothalamus. In general, however, they are much less numerous than SSVs, and in sections of most terminals just one or a few of such vesicles are visible. For this reason, LDCVs have not received much attention from cellular neurobiologists until recently.

The discovery that two types of secretory organelles can coexist in neurons has raised new important questions in the field of neurosecretion. For example: what is the biogenetic relationship between the two organelles?; is exocytosis of the two organelles controlled by the same stimulus-secretion coupling mechanism?; how are these organelles related to secretory organelles of other cells?

The present chapter summarizes work that has been carried out in our laboratory to answer some of these questions. This work, together with parallel or complementary studies carried out by other laboratories, has suggested that SSVs and LDCVs are organelles of two distinct secretory pathways involved in two distinct types of neuronal signalling.

SSVs and LDCVs have a distinct membrane composition

SSVs, which are very abundant in the brain, can be prepared with a high degree of purity (Huttner et al. 1983). This has greatly helped in the elucidation of the biochemical properties of their membranes. Several major membrane proteins which are common to all SSVs have already been purified and thoroughly characterized. Some of the major properties of these proteins are summarized below.

The synapsins. Synapsin I (Ia and Ib) and synapsin II (IIa and IIb) represent a family of highly homologous neuron-specific proteins. They are the product of two primary mRNA transcripts which are alternatively spliced to generate the a and b isoforms (Südhof et al. 1989b). They are associated with the cytoplasmic surface of SSVs (Navone et al. 1984), and recent evidence suggests that this association may involve both hydrophilic as well as hydrophobic interactions (Benfenati et al. this volume). Synapsin I has been shown also to bind actin with high affinity (Bahler and Greengard, 1987). For these reasons synapsin I is thought to act as a link protein between SSVs and the actin-based cytoskeletal matrix of nerve terminals. It may be involved in the clustering of SSVs at presynaptic sites. Recent electron microscopic studies carried out by a quick-freezing/deep-etching technique have provided additional support to this hypothesis (Hirokawa et al. 1989). The binding of synapsin II to the cytoskeleton has not been investigated so far. However, the strong similarity between synapsin II and synapsin I in the regions which are thought to interact with the cytoskeleton suggests that synapsin II might play a similar role.

Synapsin I and synapsin II are substrates for endogenous phosphorylation regulated by cAMP and Ca^{++} in mammalian brain. The state of phosphorylation of synapsin I has been shown to affect its binding to both SSVs and the cytoskeleton. Physiological and pharmacological manipulations that facilitate or promote neurotransmitter release also result in an increased state of phosphorylation of the synapsins (reviewed in De Camilli and Greengard 1986). Synapsin I and synapsin II may provide a regulated link between SSVs and the cytoskeleton, thus controlling one or more of the steps that lead(s) to synaptic vesicle exocytosis.

Synaptophysin. Synaptophysin (protein p38) is an intrinsic membrane glycoprotein of 38 kDa with four putative transmembrane domains and an extended, proline-rich, cytoplasmic carboxy-tail (Südhof et al. 1987; Leube et al. 1987). Two interesting features of this molecule include the property to bind Ca^{++} (Rehm et al. 1986) and the ability to form hexameric complexes with ion channel properties in lipid bilayers (Thomas et al. 1988). In addition, synaptophysin is a major endogenous substrate for a tyrosine kinase activity present on SSVs (Pang et al. 1988).

Synaptobrevin. Synaptobrevin is an intrinsic membrane protein of 18 kDa (Baumert et al. 1989). It has a single putative transmembrane domain with a cytoplasmic, proline-rich, amino-terminal and an extremely short lumenal carboxy-terminal (Südhof et al. 1989a). The aminoacid sequence of synaptobrevin is highly conserved through evolution. Mammalian synaptobrevin is highly homologous to a protein of the Drosophila nervous system (Südhof et al. 1989a) and is almost identical to VAMP-1 and VAMP-2, two proteins recently identified in vesicles of Torpedo (Trimble et al. 1988, Elferink et al. 1989).

Other proteins. Other characterized intrinsic membrane proteins of SSV membranes include protein p65, SV2 and protein p29 (Matthew et al., 1981; Buckley et al. 1985; Baumert et al. 1990). The primary amino acid sequence of these proteins remains to be determined. Protein p29 shares with synaptophysin immunological similarities and the property to undergo endogenous tyrosine-phosphorylation in SSVs (Baumert et al. 1990).

All of these proteins are present on virtually all SSVs irrespective of the specific neurotransmitter they contain. In the case of proteins that can exist in several isoforms (synapsin, synaptobrevin/VAMP-1), different nerve terminals may contain different isoforms or different ratios of the various isoforms (Südhof et al. 1989b; Elferink et al. 1989). In contrast, at least four of these proteins, synapsin (I and II), synaptophysin, synaptobrevin and p29 are not present at significant concentration in the membranes of LDCVs (Navone et al. 1984; Navone et al. 1986; Baumert et al. 1989; Baumert et al. 1990). The localization of p65 and SV2 in brain LDCVs has not been investigated so far.

These findings indicate the existence of major differences in the membrane composition of SSVs and LDCVs although some similarities also may exist. Homogeneous preparations of brain LDCVs have not been obtained to date. However, some information is available on the membrane composition of LDCVs of peripheral sympathetic neurons (Klein et al. 1982) and of nerve terminals of the neurohypophysis (see below). A protein that is likely to be present both on SSVs and on LDCVs is a proton pump of the vacuolar type. Furthermore, in catecholaminergic neurons, proteins involved in the transport and metabolism of catecholamines are likely to be shared by both SSVs and LDCVs (Johnson, 1987).

The existence of major differences in the composition of SSVs and LDCVs suggests an independent biogenesis of SSVs and LDCVs and speaks against the hypothesis, proposed by other investigators, that SSVs originate in nerve terminals as an endocytic by-product of exocytosed LDCVs (Lowe et al. 1988). In addition, these differences may partially account for the different traffic, life-cycle and regulated release (see below) of SSVs and LDCVs.

The special case of nerve terminals of the neurohypophysis. As mentioned above, the only known function of nerve terminals of the neurohypophysis is to secrete peptide neurohormones into the blood. Accordingly, they are densely populated by very large LDCVs. In addition, nerve terminals of the neurohypophysis also contain microvesicles which resemble SSVs of other nerve terminals. The function of these vesicles is unknown. It has been suggested that they represent endocytic vesicles involved in the retrieval of neurosecretory granule membranes following their exocytosis (Nagasawa et al. 1971). Recent studies carried out in our laboratories have shown that such microvesicles have several membrane proteins in common with SSVs of presynaptic nerve endings, and that these membrane proteins are not present at a detectable concentration in the membranes of the LDCVs which contain the neurohypophyseal hormones (Navone et al. 1989). These results demonstrate that the two types of neuronal vesicles coexist also in nerve terminals which are thought to be specialized for the secretion of neuroactive peptides. On the basis of these findings, and of the increasing evidence that all nerve terminals may secrete peptides in addition to classical neurotransmitters, we hypothesize that the two secretory pathways involving SSVs and LDCVs coexist in all neurons, and that their expression represents an obligatory and distinctive feature of neuronal differentiation.

Differential exocytosis of SSVs and LDCVs

Pharmacological studies have suggested that the relative proportion of peptide and classical neurotransmitters released from a same nerve ending varies with the frequency of stimulation, high frequency stimulation being more effective for the release of peptides (Andersson et al. 1982, Lündberg and Hökfelt, 1983). In addition, a lower LDCV/SSV ratio has been seen in some terminals after high frequency stimulation (Lynch, 1980).

A difference in the stimulus-secretion mechanisms for SSVs and LDCVs is also suggested by studies on the subtypes of Ca^{++} channels involved in neurotransmitter release. Results of these studies have raised the possibility that different types of Ca^{++} channels play a dominant role in the release of classical and peptide neurotransmitters (Rane et al. 1987; Hirning et al. 1988).

A direct demonstration that exocytosis of LDCVs and SSVs can be dissociated has been recently provided by us with experiments carried out at the frog neuromuscular junction involving the use of α-latrotoxin (Matteoli et al. 1988). Until recently, frog motor nerve terminals were thought to secrete only a classical neurotransmitter, acetylcholine, via SSVs. We have found, however, that these terminals also contain the neuroactive peptides Calcitonin-Gene-Related-Peptide (CGRP) and Substance P. These peptides are stored in the few LDCVs which are interspersed among the numerous SSVs (in resting nerve terminals the ratio of LDCVs to SSVs is about 1:100) (Matteoli et al. 1988; Matteoli et al. 1989). Secretion of these peptides at the frog neuromuscular synapses has not been directly demonstrated until now. However, the demonstration that CGRP exerts a modulatory and trophic role on muscle cells, and a modulatory role on the response of muscle to acetylcholine, strongly suggests that LDCVs release neuroactive peptides that act as physiological co-transmitters at the frog neuromuscular junction (Mulle et al. 1988; Fontaine et al. 1987; Akasu et al. 1983).

α-latrotoxin is the main toxin of black widow spider venom (Meldolesi et al. 1986) and is an agent known to trigger a massive, Ca^{++}-independent, exocytosis of SSVs and to produce a complete depletion of SSVs from nerve

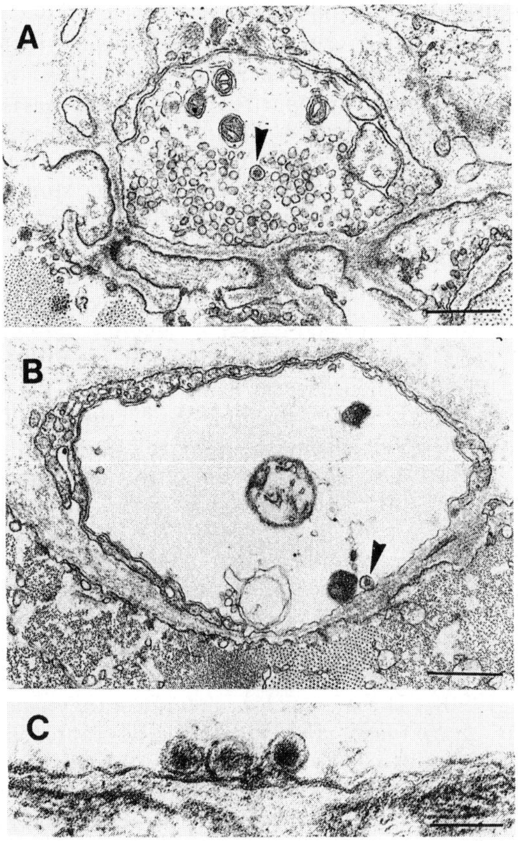

Fig.1. Differential effect of α-latrotoxin on the release of SSVs and of LDCVs at the frog neuromuscular junction. a shows a cross-section of a control nerve terminal. b and c show cross-sections of nerve terminals treated with α-latrotoxin in Ca^{++}-free solution at room temperature for 1 hr. The terminal shown in a is densely populated by SSVs. The terminals shown in b and c are completely depleted of SSVs, but LDCVs are still present. LDCVs are indicated by arrowheads in b and c. (reprinted from Matteoli et al. 1988, with permission of the National Academy of Sciences, USA) (calibration bars = a, 340 μm; b, 529 μm; c, 178 μm)

endings (Hurlbut and Ceccarelli, 1979). We found that the massive depletion of SSVs produced by the toxin is not accompanied by any relevant decrease in the LDCVs content within the same nerve terminals (fig. 1). This different effect of the toxin on the release of SSVs and LDCVs was seen both when the toxin was applied in the presence or in the absence of extracellular Ca^{++} (Matteoli et al.1988). Although α-latrotoxin represents a non-physiological stimulus, these results are consistent with the hypothesis that the exocytotic machineries for SSVs and LDCVs are at least partially different.

Strong evidence indicates that exocytosis of both SSVs and of LDCVs is triggered by a raise in cytosolic Ca^{++}. Exocytosis of the two vesicle types, however, may exhibit a different sensitivity to cytosolic Ca^{++}, or a different sensitivity to the rate of Ca^{++} rise. In addition, exocytotic sites for the two types of vesicles may have a different topological relation to sites of Ca^{++} entry. This is consistent with the observation that SSV exocytosis takes place selectively at active zones (Torri-Tarelli et al. 1985), while LDCV exocytosis takes place preferentially away from active zones

(Thureson Klein et al. 1988) (for a thorough discussion of how a rise in cytosolic Ca^{++} produced in nerve terminals by plasma membrane depolarization may result in a differential effect on SSV and LDCV exocytosis, see the review by Smith and Augustine, 1988).

Relationship of SSVs to organelles of other cells

Many peptide neurotranmsitters are also secreted by endocrine cells as hormones. Accordingly, LDCVs resemble secretory granules of endocrine cells in morphology, biochemical properties and biogenesis, and can be considered the equivalent organelles in neurons of secretory granules in endocrine cells (Johnson, 1987). SSVs, in contrast,are often thought of as organelles specific to nerve terminals. Yet, recent studies carried out by our laboratory have suggested that microvesicles related to SSVs are present in endocrine cells. We and others have found that the major intrinsic membrane proteins of SSVs identified so far, namely synaptophysin, synaptobrevin, SV2, p65 and p29 are present also in a variety of endocrine cells (Wiedenman and Franke, 1985; Navone et al. 1986; Baumert et al. 1989; Buckley and Kelly, 1985; Matthew et al. 1981; Baumert et al. 1990). Our findings that, in neurons, at least some of these proteins (possibly all of them) are not present at significant concentration in the membranes of LDCVs, prompted us to investigate their subcellular distribution in endocrine cells. So far we have investigated the subcellular distribution of synaptophysin and of p29 (Navone et al. 1986; Baumert et al. 1990).

By using electron microscopy immunocytochemistry and subcellular fractionation we have found that both proteins in endocrine cells are localized on a population of microvesicles which are scattered throughout the cytoplasm and are present at particularly high concentration in the region of the trans-Golgi network, in close proximity of centrosomes (Navone et al. 1986; Baumert et al. 1990). These vesicles undergo exocytosis, are rapidly labeled by extracellular peroxidase and most likely represent organelles which undergo exo-endocytotic cycles (Johnston et al. 1989)(fig. 2a and 2b). Since these properties, as well as their size, are reminiscent of SSVs, we refer to them as synaptic-like microvesicles (SLMVs) (De Camilli and Jahn, 1990). We did not find any significant concentration of either protein in the membranes of mature secretory granules, although a study by another group has raised the possibility that a small pool of synaptophysin might be present in the membranes of the granules (Lowe et al. 1988). One important difference between SSVs and SLMVs is that the latter do not have any synapsin associated with their membranes, since neither synapsin I nor synapsin II are present at detectable concentrations in endocrine tissues. As mentioned earlier, the synapsins might play a role in the clustering of SSVs at release sites. Lack of the synapsins from SLMVs might therefore be related to the different localization of SSVs and SLMVs in the cell cytoplasm. SLMVs are primarily concentrated at the Golgi centrosomal region of the cell rather than under the plasmalemma. The function of SLMVs remains to be determined.

These results have suggested the possibility that SSVs may represent the neuronal adaptation of an organelle present also in endocrine cells, the SLMVs. Such a finding, in turn, has raised the question of whether SLMVs may represent the endocrine cell-specific adaptation of a vesicular pathway of all cells. As a first step towards answering this question, we have studied the fate of synaptophysin when expressed by cDNA transfection in a fibroblastic cell line (Johnston et al. 1989). The rationale behind this approach was that if a related compartment exists in all cells, synaptophysin might be targeted to this organelle and be used as a tool to identify it.

We expressed synaptophysin in a fibroblastic cell line (chinese hamster ovary [CHO] cells) and subsequently investigated the fate of this protein in transfected cells by immunocytochemistry and subcellular fractionation. We found that both the pattern of glycosylation and the

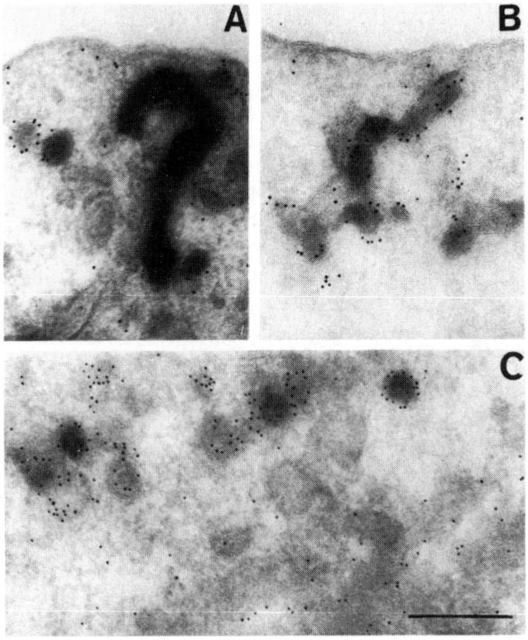

Fig. 2. Immunogold localization of synaptophysin in undifferentiated PC12 cells, which naturally express the protein (a and b) and in CHO cells which express it as a result of cDNA transfection (c). Both PC12 and CHO cells have been exposed for one hour to horseradish peroxidase before fixation to label endocytic compartments. In both cell types synaptophysin, as visualized by gold particles, is localized on microvesicles. Some of them are also positive for the endocytic tracer. Large vacuoles labeled by the endocytic tracer (probably lysosomes and large endosomes) are negative for synaptophysin immunoreactivity. Note also lack of gold labeling on the plasmalemma (from Johnston et al. 1989, reprinted with permission of IRL Press) (calibration bar = 200 nm).

half-life of the protein was similar in CHO cells and in undifferentiated PC12 cells that naturally express the protein. In addition, synaptophysin in CHO cells was found to be localized on a population of microvesicles which resemble SLMVs in several ways, including morphology, intracellular distribution and the property to become labeled by extracellular tracers (fig. 2c) (Johnston et al. 1989). To determine whether synaptophysin induces the formation of a new organelle or is targeted to a pre-existing organelle, we compared the distribution of synaptophysin with that of markers for a variety of organelles. These experiments have led to the demonstration of a striking similarity in morphology, intracellular distribution and partitioning in sucrose density gradients of synaptophysin-positive microvesicles and of the microvesicles which recycle the transferrin receptor (Johnston et al. 1989 and our unpublished observations). Currently, we are investigating whether in endocrine cells SLMVs also coincide with the vesicular pathway which recycles the transferrin receptor.

These findings suggest a possible evolution of SSVs from a recycling pathway expressed by all cells and distinct from the classical regulated secretory pathway of eukaryotic cells which involves secretory granules.

Concluding remarks

LDCVs and SSVs are secretory organelles of two distinct regulated pathways of neurons which are specialized in two distinct types of neuronal signalling (fig. 3). The pathway which operates via LDCVs is a pathway specialized for the delivery of modulatory signals. The occurrence of LDCV exocytosis primarily away from active zones suggests that the function of this secretory pathway is to modulate a microenvironment of the neuropile rather than a precise post-synaptic

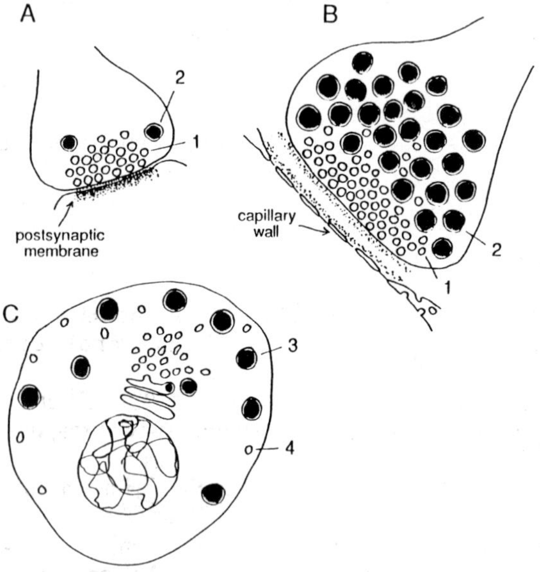

Fig. 3. Skematic drawing illustrating the relationship between secretory organelles of neurons and of endocrine cells. Nerve endings contain two types of vesicles, SSVs (1) and LDCVs (2), which represent the secretory organelles of two distinct secretory pathways. These two organelles coexist not only in typical pre-synaptic nerve endings (A), but also in nerve endings which secrete into the blood stream such as the nerve endings of the neurohypophysis (B). LDCVs are the equivalent organelles in neurons of secretory granules (3) of endocrine cells (C). SSVs are biochemically related to a population of microvesicles (4) of endocrine cells (synaptic-like microvesicles, SLMVs). The function of SSVs in nerve endings of the posterior pituitary and of SLMVs in endocrine cells remains to be determined (from Navone et al. 1989, reprinted with permission of The Journal of Cell Biology,the Rockefeller University Press)

site. The time-scale of effects produced by neuropeptides (Kuffler, 1980) is compatible with a secretory machinery which operates in a time-range more typical of endocrine secretion (seconds) than of synaptic transmission (milliseconds). This pathway appears to be the equivalent of the well established "regulated" secretory pathway of endocrine cells.

The pathway which operates via SSVs is a pathway primarily, although not exclusively, specialized for speed and topological precision, i.e. for the fast point-to point intercellular communication typical of the nervous system. SSV secretion occurs at active zones and can be turned on and off in the time-scale of a millisecond. The trigger for SSV exocytosis may be a very high, but also a very localized and transient raise in Ca^{++} concentration (Smith and Augustine, 1988). The synapsins may play an important regulatory role on this secretion by regulating availability of SSVs for exocytosis. Since SSVs can be reformed in nerve terminals by local recycling, the exocytotic rate of these vesicles can largely exceed the supply rate of new SSVs to the nerve terminal. "Fast" neurotransmitters that act on ligand-regulated ion channels typical of post-synaptic specializations are secreted via this pathway. Our findings suggest that this pathway may represent the amplification and the neuronal adaptation of a vesicular pathway which is also present in endocrine cells. In addition, they raise the possibility that such a pathway might be closely related to a recycling vesicular pathway present in all cells.

The two pathways of neuronal secretion involving SSVs and LDCVs cooperate in confirring upon the nervous system the property to propagate information at high speed and to undergo longer-lasting plastic changes.

Acknowledgments

Part of the work summarized in this manuscript has been supported by grants from MDA and from the Italian National Research Council to PDC and by the Fidia Research Foundation.

REFERENCES

Akasu, T., Kojima, M. and Koketsu, K. (1983) Substance P modulates the sensitivity of the nicotinic receptor in amphibian cholinergic transmission. Br. J. Pharmacol. **80**: 123-131.

Andersson, P. O., Bloom, S. R., Edwards, A. V. and Järhult, J. (1982) Effects of stimulation of the chorda tympani in bursts on submaxillary responses in the cat J. Physiol., **322**: 469-483.

Bähler, M., and Greengard, P. (1987) Synapsin I bundles F-actin in a phosphorylation-dependent manner. Nature, **326**: 704-707.

Baumert, M., Maycox, P. R., Navone, F., De Camilli, P., and Jahn, R. (1989) Synaptobrevin: an integral membrane protein of 18,000 Dalton present in small synaptic vesicles of rat brain. EMBO J., **8**: 379-384.

Baumert, M., Takei, K., Hartinger, J., Burger, P.M., Fischer, G., Maycox, P.R., De Camilli P. and Jahn, R. (1990) P29, a novel tyrosine-phosphorylated membrane protein present in small clear vesicles of neurons and endocrine cells. J. Cell Biol. in press.

Buckley, K. and Kelly, R.B. (1985) Identification of a transmembrane glycoprotein specific for secretory vesicles of neural and endocrine cells. J. Cell Biol. **100**: 1284-1294.

Ceccarelli, B., Hurlbut, W. P., and Mauro, A. (1973) Turnover of transmitter and synaptic vesicles at the frog neuromuscular junction J. Cell Biol., **57**: 499-524.

Ceccarelli, B. and Hurlbut, W.P. (1980) Vesicle hypothesis of release of quanta of acetylcholine. Physiol.Rev. **60**: 396-441.

Coulter, H. D. (1988) Vesicular localization of immunoreactive (Met5) enkephalin in the globus pallidus. Proc. Natl. Acad. Sci. USA, **85**: 7028-7032.

De Camilli, P., and Greengard, P. (1986) Commentary. Synapsin I: a synaptic vesicle associated neuronal phosphoprotein. Biochem. Pharm., **35**: 4349-4357.

De Camilli, P. and Jahn, R., (1990) Pathways to regulated exocytosis in neurons. Ann.Rev.Physiol. **52** in press.

Del Castillo, J. and Katz, B. (1956) Biophysical aspects of neuromuscular transmission. Prog. Biophys. Chem. **6**: 121-170.

De Robertis, E.D.P., and Bennett, H.S. (1955) Some features of the submicroscopic morphology of synapses in frog and earthworm. J. Biophys. Biochem. Cytol. **1**: 47-63.

Elferink, L.A., Trimble, W.S. and Scheller, R.H. (1989) Two vesicle-associated membrane protein genes are differentially expressed in the rat central nervous system. J. Biol. Chem. **264**: 11061-11064.

Fontaine, B., Klarsfeld, A., and Changeux, J. P. (1987) CGRP and muscle activity regulate acetylcholine sensitivity in cultured myotubes. J. Cell Biol., **105**: 1337-1342.

Heuser, J. E., and Reese, T. S. (1973). Evidence for recycling synaptic vesicle membrane during transmitter release at the frog neuromuscular junction. J. Cell Biol., **57**: 315-344.

Hirning, L. D., Fox, A. P., McCleskey, E. W., Olivera, B. M., Thayer S.A., Miller, R., and Tsien, R. W. (1988) Dominant role of N-type Ca++ channels in evoked release of norepinephrine from sympathetic neurons. Science, **239**: 57-61.

Hirokawa, N., Sobue, K., Kanda, K., Harada, A., and Yorifuji, H. (1989) The cytoskeletal architecture of the presynaptic terminal and molecular structure of synapsin I. J. Cell Biol., **108**: 111-126.

Hökfelt T., Johansson, O., Ljungdahl, Å., Lundberg, J. M., and Schultzberg, M. (1980) Peptidergic neurones. Nature, **284**: 515-521.

Hökfelt, T., Johansson, O., and Goldstien, M. (1984) Chemical anatomy of the brain. Science, **225**: 1326-1334.

Hurlbut, W.P. and Ceccarelli, B. (1979) in Advances in Cytopharmacology, Ceccarelli and Clementi eds, Raven, New York, vol3, pp 87-115.

Huttner, W. B., Schlieber, W., Greengard, P., and De Camilli, P. (1983) Synapsin I (protein I), a nerve terminal specific phosphoprotein. III Its association with synaptic vesicles studied in a highly purified synaptic vesicles preparation. J. Cell Biol., **96:** 1374-1388.

Johnson, R.G. (1987) Cellular and Molecular Biology of Hormone- and Neurotransmitter-Containing Secretory Vesicles. Ann. New York Acad. Sci. vol **493**, pp 1-590.

Johnston, P.A., Cameron, P.L., Stukenbrok, H., Jahn, R., De Camilli, P. and Sudhof, T.C. (1989) Synaptophysin expressed in CHO cells is targeted to microvesicles analogous to those of PC12 cells. EMBO J. **8**; 2863-2872.

Klein, R., Lagercrantz, H. and Zimmermann, H. (1982) Neurotransmitter vesicles. Academic Press, 1-375.

Kuffler, S.W. (1980) Slow synaptic responses in autonomic ganglia and the pursuit of a peptidergic transmitter. J. Exptl. Biol. **89**: 257-286.

Leube, R.E., Kaiser, P., Seiter, A., Zimbelmann, R., Franke, W.W., Rehm, H., Knaus, P., Prior, P., Betz, H., Reinke, H., Beyreuther, K., and Wiedenmann, B. (1987) Synaptophysin: molecular organization and mRNA expression as determined from cloned cDNA. EMBO J., **6**: 3261-3268.

Lowe, A.W., Madeddu, L., and Kelly, R.B. (1988) Endocrine secretory granules and neuronal synaptic vesicles have three integral membrane proteins in common. J. Cell Biol., **106**: 51-59.

Lundberg, J. M., and Hokfelt, T. (1983) Coexistence of peptides and classical neurotransmitters. Trends Neurosci., **6**: 325-333.

Lynch, K. (1980) Stimulation-induced reduction of large dense core vesicle numbers in cholinergic motor nerve endings. Brain Res., **194**: 249-254.

Matteoli, M., Haimann, C., Torri-Tarelli, F., Polak, J. M., Ceccarelli, B., and De Camilli, P. (1988) Differential effect of α-latrotoxin on exocytosis of ACh-containing small synaptic vesicles and CGRP-containing large dense core vesicles at the frog neuromuscular junction. Proc. Natl. Acad. Sci. USA, **85**: 7366-7370.

Matteoli, M., De Camilli, P. and Haimann C. (1989) Substance P immunoreactivity in frog motor nerve terminals. Neuroscience Abstr. **15**, 562.

Matthew, W.D., Tsavaler, L. and Reichardt, L.F. (1981) Identification of a synaptic vesicle specific membrane protein with a wide distribution in neuronal and neurosecretory tissues. J. Cell Biol. **91**: 257-269.

Meldolesi, J., Scheer, H., Madeddu, L., and Wanke, L. (1986) On the mechanism of action of alpha-latrotoxin, the presynaptic stimulatory toxin of the black widow spider venom. Trends Pharmac. Sci., **7**: 151-155.

Mulle, C., Benoit, P., Pinset, C., Roa, M. and Changeux, J.P. (1988) Calcitonin gene related peptide enhances the rate of desensitization of the nicotinic ACh receptor in cultured mouse muscle cells. Proc. Natl. Acad. Sci. USA **85**: 5728-5732.

Nagasawa, J., Douglas, W.W., and Schulz, R.A. (1971) Micropinocytotic origin of coated and smooth microvesicles (synaptic vesicles) in neurosecretory terminals of posterior pituitary glands demonstrated by incorporation of horseradish peroxidase. Nature **232**: 341-342.

Navone, F., Greengard, P., and De Camilli, P. (1984) Synapsin I in nerve terminals: selective association with small synaptic vesicles. Science, **226**: 1209-1211.

Navone, F., Jahn, R., Di Gioia, G., Stukenbrok, H., Greengard, P., and De Camilli, P. (1986) Protein p38: an integral membrane protein specific for small vesicles of neurons and neuroendocrine cells. J. Cell Biol., **103**: 2511-2527.

Navone, F., DiGioia, G., Browning, M., Greengard, P. and De Camilli P. (1989) Microvesicles of the neurohypophysis are biochemically related to small synaptic vesicles of presynaptic nerve terminals. J. Cell Biol. in press.

Palay, S.L. (1956) Synapses in the central nervous system. J. Biophys. Biochem. Cytol., 2 suppl, 193-202.

Pang, D., Wang, J., Valtorta, F., Benfenati, F., and Greengard, P. (1988) Protein tyrosine-phosphorylation in synaptic vesicles. Proc. Natl. Acad. Sci. USA, **85**: 762-766.

Rane, S., Holz, G.G. and Dunlap, K. (1987) Dihydropiridine inhibition of neuronal calcium current and Substance P release. Pflugers Arch. **409**: 361-366.

Rehm, H., Wiedenmann, B., and Betz, H. (1986) Molecular characterization of synaptophysin, a major calcium-binding protein of the synaptic vesicle membrane. EMBO, **5**: 535-541.

Robertson, J.D. (1956) The ultrastructure of reptilian myoneural junction. J. Biophys. Biochem. Cytol., **2**, 381-393.

Russell, J. T. (1987) The secretory vesicle in processing and secretion of neuropeptides. Current Topics in Membranes and Transport, **31**, 277-312.

Scharrer, E. and Scharrer, B. (1954) Hormones produced by neurosecretory cells. Recent Progr. Hormone Res., **10**:183-240.

Smith, S. and Augustine, G.J. (1988) Calcium ions, active zones and synaptic transmitter release. Trends Neurosci., **11**: 458-465.

Südhof, T. C., Lottspeich, F., Greengard, P., Mehl, E., and Jahn, R. (1987) A synaptic vesicle protein with a novel ctytoplasmatic domain and four transmembrane regions. Science, **238**: 1142-1144.

Südhof, T. C., Baumert, M., Perin, M. S., and Jahn, R. (1989a) A synaptic vesicle membrane protein is conserved from mammals to Drosophila. Neuron, **245**: 1474-1480.

Südhof, T.C., Czernik, A.J., Kao, M., Takei, K., Johnston, P., Horiuchi, A., Wagner, M., Danazir, S.D., Perin, M.S., De Camilli, P. and Greengard, P. (1989) The synapsins: mosaics of shared and unique domains in a family of synaptic vesicle phosphoprotein. Science **245**: 1474-1480.

Thomas, L., Hartung, K., Langosch, D., Rehm, H., Bamberg, E., Franke, W. W., and Betz, H. (1988) Identification of synaptophysin as a hexameric channel protein of the synaptic vesicle membrane. Science, **242**: 1050-1053.

Thureson-Klein, Å. K., Klein, R. L., Zhu, P. C., and Kong, J. Y. (1988) Differential release of transmitters and neuropeptides co-stored in central and peripheral neurons. In: "Cellular and molecular basis of synaptic transmission", Zimmermann, H. ed., Springer Verlag, Berlin., 137-151.

Torri-Tarelli, F., Grohovaz, F., Fesce, R., and Ceccarelli, B. (1985) Temporal coincidence between synaptic vesicle fusion and quantal secretion of acetylcholine. J. Cell Biol., **101**: 1386-1399.

Trimble, W. S., Cowan, D. M., and Scheller, R. H. (1988) VAMP I: a synaptic vesicle-associated integral membrane protein. Proc. Natl. Acad. Sci. USA, **85**: 4538-4542.

Wiedenmann, B. and Franke, W.W. (1985) Identification and localization of synaptophysin, an integral membrane glycoprotein of M 38,000 characteristic of presynaptic vesicles. Cell **41**: 1017-1028.

THE SYNAPTIC VESICLE MEMBRANE: ORIGIN, AXONAL DISTRIBUTION, PROTEIN COMPONENTS, EXOCYTOSIS AND RECYCLING.

Herbert Zimmermann, Walter Volknandt, Andreas Henkel, Frank Bonzelius, Alfred Janetzko and *Toku Kanaseki

AK Neurochemie, Zoologisches Institut der J.W. Goethe-Universität, Siesmayerstr. 70, D-6000 Frankfurt am Main, Federal Republic of Germany and *Tokyo Metropolitan Institute for Neurosciences, 2-6 Musashidai, Fuchu City, Tokyo, Japan.

ABSTRACT - The paper discusses functional and molecular aspects of the synaptic vesicle membrane during its life cycle. The distribution of the synaptic vesicle membrane compartment in an entire cholinergic neuron is monitored using colloidal gold labelling and a monoclonal antibody against the synaptic vesicle membrane protein SV2. This provides new insights concerning vesicle origin and fate in the various compartments of the neuron. A new synaptic vesicle membrane protein (svp25) of Mr 25,000 with properties similar to synaptophysin as well as a synaptic vesicle binding phosphoprotein of the presynaptic membrane (Mr 92,000) likely to be involved in vesicle exocytosis are described. The membrane compartment recycled on induced transmitter release contains synaptic vesicle but not plasma membrane markers and encloses both newly synthesized transmitter and a sample of extracellular medium.

Most types of neurons contain in their nerve terminals at least two types of vesicles which differ with regard to their appearance in the electron-microscope. Vesicles with an electron-dense core (dense-cored vesicles) are thought to store peptides and in some cases also neurotransmitter whereas the small electron-lucent vesicles store mainly low molecular weight substances in soluble form. The two types of vesicles may differ with regard to their origin, their molecular properties, the patterns of neuronal activation which cause release of their contents, and the synaptic release site (Walker and Agoston, 1987; Thureson-Klein et al., 1988; Zimmermann, 1988).

The electron-lucent synaptic vesicle is a specialized membrane compartment of the nerve cell accumulated in the terminal axon ramifications where it is involved in the focal release of neurotransmitter. Structural appearance, size and composition of membrane and core components may vary between individual transmitter systems. It is, however, likely that the membrane compartment of the small electron-lucent synaptic vesicle serves an identical role in the various transmitter systems and underlays the same principal mechanisms of origin, regulation and metabolic fate. This notion is supported by the increased number of membrane proteins which are found to be shared by electron-lucent vesicles in practically all types of transmitter systems (Kelly, 1988; Baumert et al., 1989).

Origin and fate of the synaptic vesicle membrane compartment monitored by immunocytochemistry

Although it is known that components of the synaptic vesicle membrane undergo orthograde and retrograde transport (Kiene and Stadler, 1987; Bööj et al., 1989),

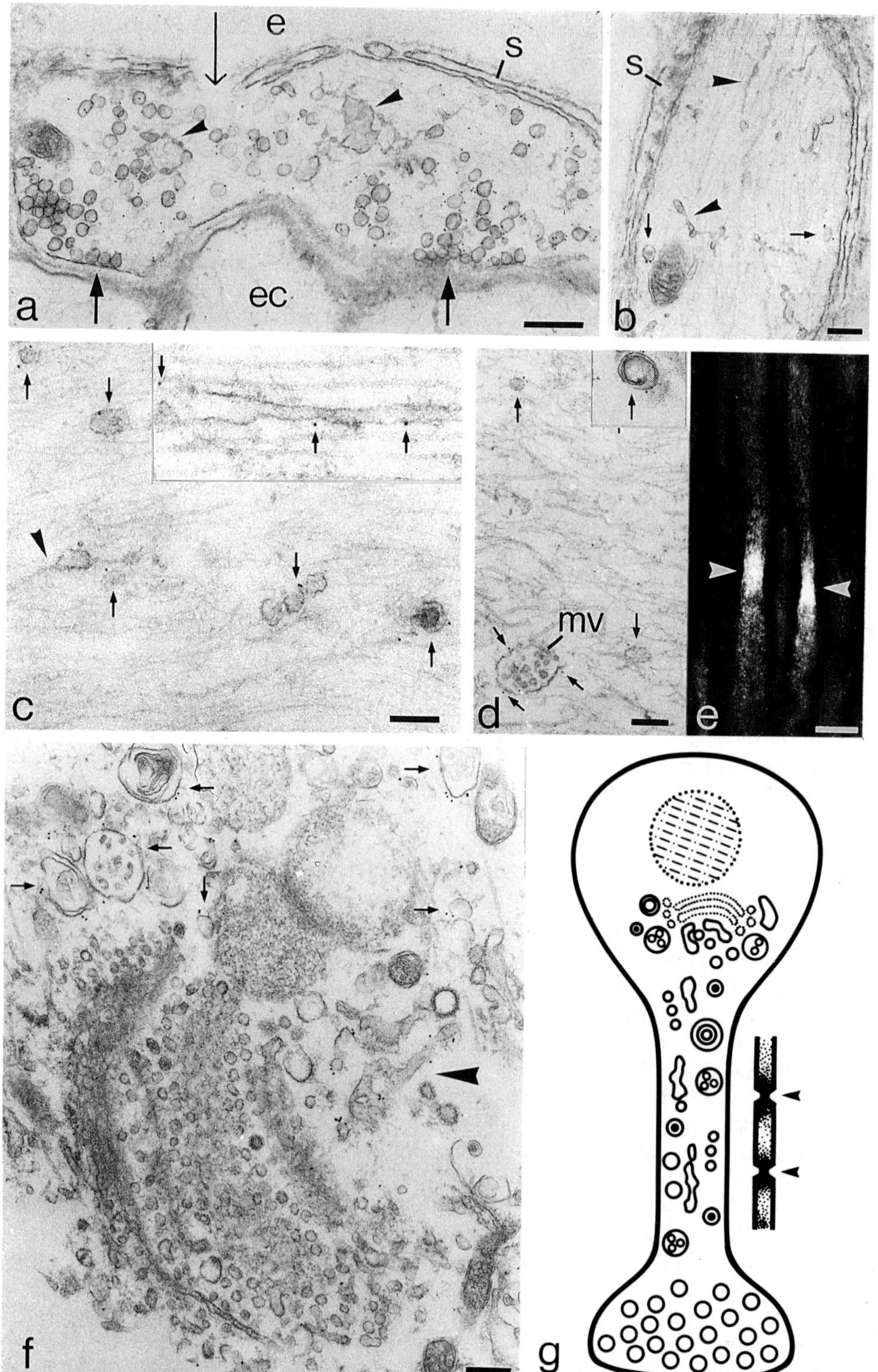
e
s
ec
a
s
b
c
mv
d
e
f
g

Fig. 1. Identification of membrane structures in the cholinergic *Torpedo* electromotor neuron which bind a monoclonal antibody against the synaptic vesicle membrane protein SV2. a) Colloidal gold labelling of nerve terminal. Binding of gold to synaptic vesicles, part of which are attached to the presynaptic membrane (arrows). Absence of labelling from elements of the axoplasmic reticulum (arrowheads). b,c,d) Labelling of a variety of axonal membrane compartments (arrows) but not of axoplasmic reticulum (arrowhead). e) Indirect immunofluorescence of axons (longitudinal section) with accumulation of labelled organelles at nodes of Ranvier (arrow heads). f) Labelling at cisternae of the *trans*-Golgi network (arrowhead) and a variety of membranous structures accumulated around the Golgi-complex (arrows). e, extracellular space between electroplaque cells; ec, postsynaptic electroplaque cell; mv, multivesicular body; s, Schwann cell process covering terminal axon branch. Bars: a,b,c,d,f = 250 nm; e = 10 μm. g) Schematic representation of intraneuronal membrane compartments with whom the synaptic vesicle compartment communicates (revealed by immunogold labelling, stippled compartments are not labelled by the antibody) and of nodal accumulation (arrow heads) of labelled membrane compartments.

---

both the site of synaptic vesicle origin and its fate after it has fulfilled its function in the nerve terminal are not clear.

Whereas synaptic vesicles are abundant in nerve terminals, corresponding membrane profiles are rare in the axon. This has led to various hypotheses regarding the origin of synaptic vesicles including their formation at nerve terminals by budding off from elements of the axoplasmic reticulum (ref. in Janetzko et al., 1989). Whereas studies using extracellular volume markers clearly revealed the retrograde axonal transport of tracers in a variety of membrane-bound organelles (Zimmermann, 1979; Feher, 1984), their relationship to the synaptic vesicle membrane compartment remains uncertain.

In order to further elucidate synaptic vesicle origin and fate we have studied the intraneuronal distribution of binding sites for a monoclonal antibody directed against a synaptic vesicle membrane protein (SV2, Buckley and Kelly, 1987, gift of Dr. Regis B. Kelly). We used the electromotor system of *Torpedo marmorata* since pericarya, axons and nerve terminals corresponding to the identical type of neuron are easily accessible. The electromotor system of electric rays is cholinergic and homologous to the vertebrate neuromuscular system. The nerve terminals in the electric organ differ, however, from terminals at neuromuscular junctions regarding the larger diameter of their synaptic vesicles, the absence of dense-cored vesicles from synaptic sites, and the absence of typical active zones involving pre- and postsynaptic specializations (Zimmermann, 1988).

Antibody-binding sites were visualized in the various compartments of the neuron using the colloidal gold technique and a preembedding protocol (Janetzko et al., 1989). In the electric organ, antibody-binding is restricted to axons and axon terminals. Synaptic vesicles are selectively labelled and may carry five or more gold particles (Fig. 1a). Only in few cases gold particles are observed at the cytoplasmic surface of the presynaptic membrane. Both, in nerve terminals and in non-synaptic parts of the axon, labelling is absent from a reticular membrane compartment likely to represent the axoplasmic reticulum (Fig. 1 a,b). This suggests that the axoplasmic reticulum is not the site of formation and presumably also retrieval of the synaptic vesicle membrane compartment.

In the axon, membrane profiles corresponding in appearance and size to synaptic vesicles are by far less frequent than in terminals. Instead, there are additional membrane-bound organelles like vesicles with a dense core, tubular structures, multivesicular bodies and lamellar bodies (Fig. 1 c,d). All these membrane compartments carry colloidal gold particles at their surface suggesting that they share all or at least part of their membrane proteins with synaptic vesicles. The axolemma, mitochondria, and elements of the axoplasmic reticulum are not labelled. Corresponding labelling of nerve terminal and axonal membrane compartments has also been obtained using an antibody against another synaptic vesicle-specific membrane protein (svp25, see below).

A variety of membrane-bound structures are involved in the retrograde axonal transport of extracellular tracers. These include multivesicular bodies, lamellar bodies and tubular membrane compartments (ref. in Janetzko et al., 1989). The widespread labelling of axonal membrane compartments observed in our study probably results from the fusion of retrogradely transported vesicles with these axonal compartments (endosomes?). It is reminiscent of the ubiquitous presence of the proton pumping ATPase in synaptic vesicles but also in other membrane-bound organelles of the cell (Cidon and Sihra, 1989). Do all these membrane compartments including the synaptic vesicles form a single cellular pool sharing their protein components?

We do not know whether the vesicles with electron-dense core represent peptide-storing granules or are lysosomal in nature.

All labelled axonal membrane compartments are accumulated intermittently at consecutive nodes of Ranvier. This can be revealed by electron-microscopical and light-microscopical (Fig. 1) immunocytochemistry (Janetzko et al., 1989; Zimmermann and Vogt, 1989). The reduction of the transverse area of the axon cylinder at the paranodes by 75% is probably involved in the nodal build up of transported organelles. The physiological implications of this phenomenon are not yet understood.

The intense labelling of the *trans*-Golgi network in the perikaryon (Fig. 1 f) suggests that this is the site of final assembly of the secretory organell "synaptic vesicle" - analogous to the formation of secretory organelles in other secretory systems. Gathered around the *trans*-side and in close proximity to the Golgi complex we find a variety of immunolabelled organelles already described for the axon: multivesicular bodies, lamellar bodies, membrane vesicles with electron-dense core of varying size and shape, but also vacuoles and peroxisomes. These organelles may be involved in the final degradation of the synaptic vesicle but possibly also in the recycling of the synaptic vesicle membrane compartment via the Golgi-complex. Fig. 1 g summarizes the observations and implies that synaptic vesicle membrane proteins may be specifically allocated to synaptic vesicles in the nerve terminal only but may be shared by a number of organelles in axon and perikaryon.

Synaptic vesicle membrane proteins

The outfit of membrane proteins enables the synaptic vesicle to fulfill all major tasks during its life cycle. These include uptake and storage of various substrates (including in some cases transmitter synthesis), the interaction with the cytoskeleton during orthograde and retrograde transport and on anchorage inside the nerve terminal, the interaction with the presynaptic plasma membrane on exocytosis, and the retrieval process after membrane fusion.

A number of these proteins have recently been identified using protein biochemical and molecular biological techniques. Although their function is often not

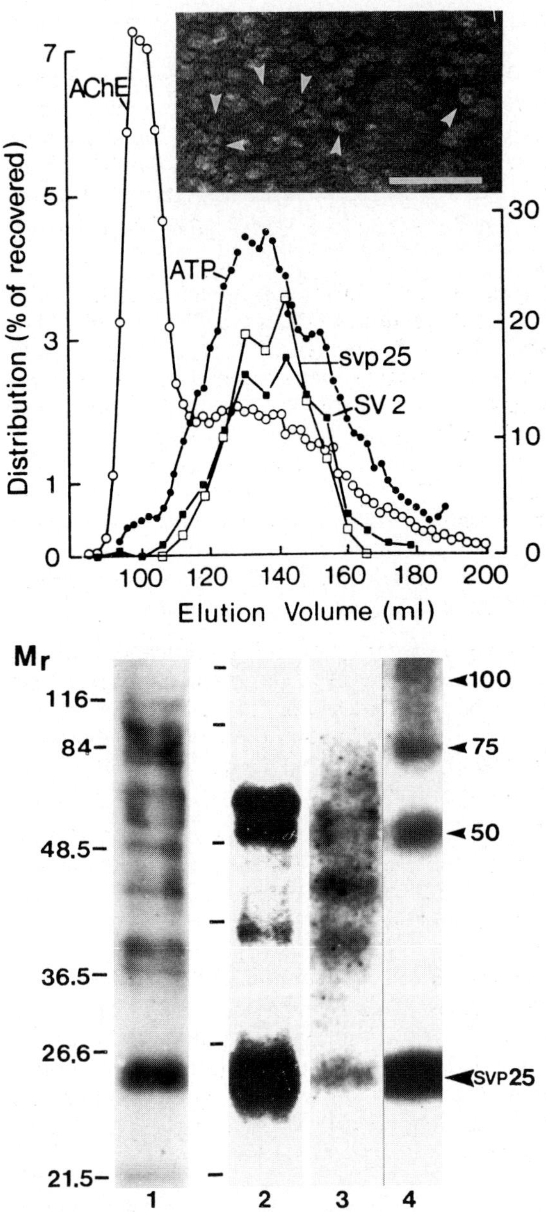

Fig. 2. Properties of svp25. Coelution with synaptic vesicles (*Torpedo* electric organ, monitored by their ATP content) and separation from acetylcholinesterase (AChE) containing larger particles on elution from a column of porous glass beads. Svp25 and SV2: distribution of the respective vesicle proteins monitored by antibody binding. Inset: Molecular complexes of svp25 with pore-like cores (arrows) visualized by negative staining; Bar = 50 nm. 1) Concanavalin A-peroxidase binding of vesicle proteins; 2) Phosphorylation of isolated svp25 in the presence of 50 μM Ca^{2+} and a cytosolic extract of the electric organ. 3) Binding of $^{45}Ca^{2+}$ to vesicle proteins; 4) Formation of homooligomers by isolated svp25 on SDS PAGE using non-reducing conditions.

known, they have proven as useful markers in cell biological studies and as diagnostic tools (Walker and Agoston, 1987; Volknandt et al., 1988; Zimmermann, 1988; Kelly, 1988). Amongst the proteins which have recently been characterized in some detail are the vesicle surface associated protein synapsin I (De Camilli and Greengard, 1986), a H^+-pumping ATPase (Cidon and Sihra, 1989), and the membrane integral protein synaptophysin (Thomas et al., 1988).

Highly purified synaptic vesicles from the *Torpedo* electric organ contain a membrane spanning glycoprotein (svp25) whose function is probably regulated by neuronal activity (Volknandt et al., 1989) (Fig. 2). On SDS PAGE svp25 migrates as a protein of Mr 25,000. It has a pI of 6.0, binds concanavalin A, is a major synaptic vesicle $^{45}Ca^{2+}$-binding protein, and becomes phosphorylated when a cytosolic extract of the electric organ containing micromolar concentrations of Ca^{2+} is added. EGTA prevents its phosphorylation. If submitted to SDS PAGE under non-reducing conditions svp25 forms homooligomers of higher molecular weight ranging to about 200 kD. On negative staining and electron-microscopical analysis svp25 displays multimolecular complexes of 7-8 nm with a pore-like core of 1-2 nm (Fig. 2 inset).

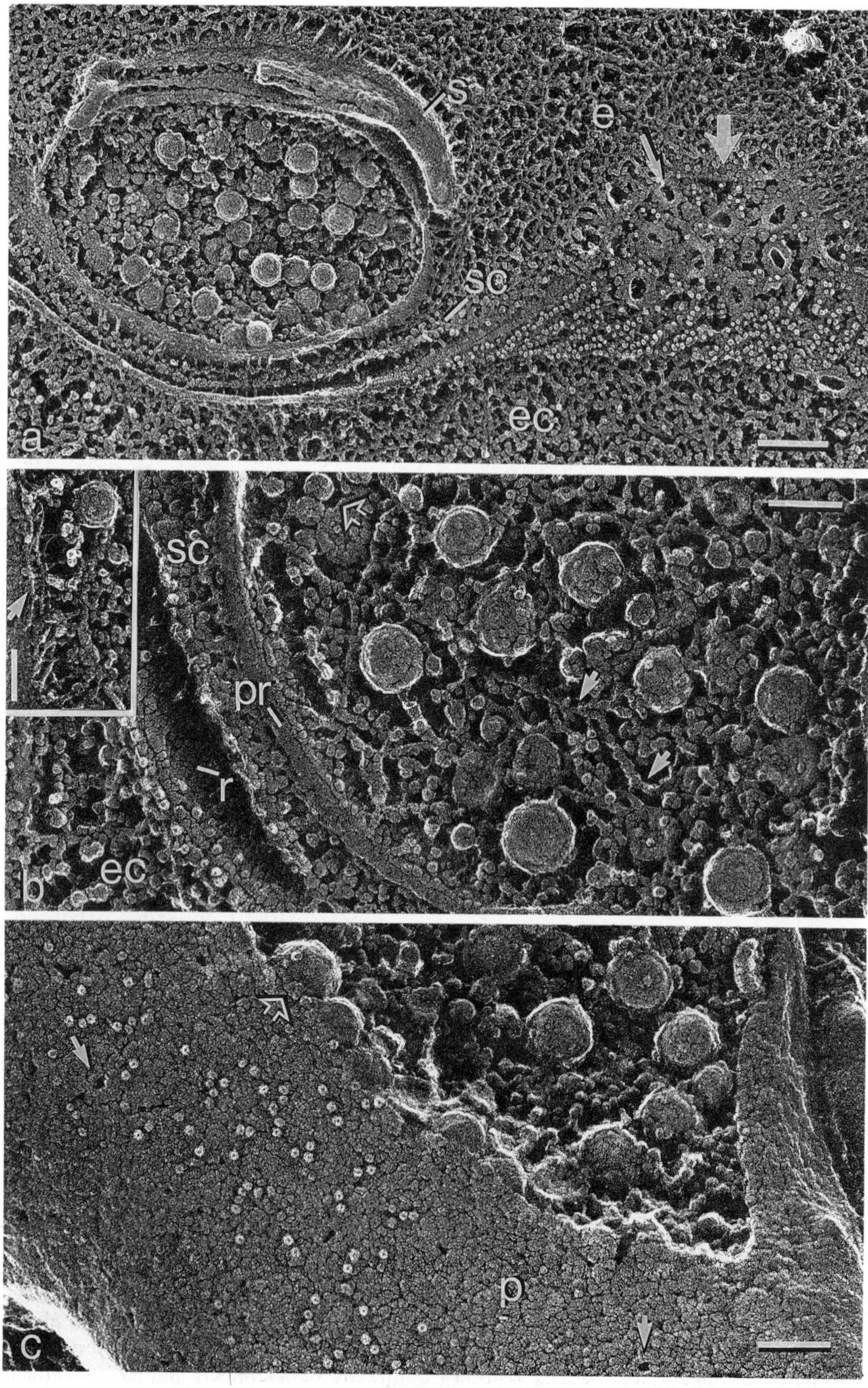
s
e
sc
ec
a
sc
pr
r
I
b
ec
p
c

Fig. 3. Molecular architecture of synaptic contact in the electric ray electric organ as revealed by quick freezing, deep etching and rotary shadowing. a) Overview with nerve terminal forming synaptic contact (*Narke japonica*). Note filaments in the cytoplasm of the postsynaptic electroplaque cell (ec) and also the filamentous character of the extracellular space (e). The basal lamina in the synaptic cleft (sc) makes filamantous attachments at the pre- and postsynaptic membranes. s, Schwann cell process covering the non-synaptic membrane of the nerve terminal. The large arrow marks a protrusion of the postsynaptic membrane with pitlike intrusions reminiscent of membrane fusion events (small arrow). This frequent postsynaptic membrane specialization may represent sites of vesicular insertion of molecular complexes (like acetylcholine receptors) into the postsynaptic membrane. b) Filaments inside the nerve terminal (*Torpedo marmorata*). Besides the narrow mesh of small interconnected filaments there are longer filaments (arrows). Filaments are connected to the presynaptic membrane (pr), to synaptic vesicles and also to the (smaller) glycogen granules (open arrow). sc, synaptic cleft with basal lamina and parallel arrays of nicotinic acetylcholine receptors (r) in a true surface view of the postynaptic membrane. ec, cytoplasm of electroplaque cell. Inset: Aspect of inner surface of presynaptic membrane with filaments attached in parallel (arrow). c) P-face view of presynaptic membrane with ring-like arrangement of intramembrane particles and direct apposition of synaptic vesicles (open arrow) (*Narke japonica*). Arrows: small holes in P-face suggestive of pulled out filamentous membrane anchors (holes are absent from the true surface of the presynaptic membrane). Bars: a = 200 nm; b,c = 100 nm.

The selective association of the protein with synaptic vesicles can also be demonstrated using a monospecific antibody and colloidal gold labelling of nerve terminals in the *Torpedo* electric organ. It is likely that a similar glycoprotein exists in synaptic vesicles isolated from either rat or bovine brain. Regarding its ability to become phosphorylated, bind Ca^{2+} and form multimolecular complexes with a pore-like core, svp25 closely resembles synaptophysin (Mr 38,000). Svp25 may serve as an ion channel, be involved in the uptake of substrates into synaptic vesicles or (as has also been suggested for synaptophysin, Thomas et al., 1988) in the process of vesicle exocytosis (comp. Fig. 4).

Morphological correlates of synaptic vesicle anchoring in the nerve terminal

Filamentous interactions of synaptic vesicles inside the axon terminal or varicosity are probably serving two mechanisms. Synaptic vesicles accumulated in the terminal are anchored within the cytoskeleton to prevent their diffusion into other parts of the axon and possibly their retrograde transport. Furthermore, in resting nerve terminals a subpopulation of synaptic vesicles is generally found in close apposition to the presynaptic membrane (comp. Fig. 4 a) implicating its immediate availability for the release stimulus. Synapsin I, actin and also fodrin (the brain analogue of spectrin) have been implicated in the nerve terminal anchorage of synaptic vesicles and in the initiation of synaptic vesicle exocytosis (De Camilli and Greengard, 1986; Walker and Agoston, 1987; Perrin et al., 1987).

A major step in understanding the structural organization of the synapse at the molecular level was the development of the quick-freeze, deep-etch and rotary replication technique (Heuser and Salpeter, 1979). Using this technique, a network of filaments can clearly be visualized in the cytoplasm of the electroplaque cell and in the presynapse (Fig. 3 a). Interestingly, a similar network also extends throughout the extracellular space between electroplaque cells.

Synaptic vesicles inside the nerve terminal are anchored within a net of filaments (Fig. 3 b). Many of these filaments are short and make contact with each other and with synaptic vesicles via knob-like endings. Several of these small filaments are often seen to converge into one common anchoring point. Other filaments are longer and proceed through the filamentous network. They may represent actin filaments (Hirokawa et al., 1989). Filaments about 200 nm long and aligned in parallel to the presynaptic membrane resemble fodrin (which is contained in these nerve terminals). Synaptic vesicles are interconnected via filaments with each other and with the presynaptic plasma membrane. They often carry knob-like particles at their surface. These may either represent large membrane intrinsic molecular complexes and/or torn off anchorage points of filaments. Since the synapsin I molecule carries a globular head region of about 14 nm, knob-like particles may represent vesicle-attached synapsin I connecting the vesicle to the cytonet.

In the electric ray electromotor synapses patches of vesicles are attached directly to the presynaptic membrane similar to results obtained at the neuromuscular junction or in brain (Couteaux and Spacek, 1988; Landis, 1988). In this case no filamentous or particulate bridges are left between the opposing membranes (Fig. 3 c). Interestingly, in P-face views of the presynaptic membrane intramembrane particles are regularly found at sites of direct synaptic vesicle apposition. They are reminiscent of intramembrane particles at the active site of the neuromuscular junction. These particles which occur in clusters and are not evenly distributed over the nerve terminal plasma membrane often form ring-like arrangements with a diamter of the size of a synaptic vesicle (ca. 100 nm). In appropriate fractions, the insertion of presynaptic cytoplasmic filaments into the presynaptic membrane forming an intramembrane particle on the P-face can directly be demonstrated. These regularly arranged intramembrane particles opposite to presynaptic vesicle attachment sites may thus represent the hydrophobic anchors of cytoplasmic filaments stabilizing the vesicles in their membrane apposition.

On the mechanism of synaptic vesicle exocytosis: Identification of a presynaptic plasma membrane associated synaptic vesicle binding protein

A major unknown in the life cycle of synaptic vesicles is the molecular cascade involved in exocytosis and membrane retrieval. Vesicle exocytosis is initiated by an increase in the concentration of free cytosolic Ca^{2+} (Augustine et al., 1987), resulting from the influx of Ca^{2+} through voltage dependent Ca^{2+} channels in close proximity to the release sites. Furthermore, activation of protein kinase C augments secretory release in neuronal and other secretory systems (Nishizuka, 1984, Haimann et al., 1987). Models of neurotransmitter release envisage the liberation of the synaptic vesicle from the cytonet possibly by Ca/calmodulin-dependent phosphorylation of synapsin I (De Camilli and Greengard, 1986). Further steps may include the binding of the synaptic vesicle to preexisting docking sites at the presynaptic plasma membrane (Fig. 4). Whether the exocytotic event at the nerve terminal involves the formation of a fusion pore (as suggested for mast cell secretion, Breckenridge and Almers, 1987) with the alignment of molecular complexes in vesicle and presynaptic membrane or whether there is direct fusion of lipids is an open question.

We have isolated a synaptic vesicle binding phosphoprotein from a fraction enriched in presynaptic plasma membranes (SPM) derived from bovine brain (Henkel and Zimmermann, 1989). This protein has an apparent Mr of 92,000 and a pI of

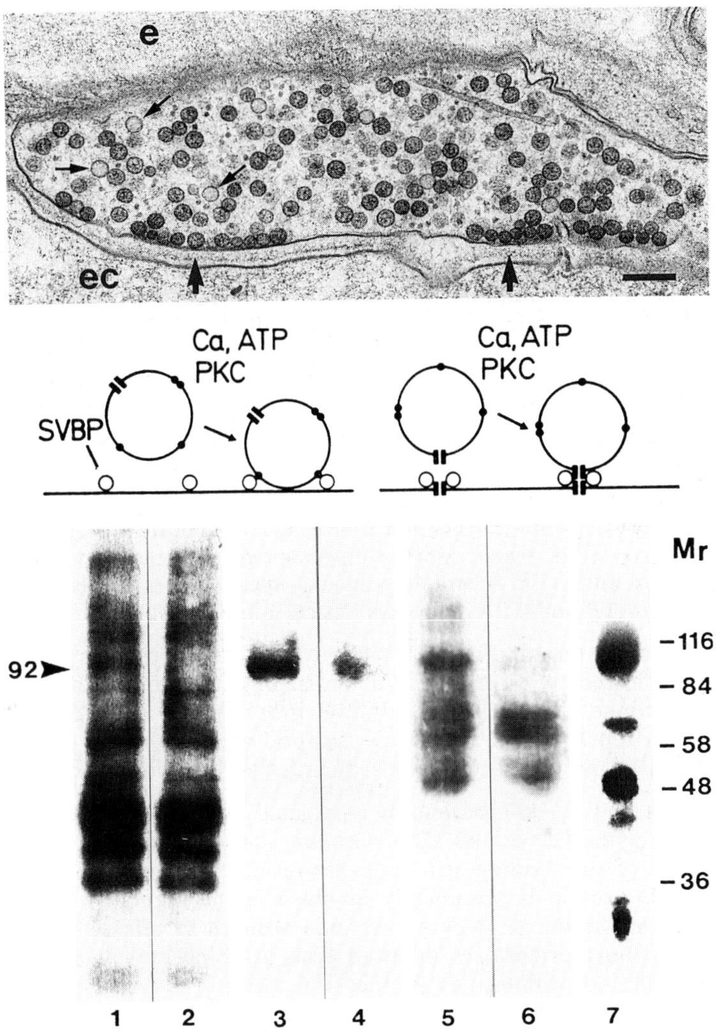

Fig. 4. Characterization of a synaptic vesicle binding protein of presynaptic plasma membranes. Top: Fine-structure of electromotor synapse in *Narke japonica* after quick freezing and freeze substitution with OsO_4. Synaptic vesicles contain dark granular material but some (small arrows) are completely electron-lucent indicative of vesicular heterogeneity. Note direct presynaptic membrane apposition of patches of vesicles (large arrows) in the resting terminal. e, extracellular space; ec, postsynaptic electroplaque cell. Bar = 250 nm. Middle: Models for the regulated binding of synaptic vesicles to the presynaptic membrane involving a synaptic vesicle binding protein (SVBP, open circle), and implicating either direct apposition of lipid domains (left) or the arrangement of molecular complexes of vesicular and presynaptic membrane for the formation of a fusion pore. Bottom: Properties of the 92 kD vesicle binding protein of bovine brain derived SPM. 1) Phosporylation of 92 kD protein on incubation of SPM in the presence of ^{32}P-ATP, EGTA (1 mM), and TPA (1 μM). 2) Lack of phosphorylation on omission of TPA. 3,4) Binding of iodinated synaptic vesicles from bovine brain to SPM-derived proteins after SDS PAGE and transfer to nitrocellulose (50 μM Ca^{2+}) (3) and on addition of TFP (20 μM)(4). 5,6) Vesicle binding under experimental conditions as in 3) but after preincubation of SPM prior to SDS PAGE, with ATP (0.5 mM) and TPA (1 μM) (5) or ATP alone (6). Part of vesicle binding to bands of Mr lower than 92 kD is presumably due to the partial degradation of the 92 kD protein on preincubation of SPM. This is supported by the observation (7) that the isolated and iodinated 92 kD protein is degraded on incubation with SPM and forms degradation products corresponding to vesicle binding bands in 5) and 6).

4.6. It binds concanavalin A, becomes phosphorylated only in the presence of the protein kinase C activator 12-O-tetradecanoylphorbol-13-acetate (TPA) (Fig. 4), and on proteolysis with *Staphylococcus aureus* V8 protease a major peptide fragment of 13 kD is formed. It does not bind calmodulin. During the isolation procedure the protein is very susceptible to hydrolysis with the formation of degradation products of Mr 74,000, 56,000 and 50,000.

The 92 kD protein was identified using two independent procedures. SPM were subjected to SDS PAGE followed by transfer to nitrocellulose. Nitrocellulose sheets were incubated with highly purified (chromatography on porous glass beads) and iodinated synaptic vesicles and the binding of vesicles to individual protein bands was monitored by autoradiography (Fig. 4). In the presence of 50 μM Ca^{2+} synaptic vesicles bind selectively to a 92 kD band. This binding is strongly reduced by the (non-specific) calmodulin antagonist trifluoperazine (TFP). When SPM are preincubated in the presence of ATP and TPA before SDS PAGE, vesicle binding to the 92 kD protein is strongly enhanced as compared to control incubations in the absence of TPA. Under these experimental conditions vesicle binding is also observed at bands of lower molecular weight. Part of these probably represent degradation products of the 92 kD component. Similar results are obtained when iodinated synaptic vesicles are bound to native SPM which were simply dotted onto nitrocellulose. Ca^{2+} significantly enhances and TFP completely blocks synaptic vesicle binding. Preincubation of SPM with ATP and TPA increases vesicle binding fourfold.

The second approach involves the binding of SPM to Affigel 10- coupled synaptic vesicle proteins. This is followed by crosslinking potential binding proteins of SPM using the reversible crosslinker dithiobis(succinimidyl-proprionate). Non-coupled proteins are removed by Triton X-100 (2%) and the synaptic vesicle binding protein can be eluted in pure form in the presence of the reducing agent dithiothreitol.

Our results suggest that the 92 kD protein is associated with the presynaptic plasma membrane. It binds synaptic vesicles after phosphorylation by protein kinase C, and the Ca^{2+} sensitivity of the binding step probably resides on the synaptic vesicle membrane. The 92 kD protein is presumably involved in the regulated exocytosis of synaptic vesicles by binding or docking synaptic vesicles to release sites at the presynaptic membrane. Furthermore, as deduced from its biochemical properties, the synaptic vesicle binding protein may be identical to the 87 kD protein described by Greengard and his group. The protein kinase C induced phosphorylation of the 87 kD protein is paralleled by augmented transmitter release (Nichols et al., 1987; Haycock et al., 1988).

Presynaptic recycling of synaptic vesicles monitored by volume and membrane markers

The exocytotic fusion of synaptic vesicles with the plasma membrane has clearly been demonstrated using the freeze fracture technique. Similarly, it has to be concluded from the stimulation induced uptake of extracellular volume markers into synaptic vesicle-like structures that transmitter release is accompanied by increased endocytosis (Zimmermann, 1979; Ceccarelli and Hurlbut 1980). Previous studies in the *Torpedo* electric organ had shown that vesicles recycled on induced transmitter release (VP_2-type) become smaller and denser than resting vesicles (VP_1-type). Therefore, they can be separated from the latter by either density gradient centrifugation or chromatography (Zimmermann 1988). Furthermore, recycled vesicles contain the majority of newly synthesized acetylcholine and ATP. From studies of this type the concept of a metabolic heterogeneity of synaptic vesicles with prefe-

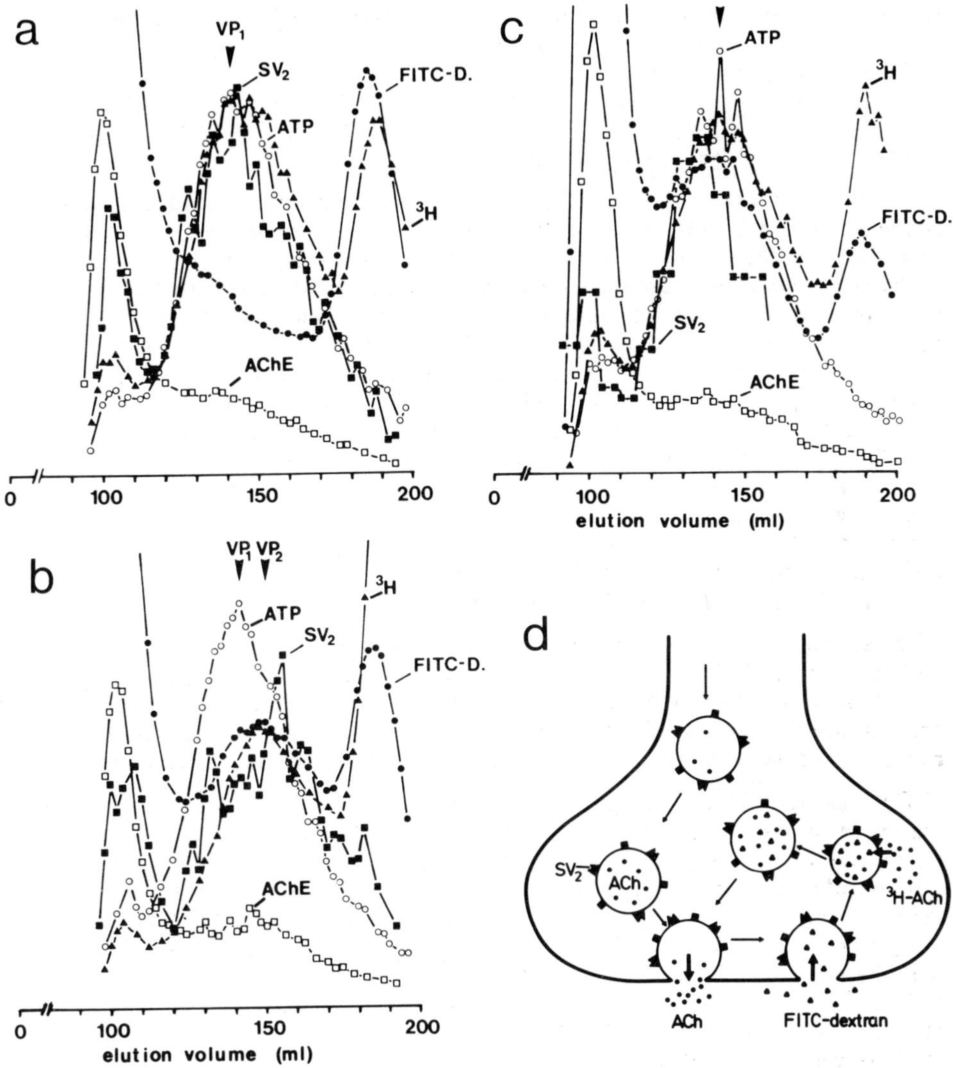

Fig. 5. Demonstration of stimulation dependent endocytosis by the synaptic vesicle membrane compartment. Separation of synaptic vesicles according to size after isolation from perfused blocks of *Torpedo* electric organ (column of porous glass beads). Perfusion (physiological saline containing ^{3}H-acetate and 2% FITC-dextran, 4 kD) under conditions of rest (a), after 1800 impulses (0.1 Hz) to the innervating nerve (b) and after subsequent recovery for 18 h (c). Means of 3 (a) 4 (b) or 2 (c) experiments. Ordinate: Percentage of marker recovered in the column effluent. Left: Void volume; Middle: vesicle peak (VP_1, VP_2); Right: Salt peak. ^{3}H, total ^{3}H, 80% of which is in the form of ^{3}H-acetylcholine within the vesicle peak. FITC-D., FITC-dextran; AChE, acetylcholinesterase; SV2, binding activity of monoclonal anti-SV2 antibody. The cartoon (d) summarizes the findings using the markers employed. It depicts endocytosis of FITC-dextran by the identified synaptic vesicle membrane compartment and subsequent refilling with newly synthesized acetylcholine.

rential release of neurotransmitter from just recycled vesicles was developed.

In the present study we have obtained further evidence that synaptic vesicles are recycled directly on induced transmitter release (Bonzelius and Zimmermann, 1989). Vesicle retrieval under conditions of modest activation of the synapse involves the uptake of extracellular volume marker (FITC-dextran) (Fig. 5). The volume marker can be identified inside isolated membrane compartments. These represent synaptic vesicles as identified by two different antibodies against vesicle-specific membrane proteins (anti-SV2, anti-svp25). Furthermore they are enriched in newly synthesized acetylcholine. Acetylcholinesterase, a marker of the presynaptic plasma membrane in *Torpedo* nerve terminals does not become accumulated in the recycled membrane compartment. This excludes a possible contribution of components of the presynaptic plasma membrane to the membrane of recycled vesicles under these experimental conditions.

Excised blocks of *Torpedo* electric organ were perfused simultaneously with the acetylcholine precursor ^{3}H-acetate and the extracellular volume marker FITC-dextran. Blocks remained either resting (Fig. 5 a), were stimulated (Fig. 5 b) or were given a rest following stimulation as in b) (Fig. 5 c). After isolation of vesicles by sucrose density gradient centrifugation, membrane compartments were further separated by size using chromatography on porous glass beads. Under resting conditions (Fig. 5 a) the synaptic vesicle marker ATP elutes as a symmetrical peak separate from the void volume (as indicated by a peak of acetylcholinesterase). Newly synthesized (radiolabelled) ACh and binding activity for the anti-SV2 antibody coelute with ATP. There is no uptake of FITC-dextran into resting VP_1-vesicles. The small shoulder of acetylcholinesterase in the range of the vesicle peak is observed independent of experimental conditions used. After stimulation (Fig. 5 b) the distribution curves of newly synthesized ACh and of antibody binding activity are shifted to the right indicating that the majority of vesicles now belong to a population of smaller size (VP_2). These VP_2-vesicles contain the extracellular volume marker FITC-dextran. After a period of recovery following stimulation (Fig. 5 c) vesicle diamters (and the corresponding markers) shift back to the original position (VP_1). The only difference to Fig. 5 a is the vesicular incorporation of FITC-dextran, indicating that recycled vesicles costore newly synthesized transmitter and a sample of extracellular volume. Fig. 5 d summarizes the findings.

REFERENCES

Augustine, G.J., Charlton, M.P. and Smith, S.J. (1987) Calcium action in synaptic transmitter release. Ann. Rev. Neurosci., **10**, 633-693.

Baumert, M., Maycox, P.R., Navone, F., De Camilli, P. and Jahn, R. (1989) Synaptobrevin: an integral membrane protein of 18 000 daltons in small synaptic vesicles of rat brain. EMBO J., **8**, 379- 384.

Buckley, K. and Kelly, R.B. (1985) Identification of a transmembrane glycoprotein specific for secretory vesicles of neural and endocrine cells. J. Cell Biol. **100**, 1284-1294.

Bonzelius, F. and Zimmermann, H. (1989) Newly synthesized ACh, extracellular volume marker and the vesicle-specific membrane marker SV2 in recycled vesicles. J. Neurochem., **52**, Suppl.: S59C.

Bööj, S., Goldstein, R., Fischer-Colbrie, R. and Dahlström, A. (1989) Calcitonin gene-related peptide and chromogranin A: Presence and intraaxonal transport in lumbar motor neurons in the rat, a comparison with synaptic vesicle antigens in immunocytochemical studies. Neuroscience, **30**, 479-501.

Breckenridge, L.J. and Almers, W. (1987) Currents through the fusion pore that forms during exocytosis of a secretory vesicle. Nature, **328**, 814-817.

Ceccarelli, B. and Hurlbut, W.P. (1980) Vesicle hypothesis of the release of quanta of acetylcholine. Physiol. Rev., **6**, 396-441.

Cidon, S. and Sihra, T.S. (1989) Characterization of a H^+-ATPase in rat brain synaptic vesicles. Coupling to L-glutamate transport. J. Biol. Chem., **264**, 8281-8288.

Couteaux, R. and Spacek, J. (1988) Specializations of subsynaptic cytoplasms. Comparison of axospinous synapses and neuromuscular junctions. in: Zimmermann, H. (ed.) Cellular and Molecular Basis of Synaptic Transmission, Berlin, Heidelberg: Springer, pp. 25- 50.

De Camilli, P. and Greengard, P. (1986) Synapsin I: a synaptic vesicle-associated neuronal phosphoprotein. Biochem. Pharmacol., **35**, 4349-4357.

Fehér, E. (1984) Electron-microscopic study of retrograde axonal transport of horseradish peroxidase. Int. Rev. Cytol., **90**, 1-29.

Haimann, C., Meldolesi, J. and Ceccarelli, B. (1987) The phorbol ester, 12-O-tetradecanoyl-phorbol-13-acetate, enhances the evoked quanta release of acetylcholine at the frog neuromuscular junction. Pflügers Arch., **408**, 27-31.

Haycock, J.W., Browning, M.D. and Greengard, P. (1988) Cholinergic regulation of protein phosphorylation in bovine adrenal chromaffin cells. Proc. Natl. Acad. Sci. USA, **85**, 1677-1681.

Henkel, A. and Zimmermann, H. (1989) Identification and characterization of a synaptic vesicle-binding protein. Biol. Chem. Hoppe-Seyler, **370**, 999-1000.

Heuser, J.E. and Salpeter, S.R. (1979) Organization of acetylcholine receptors in quick-frozen, deep-etched, and rotary- replicated *Torpedo* postsynaptic membrane. J. Cell Biol., **82**, 150- 173.

Hirokawa, N., Sobue, K., Kanda, K., Harada, A. and Yorifuji, H. (1989) The cytoskeletal architecture of the presynaptic terminal and the molecular structure of synapsin I. J. Cell Biol., **108**, 111- 126.

Janetzko, A., Zimmermann, H. and Volknandt, W. (1989) Intraneuronal distribution of a synaptic vesicle membrane protein: antibody binding sites at axonal membrane compartments and *trans*-Golgi network and accumulation at nodes of Ranvier. Neuroscience, in press.

Kelly, R.B. (1988) The cell biology of the nerve terminal. Neuron, **1**, 431-438.

Kiene, M.L. and Stadler, H. (1987) Synaptic vesicles in electromotor neurones. I. Axonal transport, site of transmitter uptake and processing of a core proteoglycan during maturation. EMBO J., **6**, 2209-2215.

Landis, D.M.D. (1988) Membrane and cytoplasmic structure at synaptic junctions in the mammalian central nervous system. J. Electron. Microsc. Techni., **10**, 129-151.

Nichols, R.A., Haycock, J.W., Wang, J.K.T. and Greengard, P. (1987) Phorbol ester enhancement of neurotransmitter release from rat brain synaptosomes. J. Neurochem., **48**, 615-621.

Nishizuka, Y. (1984) The role of protein kinase C in cell surface signal transduction and tumor promotion. Nature, **308**, 693-698.

Perrin, D., Langley, O.K. and Aunis, D. (1987) Anti-α-fodrin inhibits secretion from permeabilized chromaffin cells. Nature, **326**, 498-501.

Thomas, L., Hartung, K., Langosch, D., Rehm, H., Bamberg, E., Franke, W.W. and Betz, H. (1988) Identification of synaptophysin as a hexameric channel protein of the synaptic vesicle membrane. Science, **242**, 1050-1053.

Thureson-Klein, Å, K., Klein, R., Zhu, P.-Ch., and Kong, J.-Y. (1988) Differential release of transmitters and neuropeptides co- stored in central and pripheral neurons. in: Zimmermann, H. (ed.) Cellular and Molecular Basis of Synaptic

Transmission, Berlin, Heidelberg: Springer, pp. 137-151.

Volknandt, W., Henkel, A. and Zimmermann, H. (1988) Synaptic vesicle proteins. in: Zimmermann, H. (ed.) Cellular and Molecular Basis of Synaptic Transmission, Berlin, Heidelberg: Springer, pp. 337-350.

Volknandt, W., Schläfer, M. and Zimmermann, H. (1989). SVP_25: An integral membrane glycoprotein of synaptic vesicles. Biol. Chem. Hoppe-Seyler, **370**, 1005.

Walker, J.H. and Agoston, D.V. (1987) The synaptic vesicle and the cytoskeleton. Biochem. J., **247**, 249-258.

Zimmermann, H. (1988) Cholinergic synaptic vesicles. in: Whittaker, V.P.. (ed.) Handbook of Experimental Pharmacolcogy, Vol. 86, Berlin, Heidelberg: Springer, pp. 349-382.

Zimmermann, H. (1979) Vesicle recycling and transmitter release. Neuroscience, **4**, 1773-1804.

Zimmermann, H. and Vogt, M. (1989) Membrane proteins of synaptic vesicles and cytoskeletal specializations at the node of Ranvier in electric ray and rat. Cell Tiss. Res., in press.

Acknowledgement: This work was supported by the Deutsche Forschungsgemeinschaft (SFB 169/A10) and a fellowship of the Japanese Society for the Promotion of Science (to H. Zimmermann).

SYNAPSIN I, A NEURON-SPECIFIC PHOSPHOPROTEIN INTERACTING WITH SMALL SYNAPTIC VESICLES AND F-ACTIN

Fabio Benfenati[1,2,$], Flavia Valtorta[2,3], Martin Bähler[2] and Paul Greengard[2]

[1]Institute of Human Physiology, University of Modena, Modena, Italy, [2]Laboratory of Molecular and Cellular Neuroscience, The Rockefeller University, New York, U.S.A. and [3]CNR Center of Cytopharmacology and Center for the Study of Peripheral Neuropathies and Neuromuscolar Diseases, Department of Pharmacology, University of Milano Medical School, Milano, Italy.

Synapsin I is a neuron-specific phosphoprotein which is a substrate for cAMP- and Ca^{2+}/calmodulin-dependent protein kinases. It is specifically localized to the cytoplasmic side of small synaptic vesicles. The interaction of synapsin I with the synaptic vesicle membrane is complex in nature, since it is modulated by phosphorylation and involves binding of different domains of the molecule to phospholipid and protein components of synaptic vesicles. Synapsin I is also able to interact with actin filaments in a phosphorylation-dependent manner. Because of these properties, it has been hypothesized that synapsin I acts as a dynamic link between synaptic vesicles an the actin meshwork of the nerve terminal, thereby modulating the release of neurotransmitter.

INTRODUCTION

The reversible incorporation of phosphate into amino acid residues is now recognized as an ubiquitous process of protein modification which plays a regulatory role in a variety of cellular functions (Nestler and Greengard, 1984; Hunter and Cooper, 1985; Edelman et al., 1987). Nearly one hundred different protein kinases have been characterized so far (Hunter, 1987) and their number is constantly increasing.

Although some protein tyrosine kinases are activated directly by ligands, the majority of protein kinases are indirectly activated by extracellular signals through increases in the intracellular level of a second messenger. Complexity is added to this system by the multiplicity of possible substrates for a single enzyme and by the possibility that a single substrate is phosphorylated at the same or at distinct sites by different protein kinases.

The highest concentration of the various components of most protein phosphorylation systems (protein kinases, protein phosphatases and their substrates) is found in the central nervous system. Moreover, the central nervous system appears to contain the highest number of different substrates, some of which are neuron-specific. Among the physiological properties of neurons which are thought to be regulated by protein phosphorylation are the processes

---

[$] To whom correspondence should be addressed.

of neurotransmitter biosynthesis and release, ion channel conductance, nerve growth and differentiation and possibly short and long term memory (for review, see Nairn et al., 1985).

Some of the neuron-specific phosphoproteins appear to have a distribution limited to certain brain regions, where they are present in a single class of neurons, suggesting that they are involved in the modulation of processes which are specific to these neurons. Alternatively, there are phosphoproteins which are widely distributed throughout the nervous system, being expressed in virtually all neurons. These latter proteins are likely to be involved in the regulation of processes which are common to all neuronal cells, e.g. neurotransmitter release. One such protein is synapsin I (previously named protein I), a phosphoprotein which was originally discovered as one of the major substrates for cAMP-dependent protein kinase in the brain (Ueda and Greengard, 1977; Sieghart et al., 1978).

Synapsin I is the collective name for two closely related polypeptides, synapsin Ia and synapsin Ib, which are composed of 704 and 668 amino acid residues, respectively, in the rat. The two polypeptides are virtually identical with the exception of a small C-terminal region and arise from alternative splicing (Südhof et al, 1989). Synapsin I has been purified to homogeneity from bovine and rat brain (Ueda and Greengard, 1977; Schiebler et al., 1986) and its molecular structure has been characterized in great detail. It is a very basic (isoelectric point higher than 10) and acid-soluble protein. The synapsin I molecule is highly asymmetric, being composed of a globular, collagenase-resistant *head* region (roughly corresponding to the N-terminal and middle fragments of the molecule; Fig.1), and of an elongated, collagenase-sensitive *tail* region. The *head* region contains most of the hydrophobic amino acid residues found in the molecule, whereas the *tail* region is responsible for the basicity of the protein (Fig.1; Südhof et al., 1989).

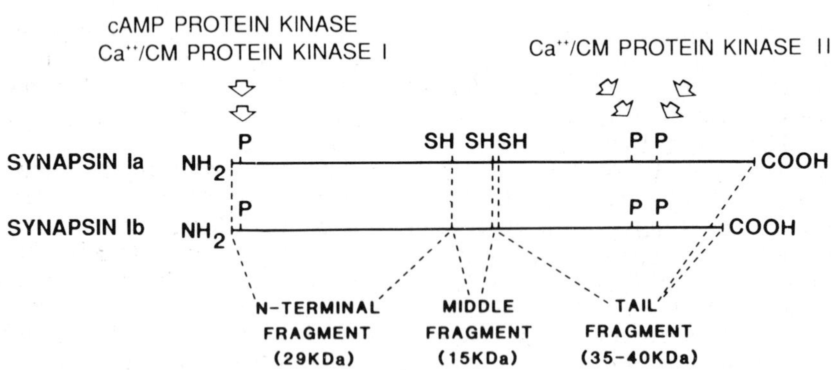

FIG.1. Schematic representation of the primary structure of synapsin Ia and Ib. The phosphorylation sites (P) and the respective protein kinases which phosphorylate them are indicated. In order to generate fragments for the structure-function analysis, synapsin I was cleaved at cysteine residues (SH) by 2-nitro 5-thiocyanobenzoic acid (NTCB; Bähler et al., 1989). The three fragments spanning the synapsin I molecule are indicated together with their apparent molecular weight on SDS-PAGE (CM = calmodulin).

Synapsin I is an excellent substrate for both cAMP- and Ca^{2+}/calmodulin-dependent protein kinases (Huttner and Greengard, 1979; Huttner et al., 1981). Cyclic AMP-dependent protein kinase phosphorylates synapsin I on a serine residue located in the *head* region (ser^9, site 1). The same residue is phosphorylated by Ca^{2+}/calmodulin-dependent protein kinase I, whereas Ca^{2+}/calmodulin-dependent protein kinase II catalyzes the incorporation of phosphate into two additional serine residues located in the *tail* region (ser^{566}, site 2 and ser^{603}, site 3) (Czernik et al., 1987; Südhof et al., 1989). Synapsin I can also be phosphorylated by protein kinase C in cell-free systems (Albert et al., 1984) and by a nerve growth factor-dependent protein kinase in PC12 cells (Romano et al., 1987); however, the physiological significance of these latter phosphorylation reactions is still uncertain.

Synapsin I is a neuron-specific protein. It is present in the central as well as in the peripheral nervous system. In the brain cortex, it constitutes about 0.4% of the total protein (Goelz et al., 1981). The small amounts of synapsin I detectable in most non-neuronal tissues can be attributed to the innervation of these tissues, as has been shown by immunocytochemistry (De Camilli et al., 1983a). Synapsin I is present in virtually all neurons irrespective of their neurotransmitter content and within neurons it is highly concentrated in the nerve terminal region. Immunoelectron microscopy as well as subcellular fractionation studies have shown that synapsin I is specifically associated with the cytoplasmic side of the membrane of small synaptic vesicles, constituting about 6% of the total protein present in a highly purified preparation of synaptic vesicles (De Camilli et al., 1983a and b; Huttner et al., 1983; Navone et al., 1984). Small amounts are also found in neuroendocrine cells. Proteins antigenically related to synapsin I have been detected in nervous tissue preparations from several vertebrate and invertebrate animal species (Sorensen and Babitch, 1984; Bixby and Reichardt, 1985; Goelz et al., 1985; Llinas et al., 1985; Volknandt et al., 1987; Valtorta et al., 1988).

The appearance of both synapsin I and of messenger RNA for synapsin I during development correlates strictly with synaptogenesis, supporting the idea that the presence of synapsin I is important for synaptic vesicle function (Lohmann et al., 1978; De Gennaro et al., 1983; Levitt et al., 1984).

Synapsin Ia and Ib are highly homologous to two other synaptic vesicle-specific phosphoproteins, synapsin IIa and IIb (originally named protein IIIa and IIIb, and collectively referred to as synapsin II; Huang et al., 1982; Browning et al., 1987). The four synapsins exhibit extensive sequence homology in the N-terminal region, but they diverge in the C-terminal region. Accordingly, phosphorylation site 1 is shared by the four polypeptides, whereas the collagenase-sensitive *tail* region containing phosphorylation sites 2 and 3 is specific for synapsin I (Südhof et al., 1989).

INTERACTION OF SYNAPSIN I WITH SYNAPTIC VESICLES AND F-ACTIN: MODULATION BY PHOSPHORYLATION

Although synapsin I penetrates into the hydrophobic core of the synaptic vesicle membrane (Benfenati et al., 1989a; see below), it

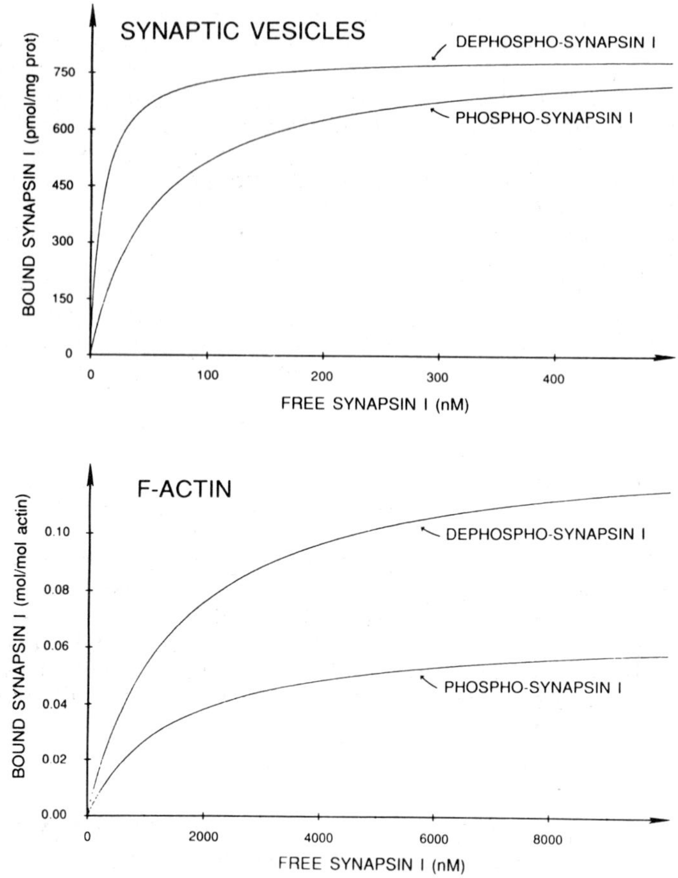

FIG.2. Binding of dephosphorylated and phosphorylated synapsin I to small synaptic vesicles (upper panel) and to F-actin (lower panel). Synapsin I was phosphorylated *in vitro* by purified protein kinases to a stoichiometry of 2.8 mol phosphate/mol synapsin I. Closely similar results were obtained with synapsin I selectively phosphorylated on the two *tail* sites by Ca^{2+}/calmodulin-dependent protein kinase II, whereas the phosphorylation of the *head* site by the catalytic subunit of cAMP-dependent protein kinase was less effective on both binding activities. The binding curves (bound vs free synapsin I concentrations) have been simulated using the mean values of the experimentally determined K_d and B_{max} (for further details see Schiebler et al., 1986 and Bähler and Greengard, 1987).

is not an integral membrane protein and can be quantitatively removed from the vesicle membrane by lowering the pH or increasing the ionic strength of the medium (Huttner et al., 1983). This property has allowed the study of the binding of exogenous synapsin I to synaptic vesicles depleted of endogenous synapsin I. Synapsin I-depleted synaptic vesicles exhibit a high affinity binding for purified dephosphosynapsin I (K_d = 10 nM at 40 mM NaCl; Fig.2, upper panel). The binding is saturable (B_{max} = 800 pmol/mg vesicle protein) and specific. The amount of synapsin I bound at saturation corresponds to the amount present in native synaptic vesicles. Phosphorylation of synapsin I by Ca^{2+}/calmodulin-dependent protein kinase II (but not by cAMP-dependent protein kinase or by Ca^{2+}/calmodulin-dependent protein kinase I) decreases the affinity of the binding five-fold without affecting the B_{max}. A similar decrease in the binding affinity can be induced by raising the ionic strength of the medium, irrespective of the state of phosphorylation of synapsin I (Schiebler et al., 1986).

Purified synapsin I is able to interact *in vitro* with various cytoskeletal proteins (spectrin, tubulin, neurofilaments and actin) (Baines and Bennett, 1985 and 1986; Goldenring et al., 1986; Bähler and Greengard, 1987; Petrucci and Morrow, 1987; Steiner et al., 1987). The affinity of synapsin I for F-actin is in the order of 1.2-1.5 μM irrespective of the state of phosphorylation of synapsin I. However, after phosphorylation by Ca^{2+}/calmodulin-dependent protein kinase II, the number of synapsin I binding sites on actin filaments is reduced by about 50% (Fig.2, lower panel). Phosphorylation by cAMP-dependent protein kinase also decreases the number of binding sites, although to a lower extent (Bähler and Greengard, 1987; Petrucci and Morrow, 1987). Electron microscopy of negatively stained specimens as well as light scattering experiments have shown that the interaction of synapsin I with actin filaments leads to the formation of bundles, suggesting that it binds to the sides of the filaments (Fig. 3). The bundling activity is reduced when synapsin I is phosphorylated by cAMP-dependent protein kinase and virtually abolished after phosphorylation of synapsin I by Ca^{2+}/calmodulin-dependent protein kinase II.

MOLECULAR CHARACTERIZATION OF SYNAPSIN I BINDING TO SYNAPTIC VESICLES AND F-ACTIN.

Synapsin I binds to synaptic vesicles with high affinity, it has a noticeable tendency to self-associate and it is able to form stable monolayers at an air-water interface (Schiebler et al., 1986; Ho et al.,

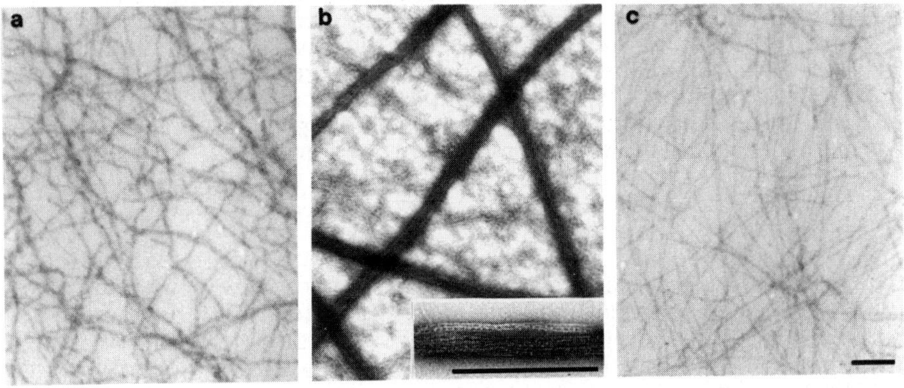

FIG.3. Phosphorylation-dependent F-actin bundling activity of synapsin I as evaluated by electron microscopy of negatively stained preparations. (a) F-actin alone (5 μM) (b) F-actin plus dephosphosynapsin I (1 μM) (c) F-actin plus fully phosphorylated synapsin I (1 μM). Bar = 0.5 μm.

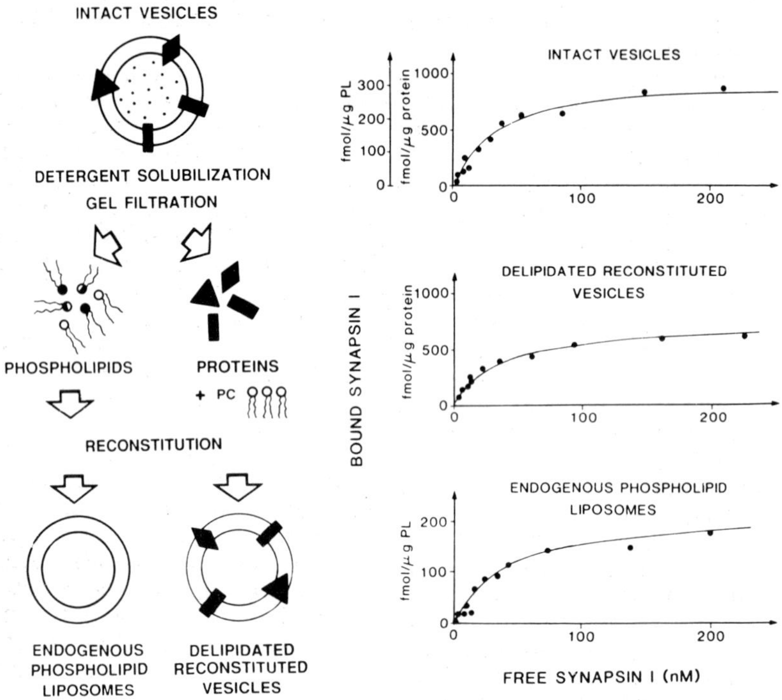

FIG.4. Demonstration of the presence of different binding components for synapsin I in the membrane of small synaptic vesicles. Purified synaptic vesicles were solubilized in an excess of sodium cholate to yield relatively pure micelles of endogenous phospholipids and of endogenous proteins. These micelles of different sizes were separated by gel filtration in the presence of detergent. Exogenous phosphatidylcholine (PC) was added to the protein-detergent micelles (PC does not interact with synapsin I) and the two pools were reconstituted by detergent removal yielding endogenous phospholipid liposomes and delipidated reconstituted vesicles. On the right, the binding of synapsin I to intact synaptic vesicles, delipidated reconstituted vesicles and endogenous phospholipid liposomes is shown. Synapsin I bound to a similar extent to both components of synaptic vesicles. The protein:phospholipid ratio (mg:mg) as experimentally determined in one synaptic vesicle preparation was 1:3.

manuscript in preparation). These observations suggest the presence of amphiphilic secondary structures in the molecule which make it extremely surface active. Vesicle phospholipids, which represent an ideal amphiphilic environment, could therefore participate in the binding of synapsin I to synaptic vesicles. An interaction of synapsin I with vesicle phospholipids has been demonstrated in the experiment shown in Fig. 4. After solubilization of highly purified synaptic vesicles in an excess of detergent, endogenous phospholipids and endogenous proteins were separated by gel filtration and reconstituted into endogenous phospholipid liposomes and delipidated reconstituted synaptic vesicles, respectively. Synapsin I binds with high affinity to both protein and phospholipid vesicles, suggesting the presence of multiple components and/or binding sites in the synaptic vesicle membrane.

The binding of synapsin I to phospholipid vesicles has also been reproduced in liposomes prepared from a mixture of exogenous phospholipids mimicking the composition of the synaptic vesicle membrane. The dissociation constant (K_d) is in the low nanomolar range (10-25 nM at 40 mM NaCl equivalent) and the average binding capacity (B_{max}) is 170 pmol/mg phospholipid; the binding is strongly dependent on the presence of negatively charged phospholipids in the membrane and is weakened by increasing the ionic strength of the medium (Benfenati et al., 1989a). It is possible that the head groups of different phospholipids form surfaces or pockets able to interact with specific amphiphilic protein domains. It is also of particular interest to note that the phospholipid distribution in the synaptic vesicle membrane is asymmetrical, the cytoplasmic leaflet being enriched in acidic phospholipids (Westhead, 1987).

By using hydrophobic probes able to covalently label the membrane-embedded domains of proteins (Brunner, 1981; Brunner and Semenza, 1981; Brunner et al., 1983; Harter et al., 1988), synapsin I has been demonstrated to interact with the hydrophobic core of the vesicle membrane (Benfenati et al., 1989a and b). Although the interaction of synapsin I with phospholipids is likely to contribute to its binding to synaptic vesicles, it is not significantly modulated by phosphorylation. The phosphorylation-dependent modulation of synapsin I binding to synaptic vesicles is therefore likely to involve an interaction with vesicle proteins.

Purified peptide fragments generated by cysteine-specific cleavage of synapsin I have been used to elucidate the domains of synapsin I involved in its interactions with synaptic vesicles and F-actin. As shown in Fig. 1, three fragments are generated: N-terminal, middle and tail fragment. An N-terminal/middle and a middle/tail fragment arise through partial cleavage. The N-terminal and middle fragments of synapsin I are hydrophobic, and the middle fragment is virtually insoluble in biological buffers.

The binding of synapsin I to protein and phospholipid components of synaptic vesicles seems to be mediated by distinct sites on synapsin I. The N-terminal fragment binds to the same extent to intact synaptic vesicles as to endogenous phospholipid liposomes (Table I). On the other hand, the tail fragment does not bind significantly to endogenous phospholipid liposomes but it does

TABLE I. Binding of the dephospho-form of synapsin I and of synapsin I fragments to synaptic vesicles and endogenous phospholipid liposomes.

PEPTIDE	SYNAPTIC VESICLES K_d (nM)	SYNAPTIC VESICLES B_{max} (pmol/mg prot)	ENDOGENOUS PHOSPHOLIPID LIPOSOMES K_d (nM)	ENDOGENOUS PHOSPHOLIPID LIPOSOMES B_{max} (pmol/mg PL)
Synapsin I	10	800	15	180
N-terminal	25	800	24	200
Tail	55	1200	--	---

interact with synaptic vesicles with fairly high affinity. This binding is dramatically impaired after phosphorylation by Ca^{2+}/calmodulin-dependent protein kinase II or exposure to high ionic strength and is totally abolished after limited proteolysis of synaptic vesicles. Moreover, in experiments involving hydrophobic labeling of vesicle-bound synapsin I followed by cysteine-specific cleavage, it was found that the derivatization is restricted to the N-terminal and N-terminal/middle fragments, with no labeling of the tail fragment. This finding further supports the idea that the N-terminal region of synapsin I is responsible for the binding to vesicle phospholipids and for the membrane penetration whereas the *tail* is the region interacting with vesicle protein(s) in a phosphorylation-dependent manner (Benfenati et al., 1989a and b). Taken together, these findings suggest that holosynapsin I may interact with synaptic vesicles as a divalent ligand binding to two distinct sites. This view is further strengthened by the observation that the simultaneous presence of the N-terminal and the tail fragments is required in order to inhibit the binding of labeled synapsin I to synaptic vesicles (Benfenati et al., 1989b).

Table II illustrates the ability of the fragments to mimick the interaction of synapsin I with F-actin. A major high affinity binding site seems to be present in the hydrophobic middle fragment of synapsin I. In fact, although the purified middle fragment has not been tested because of its poor solubility, both the N-terminal/middle and the middle/tail fragments bind F-actin with an affinity comparable to that of holosynapsin I. In contrast, the tail fragment is unable to bind at physiological salt concentrations and the N-terminal fragment binds very weakly.

In principle, the formation of bundles of actin filaments can be brought about either by the simultaneous presence of two (or more) actin-binding sites on synapsin I, so that the molecule itself can act as a bridge between actin filaments, or by self-association of two (or more) synapsin I molecules bearing only one biologically active actin-binding site. Interestingly, only the middle/tail fragment retains bundling activity suggesting that (a) the weak actin-binding site in the N-terminal region is probably biologically inactive since its presence is not necessary to achieve F-actin binding and bundling and (b) either a second actin-binding site in the middle or tail fragment is unmasked when these fragments are connected to each other or the *tail* is the region responsible for synapsin I self-association. The high hydrophilicity of the tail fragment and the

TABLE II. Interaction of the dephospho-form of synapsin I and of synapsin I fragments with F-actin.

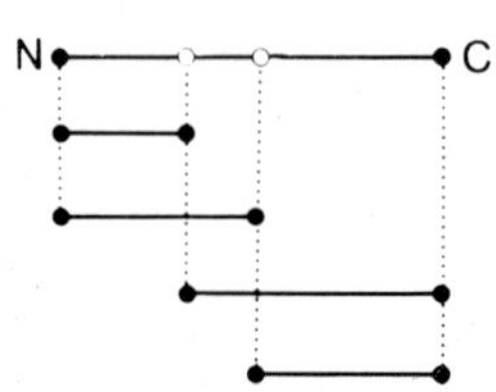

PEPTIDE	K_D FOR F-ACTIN	F-ACTIN BUNDLING
SYNAPSIN I	1.2 μM	+ + +
N-TERMINAL	168 μM	–
N-TERMINAL/MIDDLE	1.3 μM	–
MIDDLE/TAIL	0.6 μM	+ + +
TAIL	---------	–

finding that the *head* region is able to self-associate make it unlikely that the bundling phenomenon is achieved through self-association and favors the hypothesis of the two binding sites (Bähler et al., 1989).

The results of the structure-function analysis can be summarized as follows. The N-terminal-middle domain of synapsin I contains distinct sites for vesicle phospholipids and F-actin, resembling other F-actin anchoring proteins such as protein 4.1, adducin or vinculin which are also able to interact with phospholipid bilayers (Utsumi et al., 1982; Ito et al., 1983; Sato and Ohnishi, 1983; Niggli et al., 1986). On the other hand, the *tail* domain seems to be directly or indirectly responsible for the phosphorylation-dependent regulation of the interactions of synapsin I with both synaptic vesicles and F-actin. The presence of distinct binding sites for synaptic vesicles and F-actin also suggests that both interactions may occur simultaneously within the nerve terminal, with the possibility of forming a ternary complex where synapsin I acts as a dynamic link between F-actin and synaptic vesicles.

PHYSIOLOGICAL ROLE OF SYNAPSIN I IN THE NERVE TERMINAL.

The nerve terminal is virtually filled with small synaptic vesicles, but only a very limited number of them undergoes exocytosis at the arrival of one action potential. Two pools of synaptic vesicles apparently exist in the nerve terminal: a reserve pool which cannot readily interact with the presynaptic membrane and a pool which is available for the fusion process (Zimmermann and Denston, 1977). The cytoskeleton of the nerve terminal, whose major components are F-actin and spectrin (Landis et al., 1988; Hirokawa et al., 1989), may act as an anchoring system for synaptic vesicles of the reserve pool, preventing their diffusion in the cytoplasm and their spontaneous fusion with the presynaptic membrane.

Synapsin I, which is specifically associated with synaptic vesicles and is able to interact with F-actin *in vitro*, is an obvious candidate for mediating the association between synaptic vesicles and the cytoskeleton and may therefore play a relevant physiological role in the regulation of neurotransmitter release. This modulatory role seems to be brought about by changes in its phosphorylation state which in turn depend on the intracellular levels of second messengers and consequently on the activation of specific protein kinases and phosphatases. Several experimental findings support this view.

In agreement with the observation that synapsin I is an excellent substrate for cAMP-dependent and Ca^{2+}/calmodulin-dependent protein kinases *in vitro*, its phosphorylation in neuronal preparations is stimulated by a variety of physiological and pharmacological manipulations which induce an increase in the intracellular concentrations of cAMP or Ca^{2+}. Treatments such as electrical stimulation, veratridine or high extracellular potassium, which increase the flux of Ca^{2+} into the nerve terminal and induce neurotransmitter release, are associated with a prompt increase in the Ca^{2+}/calmodulin-dependent phosphorylation of synapsin I (for review, see Nestler and Greengard, 1984). It has also been shown that the repolarization is accompanied by dephosphorylation of synapsin I and that successive cycles of membrane depolarization and repolarization induce a synchronous cycle of interconversion of dephosphorylated and phosphorylated synapsin I (Forn and Greengard, 1978).

Experimental support for a role of synapsin I in the modulation of neurotransmitter release has been obtained in *in vivo* experiments where synapsin I has been microinjected into the preterminal digit of the squid giant synapse. The injection of dephosphorylated synapsin I induces a depression in the amplitude and rate of rise of the postsynaptic potentials evoked by presynaptic depolarizing steps. On the contrary, the injection of phosphorylated or heat-denatured dephosphorylated synapsin I is totally ineffective. Moreover, injection of Ca^{2+}/calmodulin-dependent protein kinase II, which phosphorylates synapsin I in the *tail* region, greatly enhances the amplitude and rate of rise of the postsynaptic potentials. These effects on the postsynaptic response are not accompanied by detectable changes in the presynaptic inward calcium current, indicating an action on the number of quanta of neurotransmitter released in response to a given Ca^{2+} influx (Llinas et al., 1985).

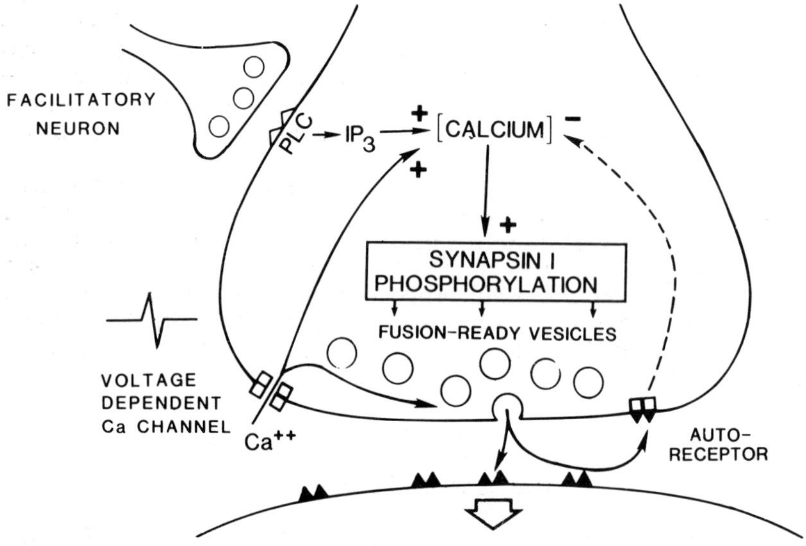

FIG.5. Mechanism by which the state of phosphorylation of synapsin I may modulate the release of neurotransmitter. Under resting conditions, most of the synaptic vesicles are cross-linked to actin filaments by dephosphosynapsin I and are not available for fusion. A secretory stimulus (e.g. an action potential) will cause an influx of Ca^{2+} in the nerve terminal, leading to exocytosis from vesicles of the available pool. At the same time, the increase in Ca^{2+} causes an increase in the state of phosphorylation of synapsin I, which results in a partial dissociation of synapsin I from the vesicle membrane and/or from F-actin and therefore in an increase in the number of synaptic vesicles available for fusion. As a result, a subsequent stimulus will cause the fusion of an increased number of synaptic vesicles and therefore the release of an increased amount of neurotransmitter.

These data strongly suggest that dephosphorylated synapsin I may provide an inhibitory constraint to the release of neurotransmitter and that this inhibitory action is abolished by phosphorylation. This inhibitory effect could be achieved by cross-linking synaptic vesicles to the F-actin meshwork of the nerve terminal. This working hypothesis is supported by the following data: (a) synapsin I binds to synaptic vesicles and to F-actin; (b) phosphorylation of synapsin I on the *tail* sites by Ca^{2+}/calmodulin-dependent protein kinase II induces an 80% decrease in the affinity for synaptic vesicles and a 50% decrease in the number of binding sites on actin filaments; (c) the structure-function analysis performed on synapsin I has identified distinct binding sites for synaptic vesicles and F-actin, consistent with the possibility of forming a ternary complex of F-actin/synapsin I/synaptic vesicle.

Within the nerve terminal, an equilibrium could be reached among free synapsin I, synapsin I bound to synaptic vesicles, synapsin I bound to F-actin and synapsin I simultaneously bound to synaptic vesicles and F-actin. Upon phosphorylation by Ca^{2+}/calmodulin-dependent protein kinase II, synapsin I tends to dissociate from synaptic vesicles and from F-actin; if such a dissociation involves a synapsin I molecule acting as a bridge in a ternary complex, the vesicle will be released from the cytoskeleton and will be incorporated into the pool of unrestrained vesicles available for fusion. Although the probability that such a dissociation of the ternary complex occurs may be rather low compared to the total number of vesicles in the reserve pool, it could be extremely significant with respect to the very limited number of vesicles forming the pool available for fusion.

This mechanism is not likely to be responsible for the fast release of neurotransmitter triggered by a single impulse, but rather it may have a modulatory and permissive role, regulating the availability of synaptic vesicles for the fusion event. Thus, synapsin I could be part of a mechanism by which the nerve terminal can finely tune the efficiency of neurotransmitter release in particular environmental conditions such as repeated stimulation or presynaptic facilitation (Fig.5).

REFERENCES

Albert, K.A., W.C.-S. Wu, A.C. Nairn, and P. Greengard (1984) Inhibition by calmodulin of calcium/ phospholipid-dependent protein phosphorylation. Proc. Natl. Acad. Sci. USA 81: 3622-3625.

Bähler, M., and P. Greengard (1987) Synapsin I bundles F-actin in a phosphorylation-dependent manner. Nature 326: 704-707.

Bähler M., F. Benfenati, F. Valtorta, A. J. Czernik, and P. Greengard (1989) Characterization of synapsin I fragments produced by cysteine-specific cleavage: identification of an N-terminal 29-kDa actin-binding fragment. J. Cell Biol. 108: 1841-1849.

Baines, A. J., and V. Bennett (1985) Synapsin I is a spectrin-binding protein immunologically related to erythrocyte protein 4.1. Nature 315: 410-413.

Baines, A. J., and V. Bennett (1986) Synapsin I is a microtubule-bundling protein. Nature 319: 145-147.

Benfenati, F., P. Greengard, J. Brunner, and M. Bähler (1989a) Electrostatic and hydrophobic interactions of synapsin I with phospholipid bilayers. J. Cell Biol. 108: 1851-1862.

Benfenati, F., M. Bähler, R. Jahn, and P. Greengard (1989b) Interaction of synapsin I with small synaptic vesicles: distinct sites in synapsin I bind to vesicle phospholipids and vesicle proteins. J. Cell Biol. 108: 1863-1872.

Bixby, J. L., and L. F. Reichardt (1985) The expression and localization of synaptic vesicle antigens at neuromuscular junction *in vitro.* J. Neurosci. 5: 3070-3080.

Browning, M. D., C-H. Huang, and P. Greengard (1987) Similarities between Protein IIIa and Protein IIIb, two prominent synaptic vesicle-associated phosphoproteins. J. Neurosci. 7: 847-853.

Brunner, J. (1981) Labelling the hydrophobic core of membranes. Trends Biochem. Sci. 6: 44-46.

Brunner, J., and G. Semenza (1981) Selective labeling of the hydrophobic core of membranes with 3-(trifluoromethyl)-3-(m-[125I]iodophenyl)diazirine, a carbene-generating reagent. Biochemistry 20: 7174-7182.

Brunner, J., M. Spiess, R. Aggeler, P. Huber, and G. Semenza (1983) Hydrophobic labeling of a single leaflet of the human erythrocyte membrane. Biochemistry 22: 3812-3820.

Czernik, A. J., D. T. Pang, and P. Greengard (1987) Amino acid sequences surrounding the cAMP-dependent and calcium/calmodulin-dependent phosphorylation sites in rat and bovine synapsin I. Proc. Natl. Acad. Sci. U.S.A. 84: 7518-7522.

De Camilli, P., R. Cameron, and P. Greengard (1983a) Synapsin I (Protein I), a nerve terminal-specific phosphoprotein. I. Its general distribution in synapses of the central and peripheral nervous system demonstrated by immunofluorescence in frozen and plastic sections. J. Cell Biol. 96: 1337-1354.

De Camilli, P., S. M. Harris, W. B. Huttner, and P. Greengard (1983b) Synapsin I (Protein I), a nerve terminal-specific phosphoprotein. II. Its specific association with synaptic vesicles demonstrated by immunocytochemistry in agarose-embedded synaptosomes. J. Cell Biol. 96: 1355-1373.

De Gennaro, L.J., W. C. Wallace, S. Kanazir, R. M. Lewis, and P. Greengard (1983) Neuron-specific phosphoproteins as models for gene expression. Cold Spring Harbor Symp. Quant. Biol. 48: 337-345.

Edelman, A.M., D.K. Blumenthal, and E.G. Krebs (1987) Protein serine/threonine kinases. Ann. Rev. Biochem. 56: 567-613.

Forn J., and P. Greengard (1978) Depolarizing agents and cyclic nucleotides regulate the phosphorylation of specific neuronal proteins in rat cerebral cortex slices. Proc. Natl. Acad. Sci. USA 75: 5195-5199.

Goelz, S.E., E. J. Nestler, B. Chehrazi, and P. Greengard (1981) Distribution of Protein I in mammalian brain as determined by a detergent-based radioimmunoassay. Proc. Natl. Acad. Sci. U.S.A. 78: 2130-2134.

Goelz, S.E., E.J. Nestler, and P. Greengard (1985) Phylogenetic survey of proteins related to synapsin I and biochemical analysis of four such proteins from fish brain. J. Neurochem., 45: 63-72.

Goldenring, J. R., R. S. Lasher, M. L. Vallano, T. Ueda, S. Naito, N. H. Sternberger, L. A. Sternberger, and R. J. DeLorenzo (1986) Association of synapsin I with neuronal cytoskeleton. Identification in cytoskeletal preparations *in vitro* and immunocytochemical localization in brain of synapsin I. J. Biol. Chem. 261: 8495-8504.

Harter, C., T. Bächi, G. Semenza, and J. Brunner (1988) Hydrophobic photolabeling identifies BHA2 as the subunit mediating the interaction of bromelain-solubilized influenza virus hemagglutinin with liposomes at low pH. Biochemistry 27: 1856-1864.

Hirokawa, N., K. Sobue, K. Kanda, A. Harada, and H. Yorifuji (1989) The cytoskeletal architecture of the presynaptic terminal and molecular structure of synapsin I. J. Cell Biol. 108: 111-126.

Huang, C-H., M. D. Browning, and P. Greengard (1982) Purification and characterization of Protein IIIb, a mammalian brain phosphoprotein. J. Biol. Chem. 257: 6524-6528.

Hunter, T. (1987) A thousand and one protein kinases. Cell 50: 823-829.

Hunter, T., and J.A. Cooper (1985) Protein tyrosine-kinases. Ann. Rev. Biochem. 54: 897-930.

Huttner, W. B., and P. Greengard (1979) Multiple phosphorylation sites in Protein I and their differential regulation by cyclic AMP and calcium. Proc. Natl. Acad. Sci. U.S.A. 76: 5402-5406.

Huttner, W. B., L. J. DeGennaro, and P. Greengard (1981) Differential phosphorylation of multiple sites in purified Protein I by cyclic AMP-dependent and calcium-dependent protein kinases. J. Biol. Chem. 256: 1482-1488.

Huttner, W. B., W. Schiebler, P. Greengard, and P. De Camilli (1983) Synapsin I (Protein I), a nerve terminal-specific phosphoprotein. III. Its association with synaptic vesicles studied in a highly purified synaptic vesicle preparation. J. Cell Biol. 96: 1374-1388.

Ito, S., D. K. Werth, N. D. Richert, and I. Pastan (1983) Vinculin phosphorylation by the src kinase. Interaction of vinculin with phospholipid vesicles. J. Biol. Chem. 258: 14626-14631.

Landis, D. M. D., A. K. Hall, L. A. Weinstein, and T. S. Reese (1988) The organization of cytoplasm at the presynaptic active zone of a central nervous system synapse. Neuron 1: 201-209.

Levitt, P., P. Rakic, P. De Camilli, and P. Greengard (1984) The emergence of cyclic guanosine 3':5'-monophosphate-dependent protein kinase immunoreactivity in developing Rhesus monkey cerebellum:

correlative immunohistochemical and electron microscopic analysis. J. Neurosci. 4: 2553-2564.

Llinas, R., T. L. McGuinness, C. S. Leonard, M. Sugimori, and P. Greengard (1985) Intraterminal injection of synapsin I or calcium/calmodulin-dependent protein kinase II alters neurotransmitter release at the squid giant synapse. Proc. Natl. Acad. Sci. U.S.A. 82: 3035-3039.

Lohmann, S.M., T. Ueda, and P. Greengard (1978) Ontogeny of synaptic phosphoproteins in the brain. Proc. Natl. Acad. Sci. USA, 75: 4037-4041.

Nairn, A. C., H. C. Jr. Hemmings, and P. Greengard (1985) Protein kinases in the brain. Ann. Rev. Biochem. 54: 931-976.

Navone, F., P. Greengard, and P. De Camilli (1984) Synapsin I in nerve terminals: selective association with small synaptic vesicles. Science 226: 1209-1211.

Nestler, E. J., and P. Greengard (1984) Protein Phosphorylation in the Nervous System. Wiley, New York. 1-394.

Niggli, V., D. P. Dimitrov, J. Brunner, and M. Burger (1986) Interaction of the cytoskeletal component vinculin with bilayer structures analyzed with a photoactivatable phospholipid. J. Biol. Chem. 261: 6912-6918.

Petrucci, T.C., and J.S. Morrow (1987) Synapsin I: an actin-bundling protein under phosphorylation control. J. Cell Biol. 105: 1355-1363.

Romano, C., R.A. Nichols, and P. Greengard (1987) Synapsin I in PC12 cells. II. Evidence for regulation by NGF of phosphorylation at a novel site. J. Neurosci. 7: 1300-1305.

Sato, S. B., and S. Ohnishi (1983) Interaction of a peripheral protein of the erythrocyte membrane, band 4.1, with phosphatidylserine-containing liposomes and erythrocyte inside-out vesicles. Eur. J. Biochem. 130: 19-25.

Schiebler, W., R. Jahn, J-P. Doucet, J. Rothlein, and P. Greengard (1986) Characterization of synapsin I binding to small synaptic vesicles. J. Biol. Chem. 261: 8383-8390.

Sieghart, W., J. Forn, R. Schwarcz, J. T. Coyle, and P. Greengard (1978) Neuronal localization of specific brain phosphoproteins. Brain Res. 156: 345-350.

Sorensen, R. G., and J. A. Babitch (1984) Identification and comparison of Protein I in chick and rat forebrain. J. Neurochem. 42: 705-709.

Steiner, J. P., E. Ling, and V. Bennett (1987) Nearest neighbor analysis for brain synapsin I. Evidence from *in vitro* reassociation assays for association with membrane protein(s) and the Mr = 68,000 neurofilament subunit. J. Biol. Chem. 262: 905-914.

Südhof, T.C., A.J. Czernik, H. Kao, K. Takei, P.A. Johnston, A. Horiuchi, M. Wagner, S.D. Kanazir, M.S. Perin, P. De Camilli, and P. Greengard (1989) The synapsins: mosaics of shared and unique domains in a family of synaptic vesicle phosphoproteins. Science 245: 1474-1480.

Ueda, T., and P. Greengard (1977) Adenosine 3':5'-monophosphate-regulated phosphoprotein system of neuronal membranes. I. Solubilization, purification, and some properties of an endogenous phosphoprotein. J. Biol. Chem. 252: 5155-5163.

Utsumi, K., E. Okimasu, Y. M. Morimoto, Y. Nishihara, and M. Miyahara (1982) Selective interaction of cytoskeletal proteins with liposomes. FEBS Letters 141: 176-180.

Valtorta, F., A. Villa, R. Jahn, P. De Camilli, P. Greengard, and B. Ceccarelli (1988) Localization of synapsin I at the frog neuromuscular junction. Neurosci. 24: 593-603.

Volknandt, W., S. Naito, T. Ueda, and H. Zimmermann (1987) Synapsin I is associated with cholinergic nerve terminals in the electric organs of Torpedo, Electrophorus, and Malapterurus and copurifies with Torpedo synaptic vesicles. J. Neurochem. 49: 342-347.

Zimmermann, H., and C. R. Denston (1977) Separation of synaptic vesicles of different functional states from the cholinergic synapses of the Torpedo electric organ. Neurosci. 2: 715-730.

SYNAPTOPHYSIN AND SYNAPSIN I AS TOOLS FOR THE STUDY OF THE EXO-ENDOCYTOTIC CYCLE

Flavia Valtorta§, Francesca Torri Tarelli, Luca Campanati, Antonello Villa and Paul Greengard*

"Bruno Ceccarelli" Center for the Study of Peripheral Neuropathies and Neuromuscular Diseases, CNR Center of Cytopharmacology, Department of Pharmacology, University of Milano Medical School, * Laboratory of Molecular and Cellular Neuroscience, The Rockefeller University, New York

Synaptophysin, an integral protein of the synaptic vesicle membrane, and synapsin I, a phosphoprotein associated with the cytoplasmic side of synaptic vesicles, represent useful markers that allow to follow the movements of the vesicle membrane during recycling. The use of antibodies against these proteins to label nerve terminals during experimental treatments which stimulate secretion has provided evidence that during the exo-endocytotic cycle synaptic vesicles transiently fuse with the axolemma, from which they are specifically recovered. When recycling is blocked, exocytosis leads to the permanent incorporation of the synaptic vesicle membrane into the axolemma and to diffusion of the vesicle components in the plane of the membrane.

INTRODUCTION

The release of quanta of neurotransmitter from nerve terminals occurs by exocytosis which involves the fusion of the synaptic vesicle membrane with the axolemma. This exocytotic event is usually followed by an endocytotic event that recovers an equivalent area of membrane from the axolemma. At the neuromuscular junction, the two processes are tightly coupled, so that the population of synaptic vesicles is maintained at nearly normal levels during long periods of intense secretion. Only at extremely high rates of secretion (which at the frog neuromuscular junction have been estimated to be in the order of thousands of quanta per second) does the coupling between the two processes become loose and the number of synaptic vesicles within the nerve terminal decreases significantly. Beside maintaining the number of synaptic vesicles constant, endocytosis also prevents the enlargement of the axolemmal surface area and maintains membrane and organelle diversity. In fact, in spite of the continuous bidirectional membrane flow which occurs during the exo-endocytotic cycle, no randomization of membrane components occurs.

At variance with what has been observed with other types of endocytosis (e.g. pinocytosis), the removal of membrane from the axolemma which follows secretion appears to be closely regulated,

---

§ to whom correspondence should be addressed

since it occurs only when triggered by exocytosis. However, the factors which control it are not known (for a recent review, see Valtorta et al., 1990).

In most systems, the pathway of recycling involves the retrieved membrane being transported to the Golgi apparatus for refilling. In the case of small synaptic vesicles which contain classical neurotransmitters this step is not necessary, since all the machinery necessary for synthetizing and loading neurotransmitters is present within the nerve terminal. Recycled synaptic vesicles can therefore move directly back to the axolemma. Using hemicholinium-3 (a blocker of choline uptake), Ceccarelli and Hurlbut (1975) showed that in electrically stimulated nerve terminals empty synaptic vesicles continue recycling, indicating that coupling of exocytosis and endocytosis does not require that synaptic vesicles are filled with neurotransmitter.

One important question in synaptic vesicle recycling concerns the mechanism which allows the maintenance of membrane specificity in spite of repeated fusion and retrieval. One possibility is that the patches of synaptic vesicle membrane maintain their identity even after their incorporation into the axolemma. A second possibility is that after exocytosis random mixing of membrane components occurs. In the latter case, the preservation of membrane specificity would imply the existence of a mechanism of molecular filtration that operates subsequently to membrane recapture. Another problem concerns the sites of endocytosis, i.e. whether vesicle recapture occurs at (or close to) the sites of exocytosis or whether the vesicle membrane is displaced along the axolemma before internalization. These problems have been examined in detail at the neuromuscular junction, and will be discussed below.

EXPERIMENTAL APPROACHES TO THE STUDY OF RECYCLING

The study of the different steps in the exo-endocytotic pathway has been approached primarily by morphological techniques. The initial demonstration of the occurrence of membrane recycling in nerve terminals was provided by the use of extracellular tracers (Holtzman et al., 1971; Ceccarelli et al., 1972 and 1973; Heuser and Reese, 1973). These authors demonstrated that after a prolonged period of intense secretion many of the synaptic vesicles present in a nerve terminal become loaded with extracellular tracers, indicating that they have undergone fusion and retrieval (see also Fig. 1 d and e).

Freeze-fracture studies have provided evidence that stimulation of neurotransmitter release is accompanied by the appearance of images of vesicle fusion on the plasmalemma. With most treatments, fusion occurs predominantly close to membrane specializations called the "active zones", but there are also exceptions to this rule (Heuser et al., 1974; Ceccarelli et al., 1979 a and b; Ceccarelli et al., 1988).

Measurements of quantal secretion combined with morphometric analyses of the ultrastructural changes occurring in stimulated nerve endings have been used to evaluate quantal release and vesicle recycling. These studies have shown that under conditions in which extracellular tracers are taken up, the number of quanta secreted exceeds the number of vesicles present at rest, indicating that recycled membranes are not degraded, but are used in successive cycles of secretion. On the contrary, when recycling is blocked, stimulation leads to depletion of both quanta and synaptic

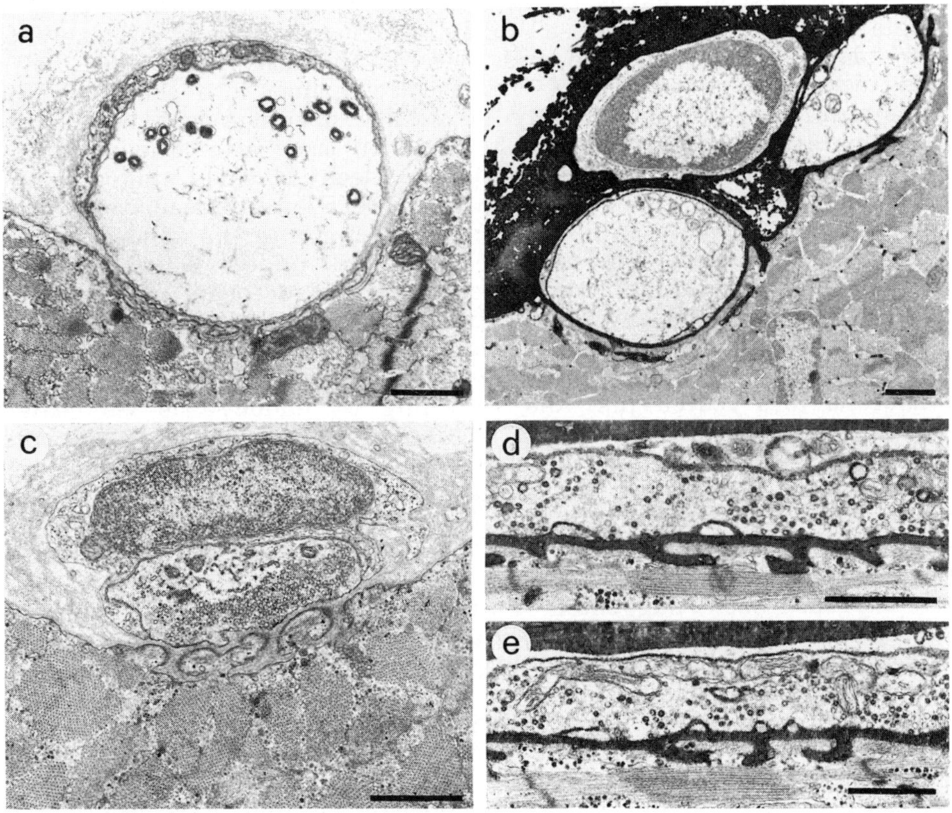

Fig. 1 Effects of α-LTx on the ultrastructure of the neuromuscular junction. (a and b) Electron micrographs of cross-sectioned terminals treated for 1 h with 0.2 μg/ml α-LTx in Ca^{2+}-free solution. The terminal branches shown in b come from an experiment in which 1.6% horseradish peroxidase and 0.5% spermwhale myoglobin were present. (c) Electron micrograph from a cross-sectioned terminal treated for 1 h with the same concentration of α-LTx in Ca^{2+}-containing Ringer's solution. (d and e) Longitudinal sections of terminals treated as in c in the presence of 1.6% horseradish peroxidase. Notice the normal appearance of the terminal in c and the depletion of synaptic vesicles and the swelling of the terminals in a and b. In d and e, most of the synaptic vesicle are loaded with horseradish peroxidase reaction product. Bars, 1 μm. (Reproduced from The Journal of Cell Biology, 1988, 107:2717-2727, by Copyright permission of the Rockefeller University Press).

vesicles (Haimann et al., 1985; Segal et al., 1985; Fesce et al., 1986; Valtorta et al., 1988a).

The quick-freezing technique, which was originally developed by Heuser et al. (1979), and subsequently improved by Ceccarelli and coworkers (Torri-Tarelli et al., 1985), has provided the best evidence for a temporal correlation between neurotransmitter release and fusion of synaptic vesicles with the axolemma. By using this technique, Torri Tarelli et al. (1985) have shown that the earliest images of vesicle fusion occur 2.5 msec after the delivery of a single shock to the nerve, a delay which corresponds precisely to the sum of conduction time and presynaptic delay. However, with this technique no images of vesicles collapsing into the axolemma were observed and the density of vesicle openings was unchanged in preparations quick frozen 2.5, 5 or 10 msec after the stimulus. These findings support the idea that, at least at early stages in the secretory process, the vesicles can be recovered immediately after their fusion, possibly without even flattening into the axolemma.

On the basis of results obtained under a variety of experimental conditions, two mechanisms have been proposed to account for the recovery of synaptic vesicles. The first implies the collapse of the fused vesicle membrane with its possible diffusion in the plane of the axolemma followed by reassembly of the vesicle membrane into coated pits and recycling by endocytosis via coated vesicles (Heuser and Reese, 1973; Gennaro et al., 1978; Lentz and Chester, 1982; Miller and Heuser, 1984). The second implies the rapid direct removal of the vesicle membrane following exocytosis without its flattening into and intermixing with the presynaptic membrane (Ceccarelli et al., 1972 and 1973; Ceccarelli and Hurlbut, 1980b; Torri-Tarelli et al., 1985).

It has been suggested that at actively secreting synapses these two mechanisms can coexist, the latter being predominant under those conditions of stimulation that allow a balance between exocytosis and endocytosis to be maintained. When the endocytotic process is outstripped by exhaustive rates of secretion, the vesicle membrane would flatten and accumulate in the axolemma, thus increasing its surface area. Endocytotic retrieval of these membranes would then occur through the coated vesicle-mediated mechanism (Meldolesi and Ceccarelli, 1981; Cooper and McLaughlin, 1983; Haimann et al., 1985; Torri-Tarelli et al., 1987).

Another possible approach to the study of recycling consists in tracing the movements of the synaptic vesicle membrane during the exo-endocytotic cycle. We performed one such study using antibodies against two synaptic vesicle proteins, synaptophysin and synapsin I.

SYNAPTOPHYSIN, A TRANSMEMBRANE PROTEIN OF SYNAPTIC VESICLES

Synaptophysin (previously referred to as p38) has been identified as a major integral membrane protein of synaptic vesicles (Jahn et al., 1985; Wiedenmann and Franke, 1985; Navone et al., 1986). It is an acidic glycopeptide with an apparent molecular weight of 38,000 daltons. Synaptophysin was initially purified from rat brain cortex, and its amino acid sequence and molecular structure have recently been elucidated (Südhof et al., 1987; Leube et al., 1987; Buckley et al., 1987). Hydrophobicity plots of the sequence suggest the presence of four transmembrane spanning regions, with both the amino- and carboxy-termini facing the cytoplasm. The carboxy terminal contains several copies of a pentapeptide repeat rich in glycine, proline and tyrosine residues, which is slightly homologous to the collagenase-sensitive tail of synapsin I. This part of the molecule is implicated in Ca^{2+} binding (Rehm et al., 1986).

Synaptophysin can be endogenously phosphorylated on tyrosine and serine residues in both purified synaptic vesicles and in synaptosomes (Pang et al., 1988a). The kinase responsible for tyrosine phosphorylation of synaptophysin is likely to be $pp60^{c\text{-}src}$, since it accounts for more than 70% of the tyrosine kinase activity in a preparation of purified synaptic vesicles (Pang et al., 1988b).

Sedimentation and cross-linking studies indicate that native synaptophysin is a disulfide-linked hexameric homo-oligomer. In reconstitution experiments, purified synaptophysin displays channel properties with a conductance similar to that of reconstituted gap junction protein (Thomas et al., 1989).

Subcellular fractionation as well as immunocytochemistry experiments indicate that within the nervous system synaptophysin has a distribution similar to that of synapsin I, being localized on synaptic vesicles from virtually all synapses so far studied. Synaptophysin is also expressed in neuroendocrine cells, where it is associated with a population of previously unidentified small vesicles which are concentrated in the Golgi region (Wiedenmann and Franke, 1985; Navone et al., 1986). The possible association of synaptophysin with endocrine secretory granules and with neuronal large dense core vesicles has been a subject of debate. Putting together the results obtained so far by several groups working on this topic, it can be concluded that synaptophysin is detected in endocrine secretory vesicles only when very sensitive biochemical methods are used (Navone et al., 1986; Lowe et al., 1988; Wiedenmann et al., 1988; Obendorf et al., 1988). These low concentrations of synaptophysin could therefore be ascribed to either membrane contamination or mis-sorting and are not likely to be physiologically significant.

SYNAPSIN I, A SYNAPTIC VESICLE-SPECIFIC PHOSPHOPROTEIN

Synapsin I (previously named Protein I) is a neuronal phosphoprotein primarily associated with the cytoplasmic surface of synaptic vesicles (Ueda and Greengard, 1977; De Camilli et al., 1983a and b; Huttner et al., 1983; Navone et al., 1984; Valtorta et al., 1988b). It exists as a doublet (synapsin Ia and synapsin Ib), having molecular weights of 86,000 and 80,000, respectively. The synapsin I molecule is highly asymmetric, consisting of a globular, collagenase-resistant hydrophobic head region and of an elongated,

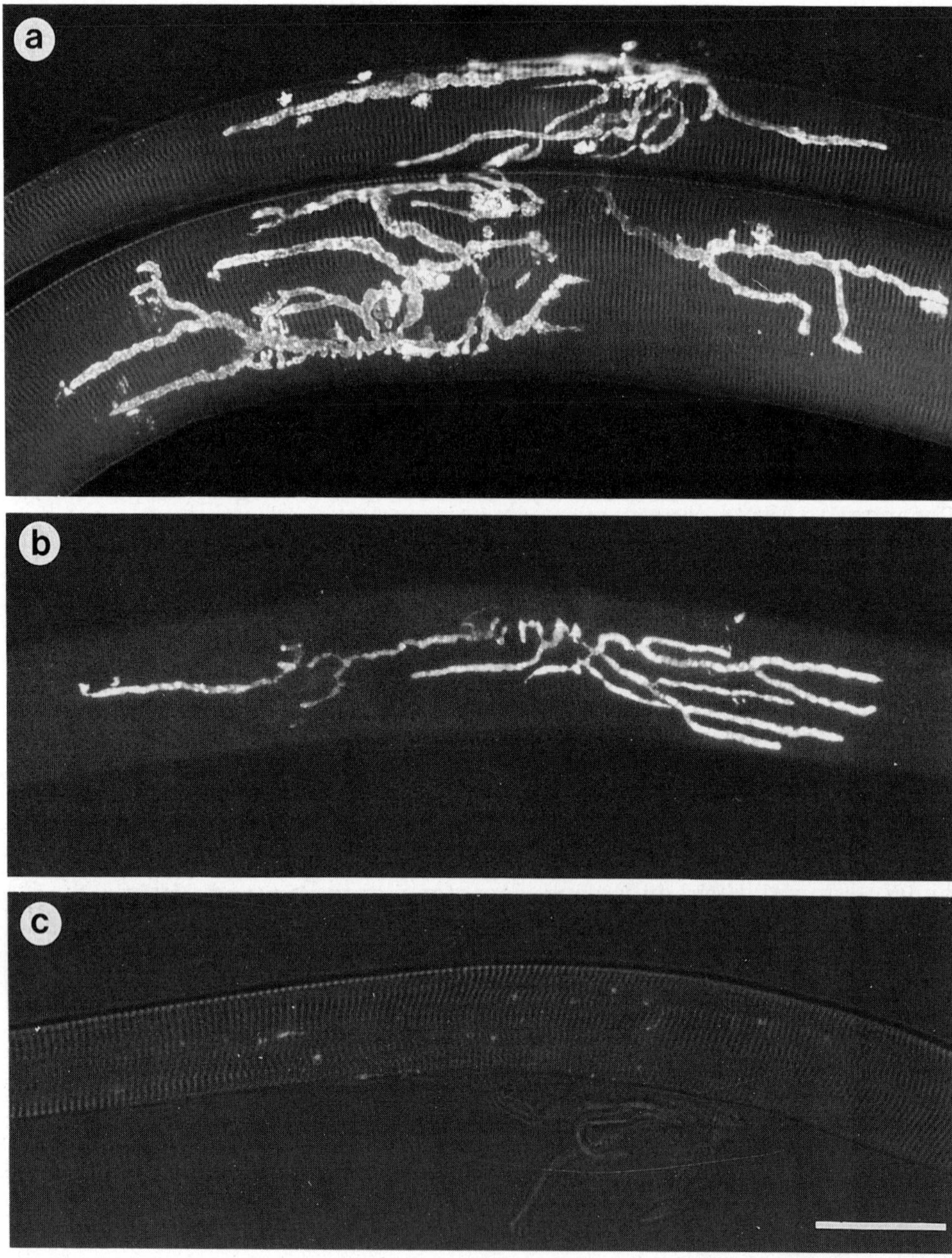

Fig. 2 Immunofluorescence for synaptophysin on single fibers teased apart from frog cutaneus pectoris muscle. The fiber shown in a is from a preparation fixed after treatment with 0.2 µg/ml α-LTx in Ca^{2+}-free medium and immunostained without detergent treatment. The fibers in b and c are from a preparation treated with 0.2 µg/ml α-LTx in Ca^{2+}- containing medium. In the case of the fiber in b, 0.1% Triton-X-100 was used prior to the application of antibodies. Bars, 50 µm.(Modified from The Journal of Cell Biology, 1988, 107: 2717-2727, by Copyright permission of the Rockefeller University Press).

collagenase-sensitive basic tail region (Ueda and Greengard, 1977; Südhof et al., 1989).

Synapsin I undergoes multisite phosphorylation. One serine residue in the collagenase-resistant head of the molecule is phosphorylated by cAMP-dependent protein kinase and by Ca^{2+}/calmodulin-dependent protein kinase I, whereas two other serine residues, located in the collagenase-sensitive tail of the molecule, are phosphorylated by Ca^{2+}/calmodulin-dependent protein kinase II (Huttner et al., 1981; Czernik et al., 1987).

The binding of synapsin I to the synaptic vesicle membrane is characterized by high affinity and saturability and is modulated by phosphorylation, the binding affinity being reduced by 5-fold upon phosphorylation of synapsin I by Ca^{2+}/calmodulin-dependent protein kinase II (Schiebler et al., 1986).

Synapsin I is also able to interact with various cytoskeletal elements (microtubules, spectrin, neurofilaments, actin; Baines and Bennett, 1985 and 1986; Goldenring et al., 1986; Bähler and Greengard, 1987; Petrucci and Morrow, 1987; Steiner et al., 1987). Its interaction with actin filaments is characterized by the formation of actin bundles. Phosphorylation of synapsin I by Ca^{2+}/calmodulin-dependent protein kinase II is associated with suppression of the actin-bundling activity (Bähler and Greengard, 1987; Petrucci and Morrow, 1987).

Experiments carried out at the squid giant synapse suggest that changes in the state of phosphorylation of synapsin I influence the amount of neurotransmitter released after a secretagogue stimulus is applied (Llinas et al., 1985). It has been proposed that synapsin I modulates neurotransmitter release by linking synaptic vesicles to the actin-based cytoskeletal network of the nerve terminal. According to this hypothesis, phorphorylation of synapsin I by Ca^{2+}/calmodulin-dependent protein kinase II leads to its dissociation from synaptic vesicles and/or actin filaments leaving the vesicles more available for fusion.

IMMUNOCYTOCHEMISTRY

Immunocytochemistry was employed to localize synaptophysin and synapsin I at the frog neuromuscular junction and to investigate the redistribution of these proteins during synaptic activity. The study of the fate of synaptophysin, an integral component of the synaptic vesicle membrane, allows one to follow the movements of the vesicle membrane during the different steps of the exo-endocytotic cycle, whereas in the case of synapsin I the same approach might provide clues to the life cycle and functional role of this protein.

As a means of stimulating neurotransmitter release we used α-latrotoxin (α-LTx), the purified active component of Black Widow Spider Venom (for review see Hurlbut and Ceccarelli, 1979; Meldolesi et al., 1986). Because of its property of exerting different effects on the exo-endocytotic process depending on the presence or absence of Ca^{2+} in the incubation media, this toxin is

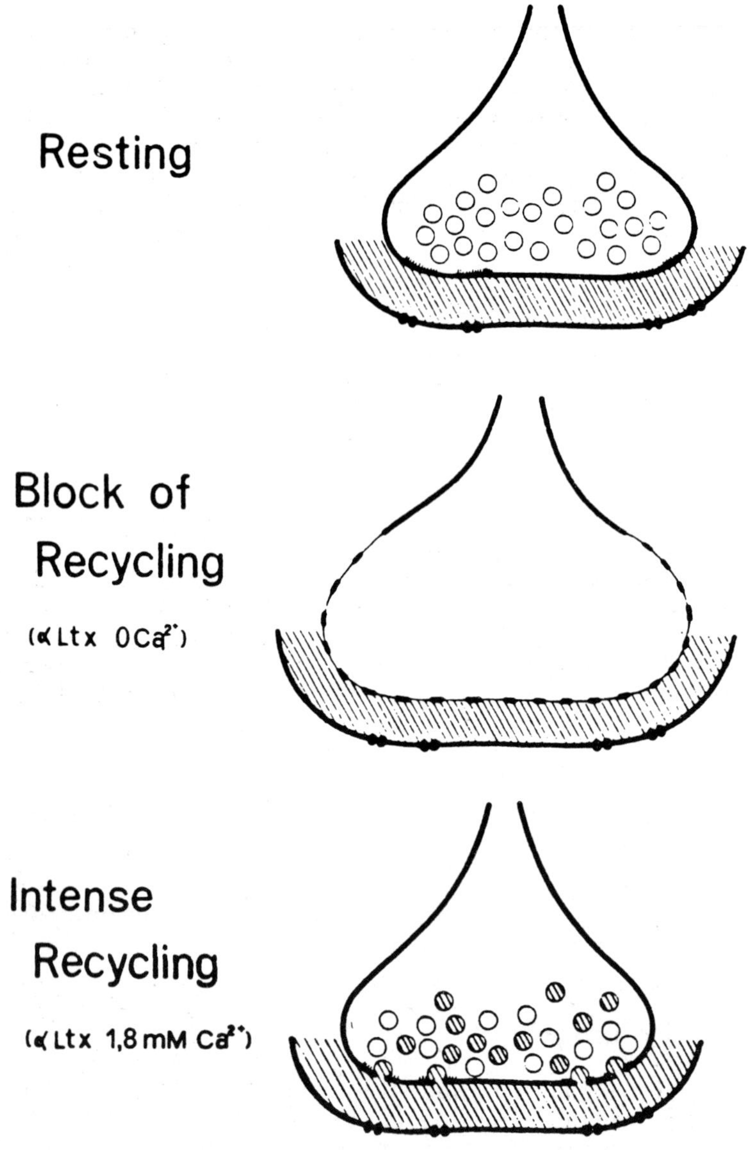

Fig. 3 Schematic drawings illustrating the neuromuscular junction ultrastructure under different conditions of stimulation. (a) In resting condition, the nerve terminal is filled with synaptic vesicles; (b) after exposure to 0.2 μg/ml α-LTx in Ca^{2+}-free medium, no vesicles can be seen in the nerve terminal which appears swollen as a result of the incorporation of synaptic vesicle membranes into the axolemma. The membranes of the vesicles have diffused in the plane of the axolemma and are therefore present also in regions distant from the sites of fusion; (c) after exposure to 0.2 μg/ml α-LTx in Ca^{2+}-containing medium, the presynaptic terminal is filled with synaptic vesicles. The hatched circles represent vesicles which have undergone recycling and are loaded with extracellular tracer reaction product.

a useful tool for studying synaptic vesicle recycling. Low doses of α-LTx, when applied in the absence of Ca^{2+}, deplete nerve terminals of both quanta of neurotransmitter and synaptic vesicles, inducing a massive but transient secretion concomitant with a block of endocytosis. When on the other hand the toxin is applied in the presence of Ca^{2+}, quantal secretion is sustained by active recycling. Under this condition high frequencies of secretion are maintained for more than one hour and the terminals maintain their complement of synaptic vesicles (Fig. 1; Ceccarelli and Hurlbut, 1980a; Valtorta et al., 1988a).

When anti-synaptophysin antibodies were used to stain nerve-muscle preparations fixed at rest, immunofluorescent images of nerve terminals were obtained only after the preparations had been permeabilized by detergent treatment. After treatment with α-LTx in Ca^{2+}-free medium, no permeabilization was necessary to obtain a bright immunofluorescent picture of the nerve terminal, indicating that intravesicular domains of synaptophysin had become exposed to the extracellular space (Figs. 2a and 4; Valtorta et al., 1988a). This result adds further support to the vesicle hypothesis of neurotransmitter release, indicating that, when secretion is stimulated in the presence of a block of endocytosis, the synaptic vesicle membrane is permanently incorporated in the axolemma. High resolution images of anti-synaptophysin immunoreactivity on ultrathin cryosections showed a uniform distribution of immunogold

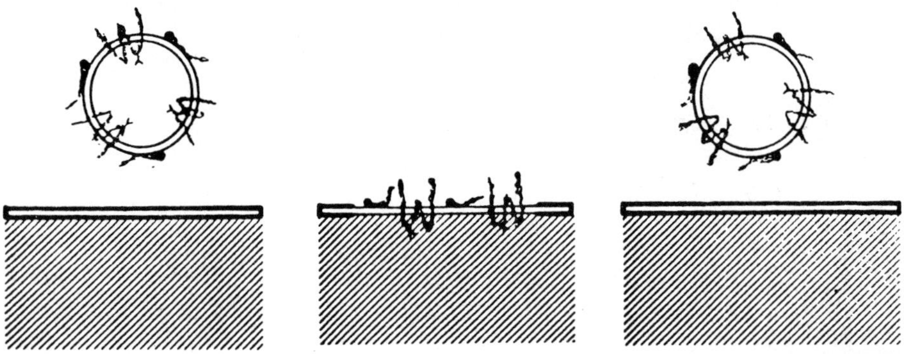

Fig. 4 Schematic drawings showing the redistribution of vesicle membrane components during the exo-endocytotic cycle. Left panel: Structural model of a synaptic vesicle with two vesicle-specific proteins, synapsin I and synaptophysin. Synapsin I is composed of a globular head and an elongated tail and is associated with the cytoplasmic side of the synaptic vesicle membrane. The synaptophysin molecule spans the vesicle membrane four times and is glycosylated in its intravesicular portion. Central panel: distribution of the synaptic vesicle membrane components after fusion. The intravesicular portion of synaptophysin is now exposed to the extracellular space. Synapsin I maintains its association with the fused vesicle membrane. Right panel: synaptic vesicle which has undergone recycling. No components of the vesicle membrane can be detected in the axolemma, suggesting a selectivity of the retrieval process.

particles along the axolemma of depleted nerve terminals: both the presynaptic membrane and the portions of the axolemma distal to the postjunctional folds were decorated (Torri Tarelli et al., 1990). This finding confirms the results obtained with immunofluorescence and indicates that, in the presence of a block of the retrieval process, the synaptic vesicle components diffuse in the plane of the nerve terminal plasma membrane after fusion (Fig.3).

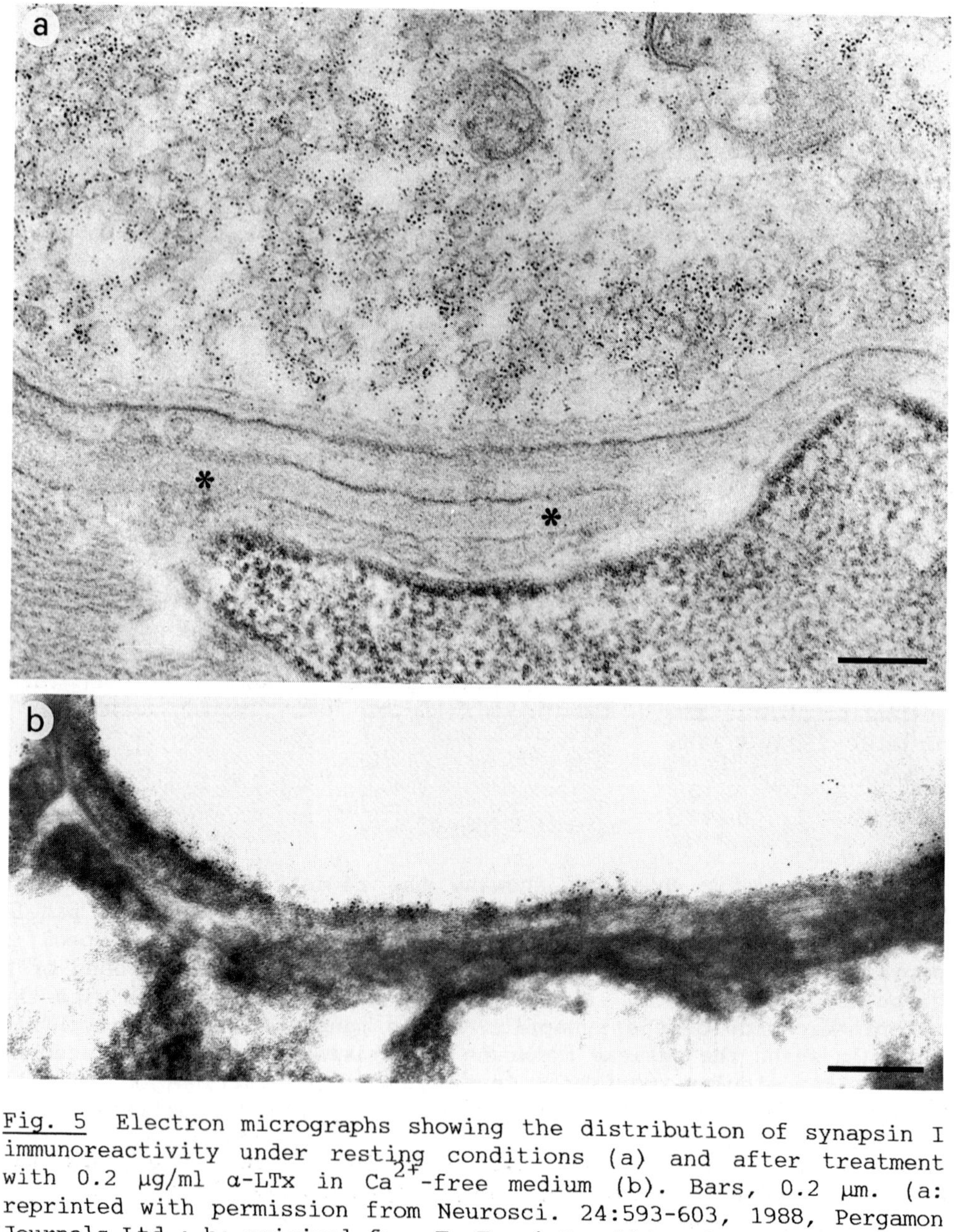

Fig. 5 Electron micrographs showing the distribution of synapsin I immunoreactivity under resting conditions (a) and after treatment with 0.2 μg/ml α-LTx in Ca^{2+}-free medium (b). Bars, 0.2 μm. (a: reprinted with permission from Neurosci. 24:593-603, 1988, Pergamon Journals Ltd.; b: original from F. Torri Tarelli and A. Villa).

Permeabilization was necessary to obtain immunofluorescence pictures of nerve terminals stimulated with α-LTx in the presence of Ca^{2+}, indicating that no relevant amounts of synaptophysin were present in the axolemma (Fig.2b and c; Valtorta et al., 1988a). These results were confirmed by ultrastructural analysis. Both at rest and after treatment with α-LTx in the presence of Ca^{2+}, immunogold particles were found to be specifically associated with the membrane of synaptic vesicles, whereas the axolemma was virtually unlabelled (Torri Tarelli et al., 1990). These results suggest that the residence time of the vesicle membrane on the surface of the nerve terminal is very short and that the retrieval mechanism is selective for vesicle components (Figs.3 and 4).

The same experimental approach, when applied to the study of the distribution of synapsin I, showed that this protein behaves in a manner similar to that of synaptophysin. After treatment with α-LTx in the presence of Ca^{2+}, synapsin I immunoreactivity appeared to be selectively associated with the membrane of synaptic vesicles, a situation similar to that observed under resting conditions (Fig.5a; Valtorta et al., 1988b; Torri Tarelli et al., 1990). These results are compatible either with a persistent association of synapsin I with the vesicle membrane during recycling or with its dissociation prior to fusion and rapid reassociation after retrieval.

Specific synapsin I labelling of the axolemma was observed in nerve terminals depleted of synaptic vesicles by treatment with α-LTx in Ca^{2+}-free medium, suggesting that under these conditions synapsin I remains associated with the vesicle membrane after fusion (Fig.3 and Fig.5b; Torri Tarelli et al., 1990). Although the mechanism by which the toxin induces secretion in Ca^{2+}-free medium is probably different from that triggered by physiological stimuli (it does not lead to an increase in cytosolic Ca^{2+} nor does it increase the state of phosphorylation of synapsin I; Meldolesi et al., 1984), this result shows that the dissociation of synapsin I from the vesicle membrane is not required in order for synaptic vesicles to undergo exocytosis.

REFERENCES

Bähler, M., and Greengard, P. (1987) Synapsin I bundles F-actin in a phosphorylation-dependent manner. Nature 326:704-707.

Baines, A. J., and Bennett V. (1985) Synapsin I is a spectrin-binding protein immunologically related to erythrocyte protein 4.1. Nature 315:410-413.

Baines, A. J., and Bennett V. (1986) Synapsin I is a microtubule-bundling protein. Nature 319:145-147.

Buckley, K.M., Floor E., and Kelly R.B. (1987) Cloning and sequence analysis of cDNA encoding p38, a major synaptic vesicle protein. J. Cell Biol. 105:2447-2456.

Ceccarelli, B., Fesce, R., Grohovaz, F., and Haimann, C. (1988) The effect of potassium on exocytosis of transmitter at the frog neuromuscular junction. J. Physiol. Lond 401:163-183.

Ceccarelli, B., Grohovaz, F., and Hurlbut, W.P. (1979a) Freeze-fracture studies of frog neuromuscular junctions during intense release of neurotransmitter. I. Effects of Black Widow Spider Venom and Ca^{2+}-free solutions on the structure of the active zone. J. Cell Biol. 81:163-177.

Ceccarelli, B., Grohovaz, F., and Hurlbut, W.P. (1979b) Freeze-fracture studies of frog neuromuscular junctions during intense release of neurotransmitter. II. Effects of electrical stimulation and high potassium. J. Cell Biol. 81:178-192.

Ceccarelli, B., and Hurlbut, W.P. (1975) The effects of prolonged repetitive stimulation in hemicholinium on the frog neuromuscular junction. J. Physiol. Lond 247:163-188.

Ceccarelli, B., and Hurlbut, W.P. (1980a) Ca^{2+}-dependent recycling of synaptic vesicles at the frog neuromuscular junction. J. Cell Biol. 87:297-303.

Ceccarelli, B., and Hurlbut, W.P. (1980b) Vesicle hypothesis of the release of quanta of acetylcholine. Physiol. Rev. 60:396-441.

Ceccarelli, B., Hurlbut, W.P., and Mauro, A. (1972) Depletion of vesicles from frog neuromuscular junctions by prolonged tetanic stimulation. J. Cell Biol. 54: 30-38.

Ceccarelli, B., Hurlbut, W.P., and Mauro, A. (1973) Turnover of transmitter and synaptic vesicles at the frog neuromuscular junction. J. Cell Biol. 57:499-524.

Cooper, N. G. F., and McLaughlin, B. J. (1983) Tracer uptake by photoreceptor synaptic terminals. J. Ultrastr. Res. 84: 252-267

Czernik, A. J.,Pang, D. T., and Greengard, P. (1987) Amino acid sequences surrounding the cAMP-dependent and calcium/calmodulin-dependent phosphorylation sites in rat and bovine synapsin I. Proc. Natl. Acad. Sci. U.S.A. 84:7518-7522.

De Camilli, P., Cameron, R., and Greengard, P., (1983a) Synapsin I (Protein I), a nerve terminal-specific phosphoprotein. I. Its general distribution in synapses of the central and peripheral nervous system demonstrated by immunofluorescence in frozen and plastic sections. J. Cell Biol. 96:1337-1354.

De Camilli, P., Harris, S. M., Huttner W. B., and Greengard, P. (1983b) Synapsin I (Protein I), a nerve terminal-specific phosphoprotein. II. Its specific association with synaptic vesicles demonstrated by immunocytochemistry in agarose-embedded synaptosomes. J. Cell Biol. 96:1355-1373.

Fesce, R., Segal, J.R., Ceccarelli, B., and Hurlbut, W.P. (1986a) Effects of Black Widow Spider Venom and Ca^{2+} on quantal secretion at the frog neuromuscular junction. J. Gen. Physiol. 88:59-81.

Gennaro, J. F., Nastuk, W. L., and Rutherford, D. T. (1978) Reversible depletion of synaptic vesicles induced by application of high external potassium to the frog neuromuscular junction. J. Physiol. Lond 280: 237-247

Goldenring, J. R., Lasher, R. S., Vallano, M. L., Ueda, T., Naito, S., Sternberger, N. H., Sternberger, L. A., and DeLorenzo, R. J. (1986) Association of synapsin I with neuronal cytoskeleton. Identification in cytoskeletal preparations in vitro and immunocytochemical localization in brain of synapsin I. J. Biol. Chem. 261:8495-8504.

Haimann, C., Torri-Tarelli, F., Fesce, R., and Ceccarelli, B. (1985) Measurement of quantal secretion induced by ouabain and its correlation with depletion of synaptic vesicles. J. Cell Biol. 101:1953-1965.

Heuser, J.E., and Reese, T.S. (1973) Evidence for recycling of synaptic vesicle membrane during transmitter release at the frog neuromuscular junction. J. Cell Biol. 57:315-344.

Heuser, J.E., Reese, T. S, Dennis, M.J., Jan, Y., and Evans, L. (1979) Synaptic vesicle exocytosis captured by quick-freezing and correlated with quantal transmitter release. J. Cell Biol. 81:275-300.

Heuser, J.E., Reese, T.S., and Landis, D.M.D. (1974) Functional changes in frog neuromuscular junctions studied with freeze-fracture. J. Neurocytol. 3:109-131.

Holtzman, E., Freeman, A. R., and L. A. Kashner (1971) Stimulation dependent alterations in peroxidase uptake at lobster neuromuscular junctions. Science 173: 733-736.

Hurlbut, W.P., and Ceccarelli, B. (1979) Use of Black Widow Spider Venom to study the release of neurotransmitter. In: Advances in Cytopharmacology, edited by B. Ceccarelli and F. Clementi, pp. 87-115. Raven Press, New York.

Huttner, W. B., and Greengard, P. (1979) Multiple phosphorylation sites in Protein I and their differential regulation by cyclic AMP and calcium. Proc. Natl. Acad. Sci. U.S.A. 76:5402-5406.

Huttner, W. B., DeGennaro, L. J., and Greengard, P. (1981) Differential phosphorylation of multiple sites in purified Protein I by cyclic AMP-dependent and calcium-dependent protein kinases. J. Biol. Chem. 256:1482-1488.

Huttner, W. B., Schiebler, W., Greengard, P., and De Camilli, P. (1983) Synapsin I (Protein I), a nerve terminal-specific phosphoprotein. III. Its association with synaptic vesicles studied in a highly purified synaptic vesicle preparation. J. Cell Biol. 96:1374-1388.

Jahn, R., Schiebler, W., Ouimet, C., and Greengard, P. (1985) A 38,000-dalton membrane protein (p38) present in synaptic vesicles. Proc. Natl. Acad. Sci. U.S.A. 82: 4137-4141.

Lentz, T. L., and Chester, J. (1982) Synaptic vesicle recycling at the neuromuscular junction in the presence of a presynaptic membrane marker. Neurosci. 7:9-20.

Leube, R. E., Kaiser, P., Seiter, A., Zimbelmann, R., Franke, W.W., Rehm, H., P., Knaus, P., Prior, P.,Betz, H., Reinke, H., Beyreuther, K.,and Wiedenmann, B. (1987) Synaptophysin: molecular organization and mRNA expression as determined from cloned cDNA. EMBO (Eur. Mol. Biol. Organ.) J. 6:3261-3268.

Llinas, R., McGuinness, T. L., Leonard, C.S., Sugimori, M., and Greengard, P. (1985) Intraterminal injection of synapsin I or calcium/calmodulin-dependent protein kinase II alters neurotransmitter release at the squid giant synapse. Proc. Natl. Acad. Sci. U.S.A. 82:3035-3039.

Lowe, A. W., Madeddu L., and R. B. Kelly (1988) Endocrine secretory granules and neuronal synaptic vesicles have three integral membrane proteins in common. J. Cell Biol. 106: 51-59

Meldolesi, J., and Ceccarelli, B. (1981) Exocytosis and membrane recycling. Phil. Trans. R. Soc. Lond B 296:55-65.

Meldolesi, J., Huttner, W. P., Tsien, R. Y. and Pozzan, T. (1984) Free cytoplasmic Ca^{2+} and neurotransmitter release: Studies on PC12 cells and synaptosomes exposed to α-latrotoxin. Proc. Natl. Acad. Sci. U.S.A. 81:620-624.

Meldolesi, J., Scheer, H., Madeddu, L., and Wanke, E. (1986) On the mechanism of action of α-latrotoxin, the presynaptic stimulatory toxin of the black widow spider venom. Trends Pharm. Sci., 7:151-155.

Miller, T.M., and Heuser, J. E. (1984) Endocytosis of synaptic vesicle membrane at the frog neuromuscular junction. J. Cell Biol. 98:685-698.

Navone, F., Greengard, P., and De Camilli, P. (1984) Synapsin I in nerve terminals: selective association with small synaptic vesicles. Science, 226:1209-1211.

Navone, F., Jahn, R., Di Gioia, G., Stukenbrok, H., Greengard, P., and De Camilli, P.(1986) Protein p38: an integral membrane protein specific for small vesicles of neurons and neuroendocrine cells. J. Cell Biol. 103:2511-2527.

Obendorf, D., Schwarzenbrunner, U., Fischer-Colbrie, R.,Laslop, A.,and Winkler H. (1988) In adrenal medulla synaptophysin is present in chromaffin granules and in a special vesicle population. J. Neurochem. 51:1573-1580

Pang, D., Wang, J.,Valtorta, F., Benfenati, F., and Greengard, P. (1988a) Protein tyrosine phosphorylation in synaptic vesicles. Proc. Natl. Acad. Sci. U.S.A. 85:762-766

Pang, D., Valtorta, F., De Marco, M. E., Brugge, J. S., Benfenati, F., and Greengard, P. (1988b) Localization of $pp60^{c-src}$ in synaptic vesicles. Abstr. Soc. Neurosci.

Petrucci, T.C., and Morrow, J. S. (1987) Synapsin I: an actin-bundling protein under phosphorylation control. J. Cell Biol. 105:1355-1363.

Rehm, H., Wiedenmann, B., and Betz, H. (1986) Molecular characterization of synaptophysin, a major calcium-binding protein of the synaptic vesicle membrane. EMBO (Eur. Mol. Biol. Organ.) J. 5:535-541.

Schiebler, W., Jahn, R., Doucet, J-P., Rothlein, J., and Greengard, P. (1986) Characterization of synapsin I binding to small synaptic vesicles. J. Biol. Chem. 261:8383-8390.

Segal, J.R., Ceccarelli, B., Fesce, R., and Hurlbut, W.P. (1985) Miniature endplate potential frequency and amplitude determined by an extension of Campbell's theorem. Biophys. J., 47:183-202.

Steiner, J. P., Ling, E., and Bennett, V. (1987) Nearest neighbor analysis from brain synapsin I. Evidence from in vitro reassociation assays for association with membrane protein(s) and the Mr = 68,000 neurofilament subunit. J. Biol. Chem. 262:905-914.

Südhof, T.C., Czernik, A. J., Kao, H., Takei, K., Johnston, P. A., Horiuchi, A.,Wagner, M., Kanazir, S. D., Perin, M. S., De Camilli, P., and Greengard, P. (1989) The synapsins: mosaics of shared and unique domains in a family of synaptic vesicle phosphoproteins. Science 245:1474-1480.

Südhof, T. C., Lottspeich, F., Greengard, P., Mehl, E., and Jahn, R. (1987) A synaptic vesicle protein with a novel cytoplasmic domain and four transmembrane regions. Science 238:1142-1144.

Thomas, L., Hartung, K., Langosch, D., Rehm, H., Bamberg, E., Franke, W.W., and Betz, H. (1988) Identification of synaptophysin as a hexameric channel protein of the synaptic vesicle membrane. Science 242: 1050-1053

Torri-Tarelli, F., Grohovaz, F., Fesce, R., and Ceccarelli, B. (1985) Temporal coincidence between synaptic vesicle fusion and quantal secretion of acetyl- choline. J. Cell Biol. 101:1386-1399.

Torri-Tarelli, F., Haimann, C., and Ceccarelli, B. (1987) Coated vesicles and pits during enhanced quantal release of acetylcholine at the neuromuscular junction. J. Neurocytol. 16:205-214.

Torri Tarelli, F., Villa, A., Valtorta, F., De Camilli, P., Greengard, P., and Ceccarelli, B. (1990) Redistribution of synaptophysin and synapsin I during α-latrotoxin induced release of neurotransmitter at the neuromuscular junction. J. Cell Biol., in press.

Ueda, T., and Greengard, P. (1977) Adenosine 3':5'-monophosphate-regulated phosphoprotein system of neuronal membranes. I. Solubilization, purification, and some properties of an endogenous phosphoprotein. J. Biol. Chem. 252:5155-5163.

Valtorta, F., Fesce, R., Grohovaz, F., Haimann, C., Hurlbut, W. P., Iezzi, N., Torri Tarelli, F., Villa, A.,and Ceccarelli, B. (1990) Neurotransmitter release and synaptic vesicle recycling. Neurosci., in press.

Valtorta, F., Jahn, R., Fesce, R., Greengard, P., and Ceccarelli, B. (1988a) Synaptophysin (p38) at the frog neuromuscular junction: its incorporation into the axolemma and recycling after intense quantal secretion. J. Cell Biol. 107:2719-2730.

Valtorta, F., Villa, A., Jahn, R., De Camilli, P., Greengard, P., and Ceccarelli, B. (1988b) Localization of synapsin I at the frog neuromuscular junction. Neurosci. 24:593-603.

Wiedenmann, B., and Franke, W. (1985) Identification and localization of synaptophysin, an integral membrane glycoprotein of M_r 38,000 characteristic of presynaptic vesicles. Cell 41:1017-1028.

Wiedenmann, B., Rehm, H., Knierim, M.,and Becker, C.M. (1988) Fractionation of synaptophysin-containing vesicles from rat brain and cultured PC12 pheochromocytoma cells. FEBS Lett. 240:71-77

VASOACTIVE INTESTINAL POLYPEPTIDE (VIP) AS A CHOLINERGIC CO-TRANSMITTER: SOME RECENT RESULTS

*V.P. Whittaker, Arbeitsgruppe Neurochemie, Max-Planck-Institut für biophysikalische Chemie, Göttingen, FRG**

The neuropeptide vasoactive intestinal polypeptide (VIP) copurifies with mammalian brain cholinergic synaptosomes when these are separated from the total brain synaptosome fraction by an immunoadsorption procedure based on an antiserum to a cholinergic-specific antigen. VIP must therefore be reckoned to be a cholinergic co-transmitter in brain. In electromotor and myenteric neurones the two transmitters are differently packaged. The frequency-dependence and pharmacology of release show that the intracellular dynamics of the storage and release processes are quite different for the two neurotransmitters. However in the ileum a portion of the vesicle-bound acetylcholine is recovered in the VIP-storing particles and this might indicate a precursor-product relationship for the two types of vesicle in this system analogous to that which has been proposed for electron-dense and electron-translucent vesicles in noradrenergic nerves.

Introduction

The phenomenon of cotransmission

In recent years it has become apparent - largely through the application of immunocytochemical techniques - that nerve terminals containing classical small-molecular-mass transmitters may often also contain neuroactive neuropeptides. This has led to the concept of co-transmission, in which a terminal may release, in addition to a classical transmitter, one or more neuropeptides. This raises a number of new problems for our understanding of synaptic transmission. We may ask, for example
- what is the function of the neuropeptide?
- how is it stored in the terminal: together with the classical transmitter in synaptic vesicles or in a separate class of storage granules?
- what is the frequency-dependence of its release and how does this compare with that of the classical transmitter?

Answers to the second and third questions may help to provide an answer to the first.

Vasoactive intestinal polypeptide - a cholinergic co-transmitter

For those of us particularly interested in cholinergic function the discovery, in recent years, that vasoactive intestinal polypeptide

---

*Postal address: Arbeitsgruppe Neurochemie, Max-Planck-Institut für biophysikalische Chemie, Postfach 2841, D-3400 Göttingen, F.R. Germany

Table I Acetylcholine and VIP contents of some tissues rich in cholinergic endings

Species and Tissue	Acetylcholine ($nmol.g^{-1}$)	VIP ($fmol.g^{-1}$)
Guinea pig		
Myenteric plexus	130 $\pm$ 20	4800 $\pm$ 600
Brain	20 $\pm$ 5	1400 $\pm$ 100
Muscle	2 $\pm$ 1	-
Torpedo		
Electric organ	920 $\pm$ 90	130 $\pm$ 16
Electric lobes	25 $\pm$ 2	820 $\pm$ 50

Values are means $\pm$ SEM of 3 or more determinations; for *Torpedo* they are porcine VIP equivalents

(VIP) is often associated with both central and peripheral cholinergic synapses is of considerable importance (reviewed by Agoston, 1988). Table I gives the acetylcholine and VIP content in several tissues of guinea pig and in the electromotor system of *Torpedo*. The myenteric plexus-longitudinal muscle preparation of guinea-pig ileum is one of the richest sources, among mammalian tissues, of cholinergic terminals; it is also a rich source of VIP; brain tissue is much less rich in both neurotransmitters, only about 5% of nerve terminals being cholinergic. Electric organ is a rich source of cholinergic nerve terminals, between 500 and 1000 times richer than muscle, from which the electrocytes are embryonically derived, while the electric lobes, prominent paired nuclei on the brain stem just caudal to the cerebellum, contain the cell bodies of the cholinergic electromotor neurones. Interestingly these structures also contain VIP-like immunoreactivity (VIPLI) (Agoston and Conlon, 1986). The values in Table I were obtained by radioimmune assay using porcine VIP as a standard, but since the displacement curves of *Torpedo* VIPLI and porcine VIP in the assay are not identical, the true values could be much higher.

Copurification of VIP with cholinergic synaptosomes

In recent years our group has identified two minor gangliosides, designated Chol-1 α and β, which are specific for cholinergic nerve terminals both central and peripheral and are conserved from *Torpedo* to mammals (Ferretti and Borroni, 1986/refs). Antisera to these gangliosides raised in sheep allow the cholinergic subpopulation of mammalian brain synaptosomes to be separated out by immunoadsorption (Agoston et al, 1988a/refs). Briefly, after addition of the antiserum in saturating amounts to the synaptosome preparation, those with attached anti-Chol-1 antibodies (i.e. the cholinergic subpopulation) selectively adhere to Sepharose beads to which a high-titre anti-sheep IgG monoclonal antibody has been attached and can be subsequently harvested. Such synaptosomes show up to an 18- to 20-fold enrichment of classical cholinergic markers, consistent with a 5-6% representation of cholinergic synaptosomes in the total synaptosome population. VIP copurifies with the cholinergic markers but with a lower enrichment factor (Table II). Lactate dehydrogenase, a general cytoplasmic marker, shows, as expected, no enrichment. It has been concluded from the enrichment factors and yields obtained that about 50% of all cholinergic synaptosomes contain VIP and 75% of all VIP-containing synaptosomes are Chol-1-positive and thus cholinergic. Such results are consistent with the conclusions of earlier immunocytochemical studies (Eckenstein and Baughman, 1984).

Table II Copurification of VIP with cholinergic markers in affinity-purified synaptosomes

Component	Purification factor	Yield %
Acetylcholine	19	-
Choline acetyltransferase	15	3.3
VIP	8	4.0
Lactate dehydrogenase	1	-

(Results are those of Agoston et al, 1988a)

The guinea-pig myenteric plexus

Isolation of two classes of storage vesicle

When cytoplasmic extracts of myenteric plexus-longitudinal muscle preparations are submitted to high-resolution centrifugal density-gradient fractionation in a zonal rotor and the various density-gradient fractions assayed after the run, acetylcholine, substance P, somatostatin and VIP are each found (Agoston et al, 1985b) to be associated with distinct populations of particles differing is size and density (Fig 1a and Table III).

The lightest and smallest particles (designated peak I) contain acetylcholine and have the typical morphology of synaptic vesicles. The particles associated with VIP (designated peak VI) were by contrast larger and denser than synaptic vesicles and a considerable proportion of them contained dense cores (Fig 1c). Interestingly, acetylcholine was bimodally distributed in the gradient; while most of it was recovered in peak I, a second peak (II) coincided with that of VIP. Attempts to dissociate peaks II and VI by exploiting possible differences in density (Fig 2a), size (Fig 2c) or osmotic fragility (Fig 1d) failed (Agoston and Whittaker, 1989). It has therefore been concluded that VIP-rich vesicles in myenteric neurones also store some acetylcholine. Putative synaptic vesicle markers, Mg-ATPase, synaptophysin and vesicle-specific proteoglycan, were also bimodally distributed in the gradient (Figs 2b and 2d) with a less dense peak coinciding with the acetylcholine-rich synaptic vesicles and a denser peak embracing the three peaks of neuropeptides (Fig 2b). This indicates that the denser neuropeptide-storing vesicles resemble synaptic vesicles in their chemical

Table III Mean diameters, densitites and neuropeptide contents of storage vesicles from the guinea-pig myenteric plexus

Peak	Substance	Diameter[a]	Density[b]	Vesicular concentration	
		(nm)	(g.ml^{-1})	units	units.(mg of protein)$^{-1}$
I	Acetylcholine	61 ± 6	1.066	nmol	34 ± 4
IV	Substance P	65 ± 3	1.123	pmol	157 ± 14
V	Somatostatin	87 ± 3	1.138	pmol	70 ± 14
II/VI	VIP+acetylcholine	110 ± 6[c]	-	-	-
	VIP	-	1.148	pmol	25 ± 4
	Acetylcholine	-	1.144	nmol	11 ± 3

[a] Mean equitorial diameter ± SD for 1120 to 1860 profiles
[b] Means of peak fractions; SDs were approximately 1% of the mean
[c] For empty and dense-cored vesicles combined (see Fig 1c)
Results are those of Dowe et al (1980) and Agoston et al (1985b)

Fig 1 *(see facing page)* ***(a)*** *Distribution of acetylcholine (ACh, peak I), substance P (SP, peak IV), somatostatin (SS, peak V) and VIP (peak VI) in a zonal density gradient after centrifugal separation of a cytoplasmic extract of guinea-pig myenteric plexus. Note the presence of a small second peak of ACh (peak II) coinciding with VIP. Results of Agoston et al (1985b).* ***(b)*** *Incorporation of newly formed d_4 ACh into the synaptic vesicle fraction after superfusion with d_4 choline and stimulation. The denser vesicles corresponding to the shoulder in the distribution of d_0 (endogenous) ACh are preferentially labelled and comprise the recycling population. Results of Agoston et al (1985a).* ***(c)*** *Size distribution of vesicles present in peaks I and VI. In the latter, the dotted lines are the observed distribution of profile diameters, the continuous lines the calculated particle size distribution. Hatched and solid blocks show the observed and calculated subpopulation of dense-cored vesicles. The electron-lucent populations probably belong to the incompletely separated SS-containing particles. For means and SDs see Table 3.* ***(d)*** *Osmotic fragility of peaks I and II/VI. ACh, filled circles and open triangles; VIP, filled triangles. Results of Agoston and Whittaker (1989).* ***(A)*** *Frequency dependence of VIP and ACh release from superfused myenteric plexus-longitudinal muscle strips. At 8 Hz, the release of both transmitters as a percentage of basal release is the same.* ***(B,C)*** *Effect of (B) hemicholinium-(HC-)3, (C) colchicine on the release of ACh and VIP from superfused myenteric plexus-longitudinal muscle strips stimulated at (B) low, (C) high frequency. Results of Agoston et al (1988b).*

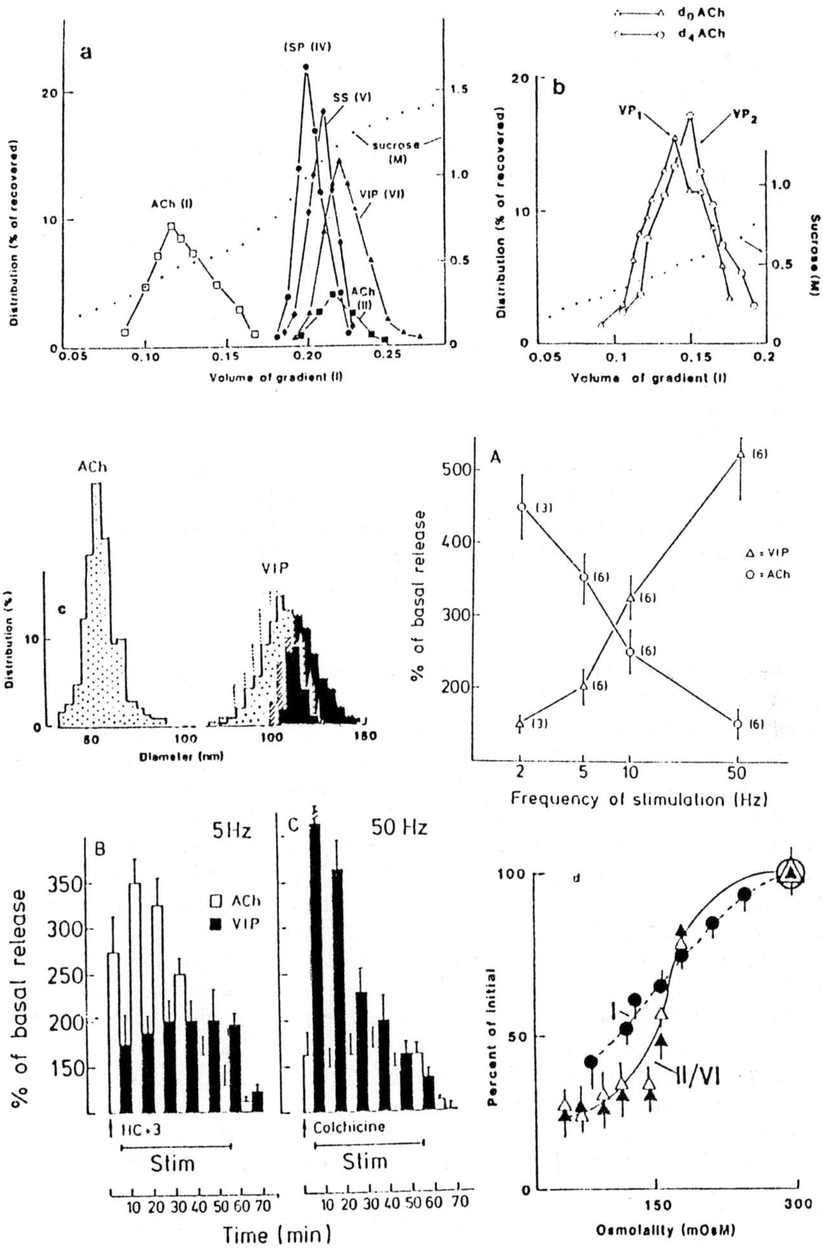
a
ACh (I)
(SP (IV)
SS (V)
sucrose (M)
VIP (VI)
ACh (II)
Distribution (% of recovered)
Volume of gradient (l)
d₀ACh
d₄ACh
b
VP₁
VP₂
Sucrose (M)
ACh
VIP
c
Distribution (%)
Diameter (nm)
A
% of basal release
Δ = VIP
O = ACh
Frequency of stimulation (Hz)
B
5Hz
C
50 Hz
ACh
VIP
Colchicine
Stim
Time (min)
d
Percent of initial
I
II/VI
Osmolality (mOsM)

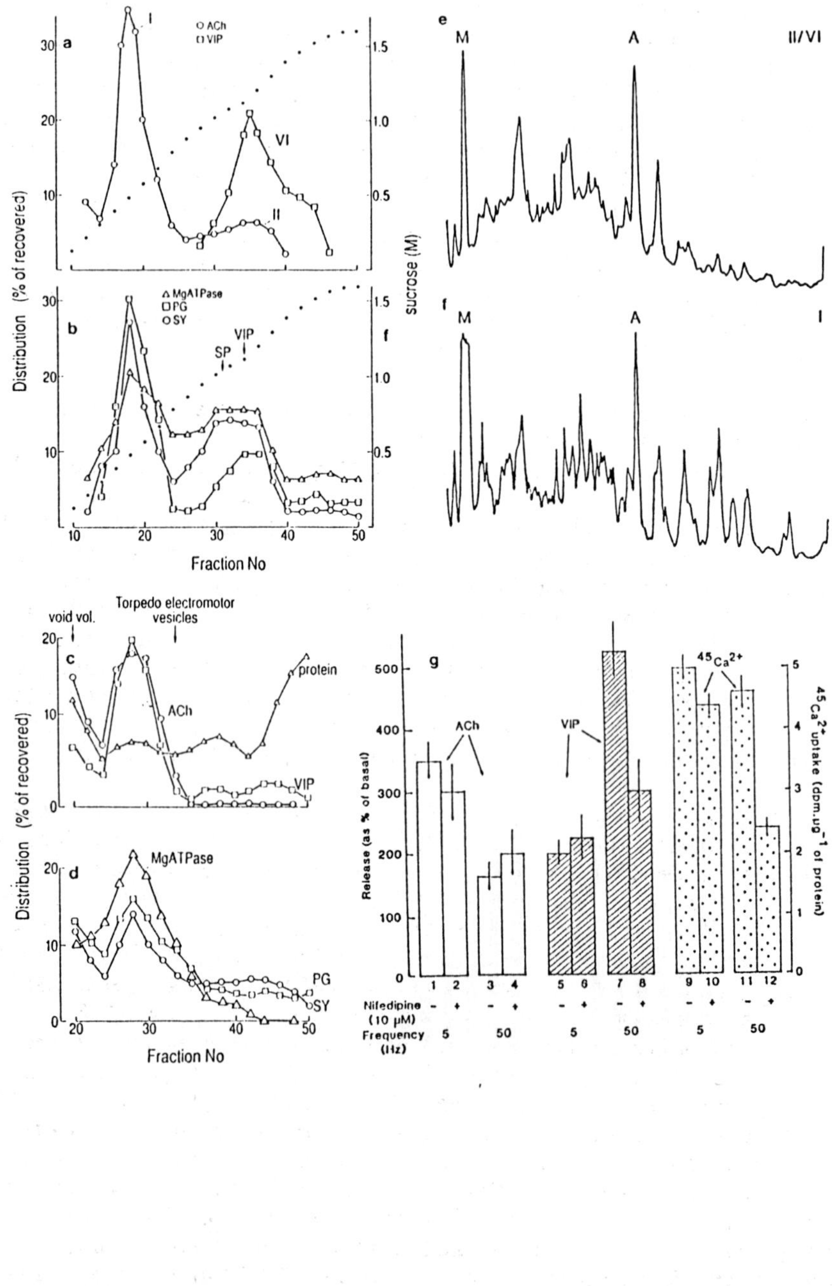
a
O ACh
□ VIP
I
VI
II
b
△ MgATPase
□ PG
O SY
SP
VIP
Distribution (% of recovered)
Sucrose (M)
Fraction No
e
M
A
II/VI
f
M
A
I
c
void vol.
Torpedo electromotor vesicles
protein
ACh
VIP
d
MgATPase
PG
SY
Distribution (% of recovered)
Fraction No
g
ACh
VIP
$^{45}Ca^{2+}$
Release (as % of basal)
$^{45}Ca^{2+}$ uptake (dpm.μg^{-1} of protein)
Nifedipine (10 μM)
Frequency (Hz)

composition and this is also borne out by similarities in their protein composition (Figs 2e and f).

Differences in intracellular dynamics

Frequency dependence of release. When strips of myenteric plexus-longitudinal muscle preparations are stimulated at different frequencies in a superfusion chamber and the release of acetylcholine and VIP monitored, a striking difference emerges between the frequency dependence of their release (Agoston et al, 1988b) (Fig 1A). Whereas the release of acetylcholine is favoured by a low (2 Hz) frequency of stimulation, VIP release is maximal at high (50 Hz) frequency. At 8 Hz, the releases (as a % of basal release) are equal. These results are similar to those previously obtained with another VIP-rich cholinergic innervation, that to the salivary gland. In such nerve terminals acetylcholine and VIP are also packaged in synaptic vesicles and dense-cored vesicles (Lundberg, 1981; Lundberg and Hökfelt, 1983).

Pharmacology of release. Figs 1B and C show the results of stimulation experiments carried out in the presence of hemicholinium-3, which, by inhibiting the uptake of choline and the resynthesis of acetylcholine, blocks vesicle recycling, and colchicine, which blocks axonal transport (Agoston et al, 1988b). In the hemicholinium experiment (Fig 1B) stimulation at low (5 Hz) frequency was selected to favour the release of acetylcholine (white blocks), though some evoked release of VIP (black blocks) does occur. Hemicholinium causes a marked diminution in acetylcholine output, leaving VIP release unaffected. In Fig 1C, the conditions (50 Hz) favoured VIP release (compare height of first black blocks with corresponding blocks in panel B), but not that of acetylcholine (compare first white blocks in the two panels; those of panel C are

Fig 2 *(see facing page)* ***(a,b)*** *Attempted separation by (a) density, (b) size of peaks II and VI. In (a) the zonal density gradient was designed to give maximum resolution in the region of peak II/VI. In (b) a single peak of acetylcholine (ACh) and VIP activity emerged with a retention volume between that of chromaffin granules ('void volume') and Torpedo electromotor synaptic vesicles.* ***(c,d)*** *The three synaptic vesicle markers, proteoglycan (PG), synaptophysin (SY) and* Mg^{2+}*-ATPase are also inseparably associated with peak II/VI.* ***(e,f)*** *Densitometriy traces of silver-stained electropherograms of the proteins of (e) synaptic vesicles (peak I) and (f) peak II/VI. Both preparations were contaminated with myosin (M) and actin (A), probably derived from the longitudinal muscle and had numerous common components.* ***(g)*** *The effect of 10 µM nifedipine on the evoked release of acetylcholine (ACh, white blocks), that of VIP (hatched blocks) and the uptake of* $^{45}Ca^{2+}$*. It will be seen that only the voltage-sensitive calcium channel activated at high (50 Hz) frequency and the high-frequency release of VIP are nifedipine-sensitive. Results are those of Agoston and Whittaker (1989) and Agoston and Lisziewicz (1989).*

much lower than the corresponding ones of panel B). The presence of colchicine, however, rapidly blocks the release of VIP while leaving that of acetylcholine unaffected. This shows that VIP release is dependent on a steady supply of VIP-containing vesicles from the cell bodies of the neurones via axonal transport whereas acetylcholine release can be sustained by local recycling without replenishment of synaptic vesicles by axonal transport, at least within this time scale. The ability of myenteric synaptic vesicles to recycle has been shown by the rapid incorporation into them of labelled (i.e. newly synthesized) acetylcholine and its subsequent release (Fig 1B) (Agoston et al, 1985a). Such highly labelled vesicles differ in density from reserve vesicles and separate from them apparently as a result of osmotic dehydration following partial loading, as has also been observed with electromotor synaptic vesicles.

The clear difference in intracellular dynamics of the acetylcholine-rich synaptic vesicles and the VIP-rich vesicles seen in these experiments is also demonstrated by differences in their response to the L-type voltage sensitive calcium-channel blocker nifedipine (Fig 2g) (Agoston and Lisziewicz, 1989). This drug has little effect on either acetylcholine (white blocks) or VIP (hatched blocks) release at low frequency (Fig 2g, blocks 1-4) but at high frequency (blocks 5-8) it markedly inhibits VIP while having little effect on acetylcholine release. Note that the increase in frequency again depressed acetylcholine release (compare blocks 1 and 5) but enhanced that of VIP (compare blocks 3 and 7). The stippled blocks (9-12) show the effect of the drug on $^{45}Ca^{2+}$ uptake at low (9 and 10) and high (11 and 12) frequencies. Ca^{2+} uptake is largely frequency independent but is much more sensitive to nifedipine at high frequency than at low frequency. We interpret this to mean that the preferred mode of Ca^{2+} entry at low frequency is via the nifedipine-insensitive N-channels but at high frequency by the nifedipine-sensitve L-channels. It would also seem that VIP release is preferentially dependent on Ca^{2+} entry through L-type channels whereas acetylcholine release is preferentially dependent on Ca^{2+} entry through N-type channels. A neat explanation of the inverse frequency dependence of acetylcholine and VIP would be to suppose that the exocytosis of the VIP-rich vesicles occurs at a different site in the terminal (where L-type Ca^{2+}-channels are concentrated) from that at which acetylcholine-rich synaptic vesicles undergo exocytosis and where N-type channels may be concentrated (Fig 3).

It has been suggested (Geffen and Livett, 1971; Lowe et al, 1988) that in the adrenergic system the membranes of dense-cored vesicles, which contain the small-molecular-mass transmitter noradrenaline as well as neuropeptides are retrieved to form small, electron-lucent vesicles which are competent to take up and release noradrenaline and recycle in the terminal. It may be that this precursor-product relationship also exists, at least in cholinergic neurones of the guinea-pig myenteric plexus, between acetylcholine-containing, VIP-rich storage particles and acetylcholine-rich synaptic vesicles, which, as we have seen, are able to recycle and thus to sustain acetylcholine release independently of axonal transport.

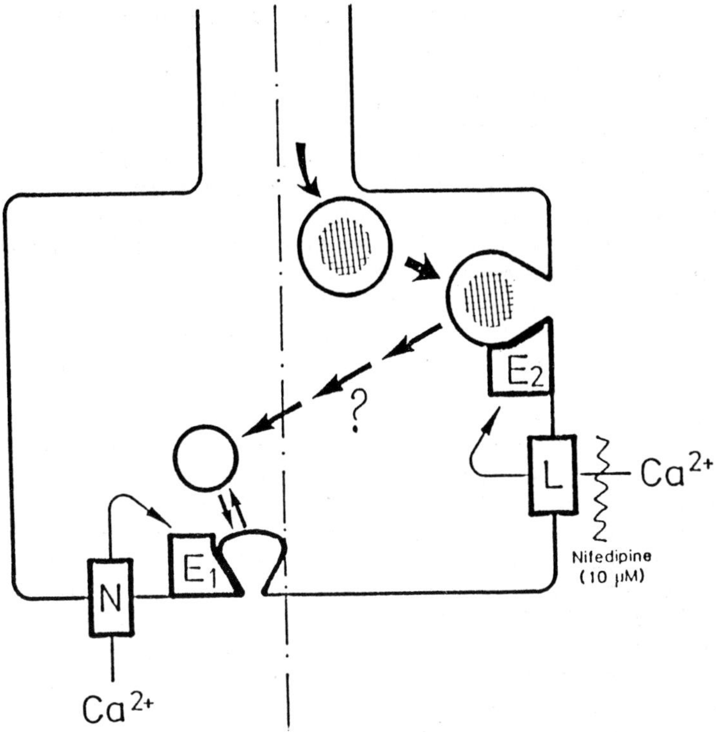

***Fig 3** Scheme showing dense-cored and recycling synaptic vesicles and their possible relationship in the cholinergic terminals of the myenteric plexus.*

The electromotor system of *Torpedo*

As already mentioned, VIPLI is present throughout the electromotor neurone. The absolute amounts have not yet been determined and the quantitative results in Figures and Tables are expressed as 'porcine VIP equivalents'.

VIPLI-containing particles separate completely from the acetylcholine-rich synaptic vesicles when a cytoplasmic extract of electric organ is separated on a zonal density gradient (Agoston et al, 1989a; Fig 4a). Both types of particle are associated with the putative stable vesicle markers synaptophysin and vesicle-specific proteoglycan (Fig 4b). Ligation of the electromotor nerve trunks causes a rise in the VIPLI content of the electromotor cell body and the axon proximal to the ligature but a fall in the distal axon and the terminals in the electric organ (Agoston and Conlon, 1986 and Table IV). This is sufficiently great after 10 days to be apparent immunohistochemically; it parallels the accumulation of proteoglycan above the ligature.

Synaptic vesicles and VIPLI-containing particles can also be separated out from axons (Agoston et al, 1989a). There is an interesting difference between them. In confirmation of Kiene and Stadler (1987), synaptic vesicles from electromotor axons are less dense than those isolated from their terminals in the electric organ; they also contain very little acetylcholine - about one-thousandth of that present in terminal synaptic vesicles (Table V). These two parameters are probably related, since in the axon, a relatively light inorganic monovalent cation may replace the denser organic cation acetylcholine. By contrast, axonal VIPLI-containing particles are essentially identical to those isolated from the terminal. Interesting also (Table V col 6, compare lines 1 and 2)

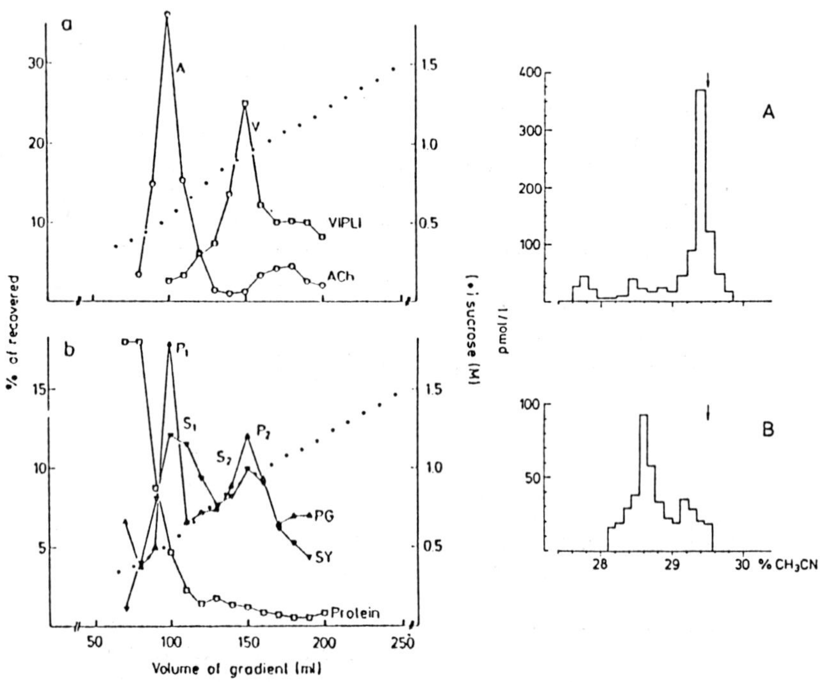

*Fig 4 (**a**) Separation of particles in cytoplasmic extracts of* Torpedo *electric organ rich in ACh and VIPLI by zonal density gradient separation. (**b**) Distribution of two putative stable synaptic vesicle markers in the same gradient, synaptophysin (SY) and vesicle-specific proteoglycan (PG). Peaks S_1 and P_1 of the two markers coincide with the ACh peak A and peaks S_2 and P_2 with the VIPLI peak V. (**A,B**) Reverse-phase analytical HPLC on Supercosil-18-DB under near isocratic conditions of the VIPLI in extracts of (A) electric lobe, (B) electric organ. The column was eluted with increasing concentrations of acetonitrile (abscissae). The arrow shows the concentration at which porcine VIP emerges from the column. Results are those of Agoston et al (1989a).*

is the lower Mg^{2+}-ATPase in axonal synaptic vesicles compared with those from the terminal. Does the ATPase get switched on in the terminal thus generating an enhanced proton gradient needed for uptake of acetylcholine there? By contrast, the Mg^{2+}-ATPase levels of axonal and terminal VIPLI-containing vesicles are essentially the same (Table V col 6, compare lines 3 and 4).

Table IV VIP-like immunoreactivity in the electromotor system of *Torpedo* and changes induced by ligation of nerve

Tissue	VIP-like immunoreactivity[a]	
	fmol.g^{-1}	% change on ligation
Electric lobe	740 ± 70	+ 84 ± 19
Electromotor nerve trunks	180 ± 30	+ 34 ± 11[b]
Electric organ	130 ± 20	- 47 ± 5
Rest of cns	550 ± 50	+ 0.5 ± 14

[a] Means of 3 expts ± SD, porcine VIP equivalents; increases are positive, decreases negative
[b] Proximal to ligature
Results are those of Agoston and Conlon (1986)

Table V Comparison of axonal and terminal synaptic and dense vesicles from *Torpedo* electromotor neurones

Site	Density	Content (units per 100 units of synaptophysin			
	(g.ml^{-1})	Acetylcholine (nmol)	VIPLI (fmol-eq)	Proteoglycan (SV-eq)	Mg^{2+}-ATPase (nmol P_i.h-1)
Synaptic vesicles					
Terminals	1.070	328	-	100	688
Axons	1.057	0.23	-	93	236
Dense vesicles					
Terminals	1.122	-	2432	84	876
Axons	1.100	-	2414	75	733

Results are those of Agoston et al (1989a)

These figures clearly indicate that the two transmitters again differ in their intracellular dynamics: they are packaged in distinct particles and at the level of axonal transport VIPLI is contained within a fully charged particle whereas synaptic vesicles only become fully charged when they reach the terminal.

In future work it will be interesting to see whether other differences in optimal frequency of release and sensitivity to drugs are similar to those found with salivary gland and myenteric plexus.

Acetylcholine in this system has not been detected in VIPLI-containing vesicles and synaptic vesicles appear, on the basis of morphological evidence, to be formed in the Golgi region of the electromotor perikarya. Another possible difference from mammalian systems is the finding that in electromotor neurones, VIPLI is subject to intravesicular modification. A comparison of the retention volumes of somatic and terminal VIPLI in reverse phase high performance liquid chromatography (HPLC) shows that a small hydrophobic sequence is cleaved off during axonal transport; whereas VIPLI isolated from electromotor cell bodies consists of a single component with a retention time close to that of porcine VIP (Fig 4A, peak and arrow), this component has all but disappeared when the storage particle reaches the terminal and has been replaced by a more hydrophilic one (Fig 4B).

Codistribution of PHI and VIP

It is now known that the 28-amino-acid peptide VIP is synthesized in the form of a propeptide precursor which is posttranslationally modified by proteolytic cleavage to generate VIP and various other fragments, the main of which is a 27-amino-acid peptide known as PHI, standing for 'the peptide with N-terminal histidine and C-terminal isoleucine amide'. VIP and PHI and the other propeptide cleavage products have been shown to coexist with VIP in a number of VIP immunopositive cells, but often not in equimolar amounts, suggesting different rates of further cleavage by tissue proteases.

We have studied the distribution of VIP- and PHI-containing particles by density and size, by applying both zonal density gradient separation and particle exclusion chromatography to cytoplasmic extracts of myenteric plexus. In all cases, the two peptides co-localized in exactly equimolar amounts (Agoston et al, 1989b). This suggests that the posttranslational modification occurs after packaging the propeptide and that any subsequent deviation from equimolarity is due to differential breakdown after release.

Conclusion

The work described here illustrates the value of a cell-biological approach to the problem of cotransmission. The results confirm the prevailing view that the classical transmitters and their accompanying neuropeptides are separately packaged in nerve terminals, within synaptic vesicles and larger, denser vesicles (which may or may not have a dense core) respectively. However, the composition of the membranes of the two particle types are similar and it is possible that at least in some terminals the membranes of dense-cored vesicles are reutilized to form synaptic vesicles.

Within the neuropeptide-storing particles, posttranslational modification occurs: in the case of VIP, equimolecular amounts of another peptide, PHI, are generated and, in the electromotor system, the VIPLI present in the particles before they leave the cell soma is further modified during axonal transport. The nature of the peptidase(s) involved is not known but it is likely that a cathepsin is involved.

The acid pH required to activate the cathepsin might well be brought about by the same ATPase as is responsible for acidifying the interior of synaptic vesicles and thus providing the driving force for acetylcholine uptake. The peptide-containing and synaptic vesicle membranes may thus use a component common to both membranes for different purposes: a good example of evolutionary thriftiness!

Acknowledgement

This work was supported by grants Co 130/1-1 and Wh 1/4-2 to V.P.W. from the Deutsche Forschungsgemeinschaft.

References

Agoston, D.V. (1988) Handb. exp. Pharm., 86, 479-533.
Agoston, D.V. and Conlon, J.M. (1986) J. Neurochem., 47, 445-453.
Agoston, D.V. and Lisziewicz, J. (1989) J. Neurochem., 52, 1637-1640.
Agoston, D.V. and Whittaker, V.P. (1989) J. Neurochem., 52, 1474-1480.
Agoston, D.V., Kosh, J.W., Lisziewicz, J. and Whittaker, V.P. (1985a) J. Neurochem., 44, 299-305.
Agoston, D.V., Ballmann, M., Conlon, J.M., Dowe, G.H.C. and Whittaker, V.P. (1985b) J. Neurochem., 45, 398-406.
Agoston, D.V., Borroni, E. and Richardson, P.J. (1988a) J. Neurochem., 50, 1659-1662.
Agoston, D.V., Conlon, J.M. and Whittaker, V.P. (1988b) Exp. Brain Res., 72, 535-542.
Agoston, D.V., Dowe, G.H.C. and Whittaker, V.P. (1989a) J. Neurochem., 52, 1729-1740.
Agoston, D.V., Fahrenkrug, J., Mikkelsen, J.D. and Whittaker, V.P. (1989b) Peptides, in press.
Dowe, G.H.C., Kilbinger, H. and Whittaker, V.P. (1980) J. Neurochem., 535, 993-1103.
Eckenstein, F. and Baughman, R.W. (1984) Nature (London), 309, 153-155.
Ferretti, P. and Borroni, E. (1986) J. Neurochem., 46, 1888-1894.
Geffen, L. and Livett, B.G. (1971) Physiol. Rev., 51, 98-157.
Kiene, M.-L. and Stadler, H. (1987) EMBO J., 6, 2209-2217.
Lowe, A.W., Madeddu, L. and Kelly, R.B. (1988) J. Cell Biol., 106, 51-59.
Lundberg, J.M. (1981) Acta Physiol. Scand. Suppl., 496, 1-57.
Lundberg, J.M. and Hökfelt, T. (1983) Neuroscience, 7, 189-222.

The Correlation between Vesicle Loss and Quantal Secretion at the Frog Neuromuscular Junction.

William P. Hurlbut

Rockefeller University 1230 York Ave. N.Y., N.Y. 10021, USA.

I first met Bruno Ceccarelli in the fall of 1970 when he came to the Rockefeller University as a post-doctoral fellow of the Muscular Dystrophy Assocation to work with Alex Mauro. This was shortly after Alex, Bart Longenecker and Allen Clark had discovered the dramatic effects of black widow spider venom (BWSV) on neuromuscular junctions in frog sartorius and cutaneous pectoris muscles (Longenecker et al., 1970; Clark et al., 1972). This venom blocked the action potential in the motor nerve terminal, and, even when applied in a Ca^{2+}-free Ringer's solution, it increased the spontaneous rate of quantal secretion by several orders of magnitude and led within about an hour to the apparent exhaustion of a terminal's store of quanta and to the loss of almost all its synaptic vesicles. Bruno had come to study the venom's actions, and it seemed to us that by using it together with extracellular tracers like horseradish peroxidase (HRP) (Graham and Karnovsky, 1966; Holtzman et al., 1972), we could test the vesicle hypothesis (Katz and Miledi, 1956; Birks et al., 1960) and measure the turnover of vesicles and quanta of transmitter at single neuromuscular junctions (Bittner and Kennedy, 1970). The basic idea was to stimulate quantal secretion, record the resulting endplate potentials (epps) and miniature endplate potentials (mepps) at a single junction, and then determine how many quanta remained in its nerve terminal by applying BWSV and counting the total number of mepps that subsequently occurred. The number of quanta stored in an unstimulated control terminal would be determined by applying BWSV to it and counting the mepps. In addition, some muscles would be fixed and their nerve terminals examined in the electron microscope to determine the number of vesicles that remained in them and to monitor their uptake of extracellular tracers.

Early Qualitative Results

Our first estimates of the number of quanta stored in unstimulated control terminals, $0.4 - 0.5 \times 10^6$ quanta/terminal, were not very exact, since individual mepps could not be resolved when the rate of secretion was at its peak (Longenecker et al., 1970; Ceccarelli et al., 1973). However, they were reasonably close to the total number of synaptic vesicles contained in such terminals ($\sim 0.9 \times 10^6$ vesicles/terminal, Heuser and Miledi, 1971), so we decided to proceed, but looked for experimental conditions which would yield clear-cut results that would not require accurate measurements of venom-induced release. Such conditions occurred when a frog cutaneous pectoris nerve-muscle preparation was stimulated indirectly at a rate of 2/s in Ringer's solution with curare. The epp at these junctions persisted through at least 2 h of continuous stimulation, though its amplitude declined by about

80%, and the terminals secreted ~ 10^6 quanta during that time (Ceccarelli et al., 1973; Ceccarelli and Hurlbut, 1975). The stimulated terminals retained about 57% of their vesicles (Torri-Tarelli et al., 1987), and many near normal sized mepps occurred if BWSV was applied (about 10 m after stimulation was stopped and all the curare had been removed). If HRP was present during the period of stimulation, many of the residual vesicles were labeled with the tracer. If the synthesis of acetylcholine (ACh) was inhibited with hemicholinium-3 (HC-3) (Schueler, 1960; Guyenet et al., 1973), then the amplitude of the epp fell almost to zero during 0.5 h of stimulation, and the terminals secreted only about 0.25 x 10^6 quanta during 2 h. Nevertheless, they still retained most of their vesicles , many of which were labelled with HRP if this tracer was present, and if BWSV was applied, the residual vesicles were lost, though few mepps occurred. These residual vesicles, therefore, contained no releasable ACh. These results showed that a normal terminal could secrete at least twice its initial store of quanta and still retain large a residual store of quanta and synaptic vesicles because the vesicles were recycled and reloaded with ACh. The vesicles could also be recycled when the synthesis of ACh was blocked, but then they were not reloaded with the transmitter. Similar results were obtained when the amount of ACh secreted from mouse diaphragms was measured by bioassay (Gorio et al., 1978).

Measurment of Mepp Rates by Fluctuation Analysis

Recently John Segal and Riccardo Fesce developed a modified procedure of fluctuation analysis (Segal et al., 1965; Fesce et al., 1986a) to measure the number of mepps that occur at junctions treated with BWSV or α-latrotoxin (α-LTx), the purified protein component of the venom that acts at vertebrate synapses (Frontali et al., 1976). This modified analytic procedure uses the variance, skew and power spectrum of the fluctuations in membrane potential at vigorously secreting junctions to determine the amplitude, rate of occurrence and time course of the mepps. Its results are more variable than those furnished by the classical procedure, which uses the mean potential instead of the skew, but they are unaffected by nonstationary mepp rates, spurious changes in the mean potential or changes in the rate of nonquantal secretion, and they are much less sensitive to the nonlinear summation of the mepps. The procedure also provides a numerical index that monitors the dispersion of mepp amplitudes and can be used to correct the results for the effects of that dispersion. We have used it to measure mepp rate and amplitude at junctions treated at room temperature with ouabain (Haimann et al., 1985), La^{3+} (Segal et al.,1985) or small doses of BWSV (Fesce et al., 1986b) and at junctions treated with large doses of α-LTx at 1-3 ^{0}C (Ceccarelli et al., 1988b), or with La^{3+} at 3-5 ^{0}C (Dekhuijzen et al., 1989). We also monitored the uptake of HRP by those terminals, estimated the number of vesicles, V_1, that remained in them at the end of the period of stimulation and estimated the number of vesicles they had recycled, V_r. V_1 was calculated from the average number of synaptic vesicles, V_s, contained in cross sections of the nerve terminals, the thickness, t, of the sections (silver-grey, ~ 40 nm), and the average length, L, of the terminals (~600 μ) (Heuser and Miledi, 1971; Letinsky et al., 1976; Valtorta et al., 1984):

$$V_l = V_s L/t(1+d/t),$$

where the factor in parentheses is a correction for the finite diameter, d, of the vesicles (Wiebel and Paumgartner, 1978). V_r was calculated from the total number of mepps that had occurred, Q_t, the number of vesicles, V_c, in control terminals (0.5-0.8 x 10^6), and V_l:

$$V_r = Q_t - (V_c - V_l).$$

The results of these experiments are summarized in Fig. 1.

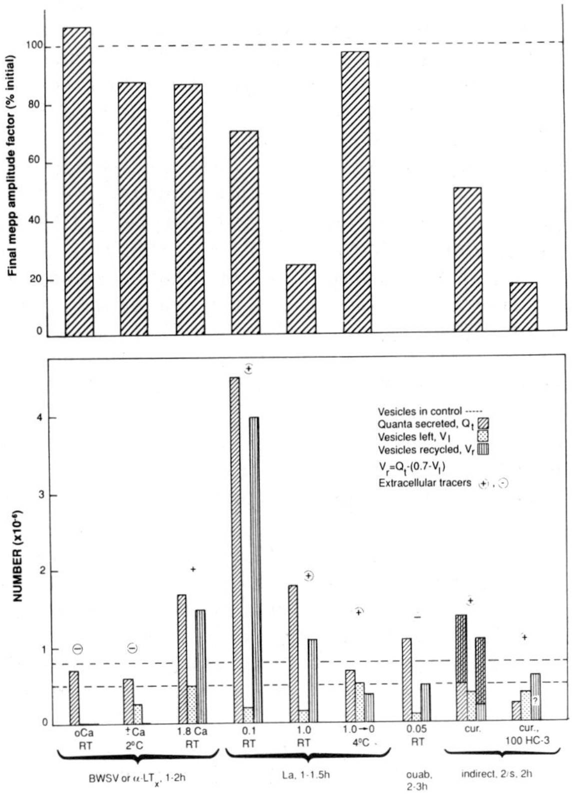

Fig. 1, lower. Measurements of the number of quanta secreted, the number of vesicles remaining and the estimated number of vesicles recycled at single neuromuscular junctions during stimulation by various means. The question mark in the last bar on the right indicates that the extent of recycling is uncertain because the recycled vesicles lacked transmitter and therefore generated no mepps.

The upper portion of this Figure shows the accompanying changes in mean mepp amplitude. Results taken from the following references: Ceccarelli et al., 1973; Ceccarelli and Hurlbut, 1975, 1980; Ceccarelli et al., 1988b; Dekhuijzen et al., 1989; Fesce et al., 1986b; Haimann et al., 1985; Heuser and Miledi, 1971; Segal et al., 1985; Torri-Tarelli et al., 1987.

When low doses of BWSV or α-LTx were applied at room temperature to junctions in Ca^{2+}-free Ringer's with 4 mM Mg^{2+}, or when large doses of α-LTx were applied at 1-3 ^{0}C to junctions in normal, or in Ca^{2+}-free Ringer's, then the number of mepps that occurred (0.6 - 0.7 x 10^6) was approximately equal to the number of vesicles lost, and HRP was not taken up. Thus recycling seemed to be blocked. Since the junctions at room temperature had ceased secreting quanta of ACh almost completely, and had lost almost all their synaptic vesicles, we have used the total number of mepps recorded from them as a measure of the number of vesicles and quanta stored in control terminals at rest. The total number of mepps recorded at the junctions subjected to the other conditions of stimulation equalled or exceeded the number of quanta stored in the controls, the mepp rate often was still very high at the end of the period of stimulation, many vesicles remained in the terminals and extracellular tracers were taken up when they were present in the bathing solutions. The dispersion in the mepp amplitudes usually increased during secretion (Kriebel and Gross, 1974; Fesce et al., 1986), but the mean amplitude changed by less than 50%, except when 1 mM La^{3+} was used (Flory and Kriebel, 1983; Kriebel and Florey, 1983; Dekhuijzen et al., 1989). However, that substance greatly reduces the sensitivity of the endplate to ACh (Magazanik and Vyskocil, 1970; Dekhuijzen et al., 1989). These quantitative results fully support the earlier qualitative ones, and they show that nerve terminals can recycle their vesicles several times and reload them with near normal levels of ACh, even at temperatures of 3-5 ^{0}C.

Correlation between Vesicle Loss and Quantal Secretion when Recycling is Blocked

These estimates of the number of recycled vesicles assumed that a quantum of ACh was released from a single vesicle. This assumption was supported by the rough equality between the number of vesicles contained in control terminals and the total number of mepps recorded at previously unstimulated junctions treated with BWSV or α-LTx in Ca^{2+}-free Ringer's solution at room temperature. However, those muscles had been fixed only after the discharge of quanta seemed to have ended, and we did not examine the time course of vesicle loss during the discharge. We also assumed an average length for the terminals in order to calculate the total number of vesicles they contained. In our recent work we have fixed muscles at various times during the quantal discharge and determined the number of synaptic vesicles that remained in randomly selected nerve terminals. We have also measured the lengths of terminals whose discharge of quanta had been recorded. This was done by injecting Lucifer yellow (Stewart, 1978) into the muscle fiber whose mepps had been recorded, staining the muscle for acetylcholinesterase (Karnovsky, 1964), and measuring in a fluorescence microscope the length of the terminal on the fluorescent fiber. We also measured the length of the sarcomeres in the injected fiber, or one of its immediately adjacent neighbors, and scaled the measured terminal length to a sarcomere length of 2.13 μ, the length in a relaxed fiber *in situ* (Gordon et al., 1966). To obtain a relatively synchronous discharge among all the terminals of a muscle, BWSV or α-LTx was applied to muscles bathed in Ringer's solution without divalent cations. The toxin binds to its receptor (Valtorta et al., 1984) under these conditions, but does not stimulate secretion, and secretion can be initiated at will by applying any one of a variety of divalent cations (Misler and Hurlbut, 1979; Misler and Falke, 1987).

Fig. 2A shows the normalized average time course of quantal secretion when 4 mM Mg^{2+} was applied to 11 junctions treated in this way at 22-23 ^{0}C. Fig. 2A also shows the normalized average number of synaptic vesicles remaining in cross sections of nerve terminals cut from muscles fixed just before (0 time), or 5, 10 or 15 m after Mg^{2+} was applied. The two time courses are clearly correlated. Fig. 2B shows the results obtained when the number of vesicles remaining per micron of terminal is plotted against the number of quanta secreted per micron. The slope of the correlation curve is -0.76 vesicles/quantum and its correlation coefficient is -0.9586. This result implies that a quantum is derived from a single vesicle, rather than several vesicles as some workers have suggested (Wernig and Motelica-Heino, 1978; Tremblay et al., 1983).

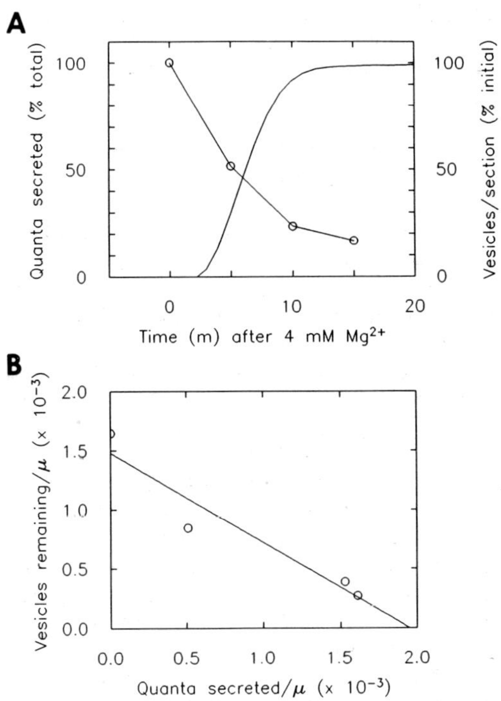

Fig. 2A. Average time course of quantal secretion at 11 junctions and the accompanying changes in the average number of synaptic vesicles remaining in cross sections of nerve terminals in frog cutaneous pectoris muscles. The muscles were treated for 25-35 m with α-LTx (0.25μg/ml) in a modified Ringer's solution with 1 mM EGTA, no divalent cations and tetrodotoxin (10^{-8}g/ml); 4 mM Mg^{2+} was added at zero time. The results are normalized to the average total secretion (0.96 ± 0.32 x 10^6 quanta/terminal) or to the average number of synaptic vesicles in terminals fixed just before Mg^{2+} was applied (132 ± 73 vesicles/section).

Fig. 2B. Results in Fig. 2A scaled to a unit length of nerve terminal and plotted against one another. The lengths of 9 of these junctions were measured, and the average total secretion per micron was 1648 quanta/μ. The secretion per micron, Q_{μ} at any given time was computed from the formula:

$$Q_{\mu} = 1648 \times (\%\ \text{total secretion}).$$

The number of vesicles remaining per micron, V_{μ}, was calculated from the formula:

$$V_{\mu} = V_s/2t,$$

where t is the section thickness (silver-grey ≃ 40 nm), and the factor 2 is a correction for the diameter of the vesicles (d ≃ t). The equation of the regression line is:

$$V_{\mu} = 1479 - 0.76\ Q_{\mu}.$$

These results, and others obtained by Bruno and his co-workers, or by other investigators (Heuser and Reese, 1973; Heuser et al., 1979), support the vesicle hypothesis and the idea that a quantum of transmitter is secreted by exocytosis when a vesicle fuses with the axolemma, usually (Heuser et al., 1974; Ceccarelli et al., 1979a), but not necessarily (Ceccarelli et al., 1979b; Ceccarelli et al., 1988a) at an active zone. The fused vesicles are quickly retrieved from the axolemma and reloaded with ACh, and under favorable conditions of stimulation a vesicle can be recycled and reloaded with ACh several times during 1-2 h at room temperature and at least once during 1.5 h at 3-5 ^{0}C. If ACh synthesis is blocked, the vesicles still recycle, but they are not reloaded with ACh and release no transmitter even if they fuse with the axolemma. If recycling is blocked, then a vesicle is lost from the axoplasm when a quantum is secreted and the vesicle's membrane is incorporated into the axolemma (Valtorta et al., 1988). I do not know why α-LTx blocks recycling, but it may act indirectly by creating ion permeable channels in the axolemma (Finkelstein et al., 1976; Fritz and Mauro, 1982; Meldolesi et al., 1986; Wanke et al., 1986), thereby changing the ion contents of the axoplasm. K^+-deficient solutions inhibit receptor-mediated endocytosis in fibroblasts (Larkin et al., 1983). I hope that the methods outlined here can be used to study the dynamics of quantal secretion in order to estimate how quickly vesicles are retrived from the axolemma and how quickly they are reloaded with ACh.

Acknowledgements

I thank Alex Mauro and for the unstinting backing he has given me at Rockefeller during the past 20 years and for introducing me to Bruno.

I am indebted to the FIDIA pharmaceutical company for their support which has allowed me to work with Bruno in Milano for 4-6 weeks each summer since 1972. I thank Professors Mantegazza and Clementi and the Department of Cytopharmacology for their hospitality over those years and for providing me with living quarters. I am grateful to Bruno's students and co-workers for their contributions to this work: Alfredo Gorio, Fabio Grohovatz, Riccardo Fesce, Claudia Haimann, Flavia Valtorta, Numa Iezzi, Franco Crippa, Paulo Tinelli and Ulla Bøstrup, and to Stanley Misler, who worked with me while he was a graduate student at New York University. I am pleased to acknowledge the unfailing generosity of Jacopo Meldolesi who willingly provided all the α-latrotoxin we used during the past several years.

I owe special thanks to Serenella Ceccarelli for providing a second home for me in Milano. My wife, Helen, and I hope we will have an opportunity to do the same for her someday in New York.

My research has been supported by grants from the NIH, the NSF, the Muscular Dystrophy Association and currently by USPHS grant #2R01 NS18354.

REFERENCES

Birks, R., Huxley, A.H. and Katz, B. (1960). The fine structure of the neuromuscular junction of the frog. J. Physiol. (Lond.). **150**: 134-144.

Bittner, G.D. and Kennedy, D. (1970). Quantitative aspects of transmitter release. J. Cell Biol. **47**: 585-592.

Ceccarelli, B., Fesce, R., Grohovaz, F. and Haimann, C. (1988a). The effect of potassium on exocytosis of transmitter at the frog neuromuscular junction. J. Physiol. (Lond.). **401**: 163-183.

Ceccarelli, B., Grohovaz, F. and Hurlbut, W.P. (1979a). Freeze-fracture studies of frog neuromuscular junctions during intense release of transmitter. I. Effects of black widow spider venom and Ca^{2+}-free solutions on the structure of the active zone. J. Cell Biol. **81**: 163-177.

Ceccarelli, B., Grohovaz, F. and Hurlbut, W.P. (1979b). Freeze-fracture studies of frog neuromuscular junctions during intense release of neurotransmitter. II. Effects of electrical stimulation and high potassium. J. Cell Biol. **81**: 178-192.

Ceccarelli, B. and Hurlbut, W.P. (1975). The effects of prolonged repetitive stimulation in hemicholinium on the frog neuromuscular junction. J. Physiol. (Lond.). **247**: 163-188.

Ceccarelli, B. and Hurlbut, W.P. (1980). Ca^{2+}-dependent recycling of synaptic vesicles at the frog neuromuscular junction. J. Cell Biol. **87**: 297-303.

Ceccarelli, B., Hurlbut, W.P. and Iezzi, N. (1988). The effect of α-latrotoxin on the frog neuromuscular junction at low temperature. J. Physiol. (Lond.). **402**: 195-217.

Ceccarelli, B., Hurlbut, W.P. and Mauro, A. (1973). The turnover of transmitter and synaptic vesicles at the frog neuromuscular junction. J. Cell Biol. **57**: 499-524.

Clark, A.W., Hurlbut, W.P. and Mauro, A. (1972). Changes in the fine structure of the neuromuscular junction of the frog caused by black widow spider venom. J. Cell Biol. **52**: 1-14.

Dekhuijzen, A., Iezzi, N. and Hurlbut, W.P. (1989). A re-examination of the effects of lanthanum on the frog neuromuscular junction. Pflug. Arch. **414**: 683-689.

Del Castillo, J. and Katz, B. (1956). Biophysical aspects of neuro-muscular transmission. Prog. Biophysics Biophys. Chem. **6**: 121-170.

Fesce, R., Segal, J.R., Ceccarelli B. and Hurlbut, W.P. (1986b). Effects of black widow spider venom and Ca^{2+} on quantal secretion at the frog neuromuscular junction. J. Gen. Physiol. **88**: 59-81.

Fesce, R., Segal, J.R. and Hurlbut, W.P. (1986a). Fluctuation analysis of nonideal shot noise. Application to the neuromuscular junction. J. Gen. Physiol. **88**: 25-57.

Finkelstein, A., Rubin, L.L. and Tzeng, M. C. (1976). Black widow spider venom: effect of purified toxin on lipid bilayer membranes. Science (Wash. DC). **193**: 1009-1011.

Florey, E. and Kriebel, M.E. (1983). Changes in acetycholine concentration, miniature end-plate potentials and synaptic vesicles in frog neuromuscular preparations during lanthanum treatment. Comp. Biochem. Physiol. **75C**: 285-294.

Fritz, L.C. and Mauro, A. (1982). The ionic dependence of black widow spider venom action at the stretch receptor neuron and neuromuscular junction of crustaceans. J. Neurobiol. **13**: 385-401.

Frontali, N., Ceccarelli, B., Goria, A., Mauro, A., Siekevitz, P., Tzeng, M.-C. and Hurlbut, W.P. (1976). Purification from black widow spider venom of a protein factor causing the depletion of synaptic vesicles at the neuromuscular junction. J. Cell Biol. **68**: 462-479.

Gordon, A.M., Huxley, A.F. and Julian, F.J. (1966). The variation in isometric tension with sarcomere length in vertebrate muscle fibers. J. Physiol. (Lond.). **184**: 170-192.

Gorio, A., Hurlbut, W.P. and Ceccarelli, B. (1978). Acetylcholine compartments in mouse diaphragm: a comparison of the effects of black widow spider venom, electrical stimulation and high concentrations of potassium. J. Cell Biol. **78**: 716-733.

Graham, R.C. and Karnovsky, M.J. (1966). The early stages of absorption of injected horseradish peroxidase in the proximal tubule of the mouse kidney: Ultrastructural cytochemistry by a new technique. J. Histochem. Cytochem. **14**: 291-302.

Guyenet, P., Lefresne, P., Rossier, J., Beaujovan, J.C. and Glowinski, J. (1972). Inhibition by hemicholinium-3 of [^{14}C]acetylcholine synthesis and [^{3}H]choline high affinity uptake in rat striated synaptosomes. Mol. Pharm. **9**: 630-639.

Haimann, C., Torri-Tarelli, F., Fesce, R. and Ceccarelli, B. (1985). Measurement of quantal secretion and its correlation with depletion of synaptic vesicles. J. Cell Biol. **101**: 1953-1965.

Heuser, J. and Miledi, R. (1971). Effect of lanthanum ions on function and structure of frog neuromuscular junctions. Proc. Roy. Soc. Lond. (Biol.). **179**: 247-260.

Heuser, J. and Reese, T. (1973). Evidence for recycling of synaptic vesicle membrane during transmitter release at the frog neuromuscular junction. J. Cell Biol. **57**: 315-344.

Heuser, J., Reese, T.S., Dennis M., Jan, Y., Jan, L. and Evans, L. (1979). Synaptic vesicle exocytosis captured by quick freezing and correlated with quantal transmitter release. J. Cell Biol. **81**: 275-300.

Heuser, J., Reese, T. and Landis, D.M.P. (1974). Functional changes in frog neuromuscular junctions studied with freeze-fracture. J. Neurocytol. **3**: 109-131.

Holtzman, E., Freeman, A.R. and Kashner, L.A. (1971). Stimulation dependent alterations in peroxidase uptake at lobster neuromuscular junctions. Science (Wash. DC). **176**: 733-736.

Karnovsky, M.J. (1964). The localization of cholinesterase activity in the rat cardiac muscle by electron microscopy. J. Cell Biol. **23**: 217-232.

Kriebel, M.E. and Florey, E. (1983). Effect of lanthanum ions on the amplitude distributions of miniature endplate potentials and on synaptic vesicles in frog neuromuscular junctions. Neurosci. **9**: 535-547.

Kriebel, M.E. and Gross, C.E. (1974). Multimodal distribution of frog miniature endplate potentials in adult, denervated, and tadpole leg muscle. J. Gen. Physiol. **64**: 85-103.

Larkin, J.M., Brown, M.S., Goldstein, J.L. and Anderson, R.G.W. (1983). Depletion of intracellular potassium arrests coated pit formation and receptor-mediated endocytosis in fibroblasts. Cell. **33**: 273-285.

Letinsky, M.S., Fishbeck, K.H. and McMahan, U.J. (1976). Precision of reinnervation of original post-synaptic sites in frog muscle after a nerve crush. J. Neurocytol. **5**: 691-718.

Longenecker, H.E., Hurlbut, W.P., Mauro, A., Clark, A.W. (1970). Effects of black widow spider venom on the frog neuromuscular junction. Nature. **225**: 701-705.

35. Magazanick, L.G. and Vyskocil, F. (1970). Dependence of acetylcholine desensitization on the membrane potential of frog muscle fiber and on the ionic changes in the medium. J. Physiol. (Lond.). **210**: 507-518.

Meldolesi, J., Scheer, H., Madeddu, L. and Wanke, E. (1986). Mechanism of action of α-latrotoxin: the presynaptic stimulatory toxin of the black widow spider venom. Trends Pharmacol. Sci. **7**: 151-155.

Misler, S. and Falke, S.C. (1987). Dependence upon multivalent cations of quantal release of transmitter induced by black widow spider venom at the frog neuromuscular junction. Am. J. Physiol. **253C**: 469-476.

Misler, S. and Hurlbut, W.P. (1979). Action of black widow spider venom on quantized release of acetylcholine at the frog neuromuscular junction: Dependence upon external Mg^{2+}. Proc. Natl. Acad. Sci. USA. **76**: 991-995.

Schueler, F.W. (1960). The mechanism of action of the hemicholiniums. Int. Rev. Neurobiol. **2**: 77-97.

Segal, J.R., Ceccarelli, B., Fesce, R. and Hurlbut, W.P. (1985). Miniature endplate potential frequency and amplitude determined by an extension of Campbell's Theorem. Biophys. J. **47**: 183-202.

Stewart, W.W. (1978). Functional connections between cells as revealed by dye-coupling with a highly fluorescent naphthalamide tracer. Cell. **14**: 741-759.

Torri-Tarelli, F., Haimann, C. and Ceccarelli, B. (1987). Temporal coincidence between synaptic vesicle fusion and quantal secretion of acetylcholine. J. Neurocytol. **16**: 205-214.

Tremblay, J.P., Laurie, R.E. and Colonnier, M. (1983). Is the MEPP due to the release of one vesicle or to the simultaneous release of several vesicles at one active zone? Brain Res. Rev. **6**: 299-314.

Valtorta, F., Jahn, R., Fesce, R., Greengard, P. and Ceccarelli, B. (1988). Synaptophysin (P38) at the frog neuromuscular junction: its incorporation into the axolemma and recycling after intense quantal secretion of neurotransmitter. J. Cell Biol. **99**: 124-132.

Valtorta, F., Madeddu, L., Meldolesi, J. and Ceccarelli, B. (1984). Specific localization of the α-latrotoxin receptor in the nerve terminal plasma membrane. J. Cell Biol. **99**: 124-132.

Wanke, E., Ferroni, A., Gattanini, P. and Meldolesi, J. (1986). αLatrotoxin of the black widow spider venom opens a small, non-closing cation channel. Biochem. Biophys. Res. Commun. **134**: 320-325.

Weibel, E.R. and Paumgartner, D. (1978). Integrated steriological and biochemical studies on hepatic membranrs. II. Correction of section thickness effects on volume and surface density measurements. J. Cell Biol. **77**: 584-597.

Wernig, A. and Motelica-Heino, I. (1978). On the presynaptic nature of the quantal subunit. Neurosci. Let. **8**: 231-234.

THE ROLE OF COATED VESICLES IN RECYCLING OF SYNAPTIC VESICLE MEMBRANE

John Heuser

Department of Cell Biology & Physiology
Washington University School of Medicine
St. Louis, Missouri 63110

ABSTRACT

The uptake of extracellular tracers into synaptic nerve terminals has been a phenomenon of persistent interest. Uptake is into synaptic vesicles, hence vesicles spend part of their life in continuity with the plasma membrane, as expected if exocytosis underlies the quantal discharge of neurotransmitters. However, exactly how or when synaptic vesicles acquire extracellular tracers has not been unambiguously determined. Two schools of thought have developed, one holding that vesicles acquire tracers directly via a reversible exo/endocytotic sequence in which they consistently maintain their biochemical identity during their transient continuity with the plasma membrane, the other holding that synaptic vesicles acquire tracers indirectly, via the formation of clathrin-coated vesicles which are spatially and temporally separate from exocytosis and reverse a temporary loss of the vesicles' individual identity upon merger with the plasma membrane. Efforts to distinguish between these two alternatives have generated an interesting diversity of electron microscopic experiments, many of which are reviewed here. However, definitive determination of which view is correct may ultimately require direct visualization of synaptic vesicle turnover in living nerve terminals. To this end, we here review the results of visualizing endocytosis in tissue cultured cells, where light microscopy can provide sufficient resolution to reveal membrane dynamics in living cells. This has allowed visual discrimination of two different types of endocytosis, one clathrin-mediated (coated vesicle formation) and the other actin-mediated (macropinocytosis). Current work is also reviewed which aims at determining experimental methods for inhibiting each type of endocytosis selectively. Hypertonicity and severe cytoplasmic acidification turn out to inhibit coated vesicle formation, while cytochalasin D and mild cytoplasmic acidification selectively inhibit macropinocytosis. Applied to nerves, these various treatments affect synaptic vesicle turnover in a manner that supports the notion that synaptic vesicle membrane recycles via the "indirect" route of coated vesicle formation.

INTRODUCTION: BRUNO CECCARELLI'S LEGACY

Bruno Ceccarelli was one of the few adventurers who attempted to analyze the membrane dynamics of neuronal synapses by utilizing electron microscopy (EM). Thus, he was relegated to working with static images, which are often difficult to interpret when representing liquid structures like biological membranes, particularly because membranes react only slowly and imperfectly with standard EM fixatives. In contrast, the membrane events that occur during synaptic transmission are extremely rapid and fleeting. Faced with such difficulties, pure physicists have studied fluid dynamics by adding boluses of dye to their fluids and then directly monitoring changes in the dye's distribution over time. Ceccarelli often pointed out in his publications how informative it would be if a similar approach could be developed for synaptic membranes, and he dreamed of the day that specific EM markers of synaptic vesicle membrane would be forthcoming. Sadly, he did not live to see that day, though he and his colleagues' most recent work with light microscopic immunocytochemistry is clearly approaching that goal (Valtorta et al., 1988b; see also Valtorta et al., in this Volume). Still, those of us who wish to carry on this inquiry continue to struggle with the analysis of static electron micrographs in which all membranes usually look very much the same.

In coping with these difficulties, Ceccarelli made the wise choice to concentrate his structural analyses on a type of synapse that is uniquely amenable to physiological control and monitoring and can even be monitored during the time it is being fixed for EM. That is the frog neuromuscular junction, which is readily accessible in standard dissections of cutaneous pectoris or sartorius muscles (Birks et al., 1960). Ceccarelli thus included, both in his international collaborations and in the organization of his own laboratory, top-notch electrophysiologists who could help him to determine quantal secretion rates at individually identified neuromuscular junctions during experimental treatment and during chemical fixation. Also, he perfected the techniques of doing electron microscopy on frog muscles to a point where his images were as true-to-life as possible. In this way, he put himself in the ideal position to do structure/function analyses of membrane dynamics at a prototypical synapse.

This led him to a long series of reports, spanning more than 20 years, which described structural changes that accompany a variety of physiological and pharmacological manipulations of the frog neuromuscular junction. These fully established Ceccarelli as the world's leading expert on the electron microscopy of synapses. Nevertheless, Ceccarelli never fully overcame the intrinsic difficulties involved in studying rapid membrane dynamics, so we are left with a rich legacy of unsolved questions about synaptic vesicle membrane turnover. These will be the topic of this brief review, which is dedicated with great fondness to Ceccarelli's memory and written by a person who inevitably respected Ceccarelli's approach because he followed it in his own work as closely as possible.

ACCEPTED AND CONTROVERSIAL ASPECTS OF SYNAPTIC STRUCTURAL DYNAMICS

Few investigators today question the basic notion that synaptic transmission is mediated by discharge of synaptic vesicles, whose small size "quantizes" this discharge into multiple small boluses of neurotransmitter. An overwhelming body of EM data, Ceccarelli's as well as other's, further indicate that quantal discharge involves synaptic vesicle fusion with the plasma membrane, otherwise known as exocytosis (Couteaux & Pecot-Dechavassine, 1970; Heuser & Miledi, 1971; Ceccarelli et al., 1972, 1973; Heuser & Reese, 1973). The uncertainties and disagreements begin when attempting to determine the structural sequellae of exocytosis. The problem can be stated thusly: what happens to synaptic vesicle membrane after fusion with the plasma membrane? Ceccarelli et al.'s demonstrations of how many quanta can be discharged from a frog motor nerve terminal (around 2-3 x 10^6) compared to its initial stock of synaptic vesicles (around 0.5 x 10^6) indicated that each individual vesicle must discharge over and over again (Ceccarelli et al., 1972, 1973; see also Segal et al., 1985; Fesce et al., 1986; and Hurlbut's article in this Volume). This simple fact indicates that after discharge each vesicle must be recovered from the plasma membrane, reloaded with transmitter, and readied for re-use. Stimulation-dependent uptake of the extracellular tracer horseradish peroxidase (HRP), a phenomenon long studied by Ceccarelli and colleagues (Ceccarelli et al., 1972, 1973, 1979b) as well as ourselves (Heuser & Reese, 1973; Heuser, 1976), has generally been accepted as the prime manifestation of such synaptic vesicle recycling. Yet Ceccarelli himself remained cautious about this phenomenon, never feeling fully certain that HRP-loaded vesicles would necessarily rejoin the pool of available quanta, as opposed to being removed from circulation by fusion with lysosomes.

Ceccarelli's patient agnosticism on such matters was reflected also in his persistent reservations about several of the interpretations that we offered for the structural changes we observed at the frog neuromuscular junction (Heuser & Reese, 1973; Heuser, 1976). We argued, largely because we observed bulk shifts of membrane from vesicles to plasma membrane during stimulation and reverse shifts of surface membrane into intracellular "cisternae" after stimulation (Heuser & Reese, 1973), that vesicle recycling occurred by the scheme outlined in Fig. 1. In this view, synaptic vesicles would collapse after exocytosis and then totally mix into the plasma membrane, so that in order to be regenerated they would subsequently have to be regathered or segregated out of the rest of the plasma membrane before being re-internalized. This segregation and internalization event was, we proposed, the role of coated vesicles. These we felt were unusually abundant at the neuromuscular junction and in a prime position for retrieving vesicle membrane from the plasma membrane.

This is where we and the Ceccarelli school disagreed most heartedly. Throughout all of their publications, they pointed out how their observations were more consistent with a mechanism in which new vesicles formed directly from the synaptic membrane, in just the same spots as which they discharged, (hence by a direct reverse of exocytosis), rather than indirectly as the last step in a series of transformations involving intraterminal membrane compartments. What follows in this article is a brief review of the specific experiments that Ceccarelli and colleagues cited as being inconsistent with the idea that coated vesicles are required for retrieval of synaptic vesicle membrane (Fig. 1), experiments which they instead interpreted as indicating direct synaptic vesicle retrieval from the plasma membrane.

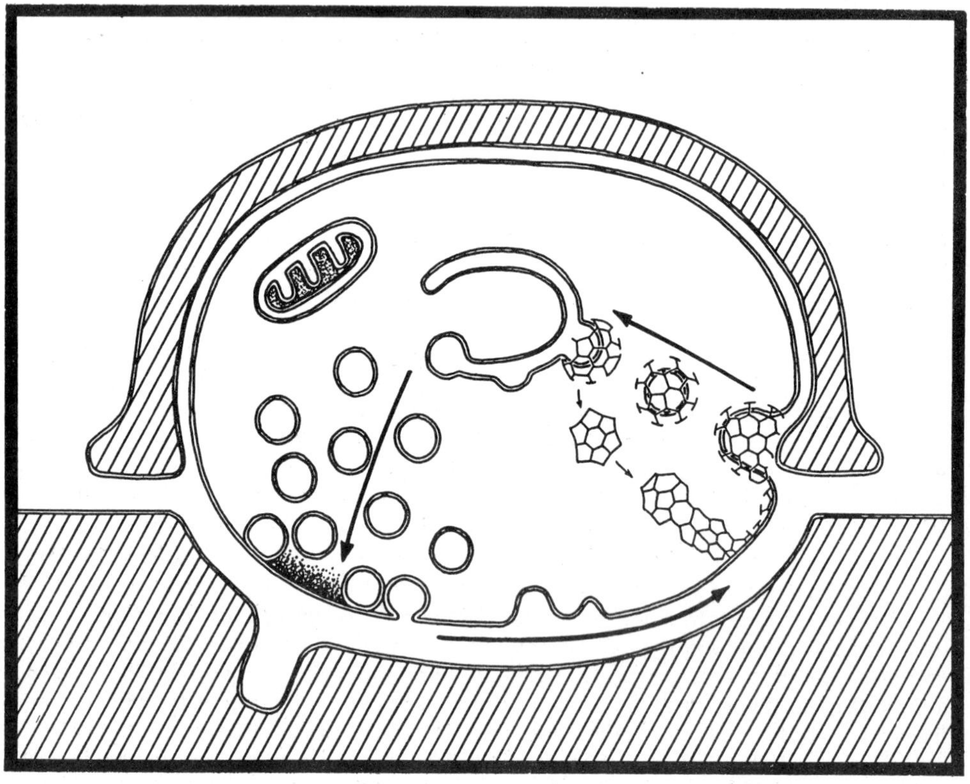

Figure 1: Diagram of our hypothesis of synaptic membrane recycling (Heuser & Reese, 1973). In the original study, the legend stated: "Synaptic vesicles discharge their content of transmitter by coalescing with the plasma membrane at specific regions adjacent to the muscle; then equal amounts of membrane are retrieved by coated vesicles arising from regions of the plasma membrane adjacent to the Schwann sheath; then, coated vesicles lose their coats and coalesce to form cisternae which accumulate in regions of vesicle depletion and slowly divide to form new synaptic vesicles". Points of subsequent and continuing controversy include: (1) whether synaptic vesicles open transiently and reversibly, instead of completely coalescing with the plasma membrane; (2) whether coated vesicle formation is abundant and fast enough to keep pace with synaptic vesicle discharge; and (3) whether cisternae are the products of coated vesicle coalescence or are direct extensions of the plasma membrane that remain continuous with it. These controversial points are discussed in the text. Reprinted with permission from Heuser & Reese, 1973.

THIN-SECTION ANALYSES OF SYNAPTIC VESICLE EXO/ENDOCYTOSIS

First, in the days before freeze-fracture EM, when all structural analyses were done on thin-sectioned muscles, Ceccarelli and colleagues were unable to find large changes in coated vesicle abundance during or after prolonged transmitter release, regardless of whether they produced the release by long slow nerve stimulation, by a brief period of intense nerve stimulation, or by direct K^+ depolarization of the nerve terminals (Ceccarelli et al., 1972, 1973). Though they later confirmed our description of a modest increase in coated vesicle abundance after intense stimulation (Torri-Tarelli et al., 1987), they did not feel this increase was sufficient to explain the tremendous enhancement of vesicle membrane turnover that must accompany intense transmitter release. Still, remaining open-minded on this point, they concluded one paper (Ceccarelli et al., 1979b) by saying: "However, if coats were associated with vesicles for only a small fraction of the time required for endocytosis, then one would not expect them to become very numerous even if endocytosis was accelerated."

Ceccarelli and colleagues hit on the key problem here: namely, that the abundance of transient structures in the cell, when seen in static electron micrographs, will depend upon their rate of occurrence as well as on their lifetime. For example, if stimulation of synaptic vesicle discharge led to an increased rate of coated pit formation but a commensurate reduction in how long it took each coated pit to pinch off from the plasma membrane to become a coated vesicle, then the overall abundance of coated pits would not increase even if endocytosis was accelerated. In fact, we once proposed that coated vesicles on the nerve terminal may remain "poised", in readiness for endocytosis at all times, but may only go ahead and pinch off when synaptic vesicle membrane is added to the surface. (They would behave this way if, for example, a lack of extra surface membrane kept them "poised", until synaptic vesicle exocytosis provided the extra membrane they need to pinch off.) In fact, that seems to be the behavior of coated pits in the insect oocytes where they were first discovered (Roth & Porter, 1964). In that cell type, coated pits are more abundant before a blood meal stimulates lipoprotein endocytosis; thereafter, coated pits become less abundant because they begin to pinch off from the oocyte surface and time is spent recycling their clathrin back to the plasma membrane.

Perhaps some of the disagreements that developed about the role of coated vesicles at the synapse arose from ambiguities in whether different groups were measuring the same structures. No one in the early days of thin sectioning made a clear distinction between coated pits and coated vesicles, yet it later became clear that the lifetime of a free coated vesicle in the cytoplasm may be so brief (because its coat may fall off so fast) that no one was seeing <u>free</u> coated vesicles at all, only coated pits with longer or shorter "necks" (i.e., longer or shorter membranous attachments to the axolemma). This realization led some investigators to question for a while whether coated vesicles ever pinch off from the plasmalemma at all (for example, Willingham & Pastan, 1980), although the prevailing view today is that they do indeed pinch off. Thus, the issue boils down to whether the rate of coated vesicle formation at the neuromuscular junction could ever keep pace with the rate of synaptic vesicle discharge. We have consistently maintained that it can (Heuser & Reese, 1973; Miller & Heuser, 1984), and would only add here that regardless of whether or not coated pits become more abundant during stimulation, the resting abundance of coated pits (namely, 1-4/μm^2 of nerve terminal plasma membrane; cf. Heuser & Reese, 1973; Miller & Heuser, 1984; Torri-Tarelli et al., 1987) would be sufficient to account for the typical rate of vesicle turnover that synapses can sustain for long periods of time (namely, 4 vesicles/μm^2/min; cf. Ceccarelli et al., 1973, 1979b; Haimann et al., 1985; Segal et al., 1985; Fesce et al., 1986; Torri-Tarelli et al., 1987), so long as each coated pit pinched off about once per minute. This is about the rate at which coated vesicles are thought to form in fibroblasts and other cells (Davoust et al., 1987; Sandvig et al., 1987; Heuser, 1989a), which is consistent with the idea that coated vesicles are centrally involved in the re-internalization of synaptic vesicle membrane.

Two other factors that led us to this view were, first, that the accumulations of membrane that occur during intense stimulation of transmitter release do not occur at the "active zones" where vesicles initially discharge (Couteaux & Pecot-Dechavassine, 1970, 1974), but elsewhere, typically beneath the Schwann cell covering of the nerve terminal (Heuser & Reese, 1973; Haimann et al., 1985; Torri-Tarelli et al., 1987; Ceccarelli et al., 1989); and second, that the maximum numbers of coated pits are seen on these membrane accumulations (Heuser & Reese, 1973; Miller & Heuser, 1984; Haimann et al., 1985; Ceccarelli et al., 1989). This would require bulk flow of membrane from the initial sites of exocytosis to different sites of endocytosis. This would provide sufficient time for membrane mixing which would generate the need to re-segregate synaptic vesicle components into structures like coated pits.

FREEZE-FRACTURE ANALYSES OF SYNAPTIC VESICLE EXO/ENDOCYTOSIS

With the advent of freeze-fracture of the neuromuscular junction (Dreyer et al., 1973; Peper et al., 1974), electron microscopists had the opportunity to analyze the above two alternatives more definitively. Freeze-fracture provided vast, panoramic, en face views of the plasma membrane, in place of the narrow thin sections previously available. Questions of where and how many membrane fusion events were occurring finally became experimentally accessible. Ceccarelli promptly adopted this technical approach and developed it to as high a level of excellence as he had for thin-section EM, thus was in a position to further test the above alternatives. For example, the scheme in Fig. 1 was based on our feeling that the retrieval of vesicle membrane was spatially separate from exocytosis (Heuser & Reese, 1973), as well as temporally separate (Miller & Heuser, 1984). However, when

Ceccarelli and colleagues compared the freeze-fracture appearance of nerves that were stimulated intensively right up until the moment of fixation (in which exocytosis should have been going on more rapidly than endocytosis) versus nerves rested for 1/2-1 min before fixation (in which exocytosis should have subsided but endocytosis should have been continuing at a high rate in compensation for the excess of membrane still left on the cell surface), they observed no structural differences! Both conditions displayed plasma membrane "dimples" (the freeze-fracture appearance of fused vesicles, whether coated or not) in greatest abundance immediately beside the active zones and in lesser abundance elsewhere (Ceccarelli et al., 1979b).

Since no one has ever seen coated vesicle formation immediately beside the active zones (Heuser & Reese, 1973; Miller & Heuser, 1984), we would have predicted that the fused vesicles Ceccarelli et al. found at the active zones were be synaptic vesicles caught in the act of discharge, while the "dimples" they found elsewhere were coated pits caught in the act of endocytosis. If this were so, however, the dimples beside the active zones ought to have disappeared as soon as nerves were allowed to rest. Ceccarelli and colleagues concluded that because those dimples did not disappear, they must have represented new vesicles caught in the process of reforming, at one in the same spot where they had formerly discharged (Ceccarelli et al., 1979b). Furthermore, related experiments suggested to them that the population of plasmalemmal "dimples" they observed at some distance from the active zones were not coated pits engaged in endocytosis, but instead "ectopic" or displaced exocytotic events. This idea emerged from experiments in which they bathed frog muscles in 20 mM K^+ to depolarize their nerve terminals directly. This produced freeze-fracture "dimples" all over the nerve terminal surfaces, with no obvious predilection for the active zones (Ceccarelli et al., 1979b). This uniform distribution was interpreted suggesting that prolonged depolarization in K^+ disorganized the release machinery and activated "latent" or ectopic release sites (Ceccarelli et al., 1979b).

As for the alternative we would favor (namely, that the "ectopic" dimples might instead have been sites of endocytosis), Ceccarelli et al. (1979b) reinterated that they saw no increase in coated vesicle abundance in K^+ depolarized nerve terminals, and went on in experiments published several years later to explore the K^+-effect in more detail (Ceccarelli et al., 1988 and Grohovaz et al., the present Volume). Then, they added the experiment of placing a frog muscle into 20 mM K^+ at the same time as it went into the EM fixative, rather than into K^+ 15 or 60 minutes before fixation. This led to a massive burst of transmitter discharge during fixation, but in this case a clear-cut preponderance of vesicle openings immediately beside the active zones. This is the distribution that is consistently observed when vesicle discharge is "freshly" evoked, whether by nerve stimulation or by toxins (Heuser et al., 1974; Heuser, 1977; Ceccarelli et al., 1979; Heuser et al.,

1979; Heuser & Reese, 1981; Torri-Tarelli et al., 1985). Thus, it appears that time has to be spent in high K^+ before frog nerves will develop "ectopic" vesicle openings. (This observation is reiterated and expanded in the report of Grohovaz et al. in the present Volume).

Still, we could interpret even the more recent K^+-results as suggesting that "ectopic" fusion sites are not vesicles discharging but coated vesicles forming, since it takes time for the latter process to get started after transmistter discharge begins (Heuser & Reese, 1981; Miller & Heuser, 1984) just as it takes time for the 'ectopic' sites to appear. This argument Ceccarelli and colleagues countered in the course of additional K^+-depolarization experiments that utilized sophisticated physiological monitoring of quantal discharge rates throughout fixation (Ceccarelli et al., 1988 and Grohovaz et al., the present Volume). They found that 20 mM K^+ in the fixative provokes even more discharge when nerves are pretreated with 1, 5, 15 or 30 min of K^+ than when they are not so pretreated. Yet, as described above, the abundance of "dimples" at the active zones of such pretreated nerves is much less. Hence, the only way Ceccarelli et al. could account for the final massive burst of exocytosis in K^+-pretreated nerves was to imagine that most of the "ectopic" vesicle fusions were also discharge events. This led Ceccarelli and colleagues to reinforce their conclusion that K^+ depolarization leads to a progressive inactivation of "active zone" discharge sites and a progressive increase in "ectopic" vesicle fusion sites (Ceccarelli et al., 1988 and Grohovaz et al., the present Volume). On this point, one is reminded of their earlier images of total active zone displacement after 1 hr in 20 mM K^+ (Ceccarelli et al., 1979b). This interesting observation deserves to be confirmed. One wonders whether future experiments will reveal a fundamental K^+-sensitivity in the membrane structures that allow active zones to be "hot spots" of vesicle discharge and also allow them to be spots of attachment of nerve to muscle.

FUTURE DIRECTIONS OF INQUIRY THAT MAY RESOLVE THE CURRENT CONTROVERSY

Without Ceccarelli's inspiring and insightful input into this field, it is doubtful that the above differences of interpretation on vesicle recycling will soon be resolved. However, he contributed several ancillary observations to the scientific literature that are likely to germinate future experiments that may help toward a resolution. Of particular interest is a report in which he and colleagues showed that ouabain stimulates transmitter release yet abolishes vesicle recycling, so that only one full round of quantal discharge occurs (Haimann et al., 1985). Interestingly, terminals so treated end up with deep plasma membrane involutions studded with coated pits (Fig. 2). Here, coated pit abundance has increased possibly as much as 15 fold, even though vesicle recycling is clearly blocked. [The actual tabulated data in Haimann et al. (1985) describe an increase in "coated vesicles" from $0.4 \pm 0.2/\mu m^2$ in controls to $2.3 \pm 0.7/\mu m^2$ in ouabain, a roughly 6-fold increase in the mean value which would increase to 15-fold if the upper and lower values of the standard errors happened to be more representative. In Torri-Tarelli et al. (1987) these values were revised to 0.3 ± 0.2/μm^2 (control) and 1.5 ± 0.5/μm^2 (ouabain minus Ca), again a 5-fold increase.]

In a similar vein, Ceccarelli and colleagues recently reported that isotonic K^+-propionate (KPr) also arrests synaptic vesicle recycling and limits nerve terminal discharge to one full round of quanta (Ceccarelli et al., 1989). Again in this situation, nerve terminals end up with extensive invaginations of the plasma membrane studded with many coated pits (Ceccarelli et al., 1989). The inhibition of vesicle recycling in the latter instance was thought to be due to chloride deprivation, however, it may turn out that both means of inhibition operate via a common mechanism of cytoplasmic acidification (Roos & Boron, 1981). The reasoning here is as follows: ouabain causes an accumulation of intracellular sodium, while application of isotonic KPr effectively eliminates external sodium. Either one of such conditions (high Na_i or zero Na_e) will shut down any Na:H antiporters that might exist in the

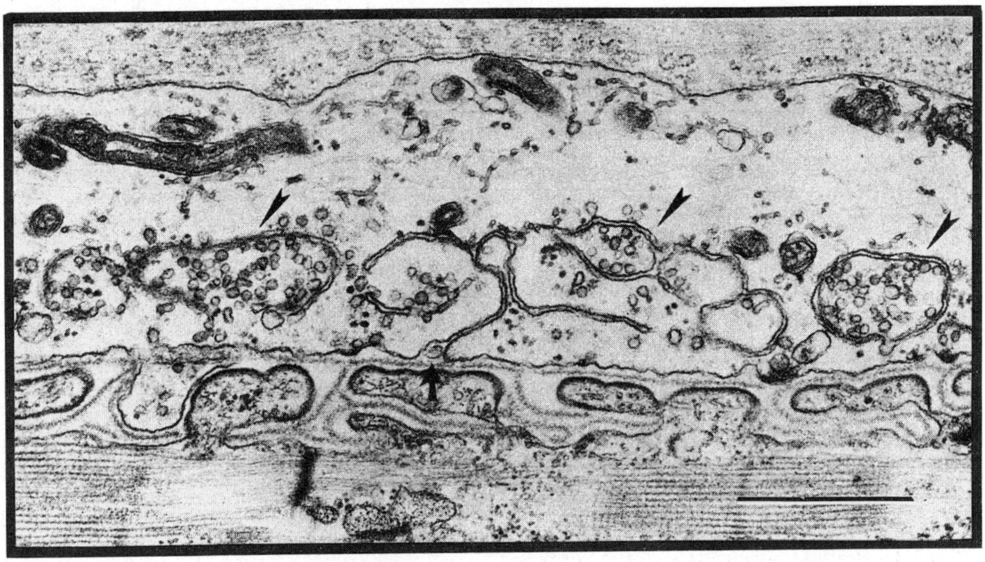

Figure 2: Longitudinal section of a frog motor nerve terminal, OsO_4 fixed after 3 hr exposure to 50 μM ouabain in Ca free-Ringer's containing 1 mM EGTA and 4 mM Mg^{++}. This treatment was long enough to go beyond the massive discharge of transmitter quanta provoked by ouabain. Accompanying the profound exhaustion of synaptic vesicles occurring at that point is the formation of many deep invaginations of the plasma membrane. These appear to be studded with coated pits, which would be interpreted in light of the scheme in Fig. 1 as indicating an inhibition of synaptic vesicle recycling at the stage of coated pit "budding". Other more recent studies on cultured cells suggest that ouabain may inhibit coated vesicle formation and hence synaptic vesicle recycling by acidifying the cytoplasm (Heuser, 1989a,b). Bar, 1.0 μm. Reprinted with permission from Haiman et al., 1985.

nerve plasma membrane. In most cells, these antiporters are vital for maintaining normal intracellular pH, in that they prevent acidification by electroneutrally moving protons <u>out</u> in exchange for sodium <u>in</u> (Roos & Boron, 1981). When Na:H antiporters are blocked, cells become acidic simply due to their ongoing metabolism. (Moreover, in the case of isotonic KPr, Ceccarelli et al. (1989) also noted that the protonated form of the anion is likely to be membrane-permeant and thereby further acidify the nerve terminal by directly transporting protons into it.) Thus, it seems highly likely that future experiments will confirm that cytoplasmic acidification blocks synaptic vesicle recycling.

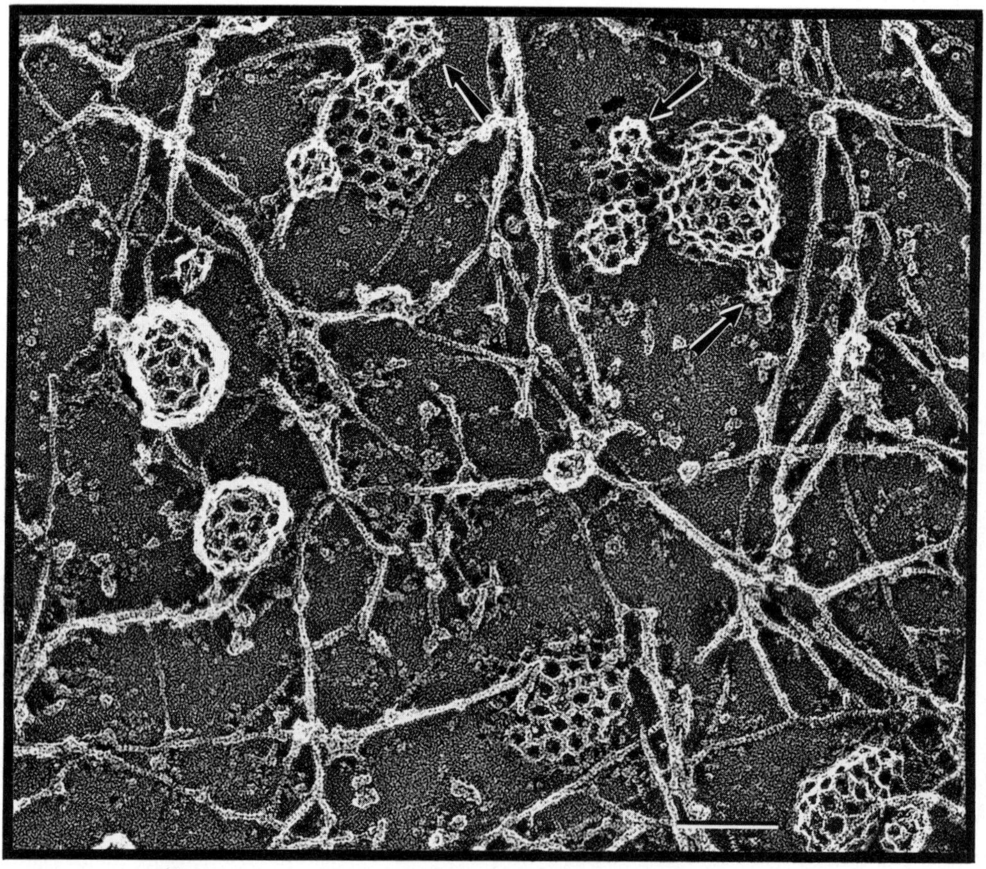

Figure 3: Survey view of a human fibroblast acidified by nigericin treatment at pH 6.3 for 2 min at 37°C. This results in several changes in coated pits, including excessive rounding as well as the development of adjacent foci of extremely intense curvature (a few of the typical clathrin "buds" are indicated by the arrows). In spite of this pH-induced tendency for clathrin lattice polymerization and increased curvature, such coated pits are "paralyzed", in that they are unable to pinch off from the plasma membrane. As a result, all endocytosis stops at low cytoplasmic pH. Bar, 0.1 μm. Reprinted with permission from Heuser, 1989a).

Presuming for the moment that acidification does occur in ouabain or KPr, we may then ask at what step this blocks vesicle recycling. The accumulation of coated pits seen in both of the above studies is, we think, an important lead. Recent work on various tissue cultured cells has shown that these, cytoplasmic acidification blocks coated vesicle formation at the coated pit stage. This is noticeable because it leads to an accumulation of fully-formed coated pits which for some reason are unable to pinch off from the plasma membrane (Davoust et al., 1987; Sandvig et al., 1987; Heuser, 1989; cf. Fig. 3). Ceccarelli and colleagues' pictures of ouabain or isotonic KPr-treated nerve terminals also show the same sort of accumulation of fully-formed coated pits (Fig. 2), which is consistent with a blockage of vesicle recycling at the stage of coated vesicle formation. Likewise, the images of nerves stimulated with black-widow spider venom in the absence of external Ca^{++}, which again blocks vesicle recycling, also show a 15X increase in coated pits on the plasmalemma (Fesce et al., 1986; Torri-Tarelli et al., 1987). It will be interesting to learn whether under these conditions, the venom also causes acidification of the nerve terminal axoplasm.

CONCLUSIONS

At this date, any generalizations concerning a central role for coated vesicle formation in synaptic vesicle recycling are still tentative and we think it best to end this brief retrospective with a statement from Ceccarelli and Hurlbut's influential review, a statement as true today as when it was first published 10 years ago: "There is evidence that more than one endocytotic process occurs on nerve endings at synapses..., and coats may be important only in processes that do not play a role in the retrieval of synaptic vesicles. Small numbers of coated vesicles are commonly observed on resting terminals and these coated vesicles may be involved in endocytotic activity unrelated to the retrieval of synaptic vesicles. The increased numbers of coated vesicles have been found on terminals subjected to massive stimulation. They may have been prominent in these preparations because the normal recovery processes had been fatigued or depressed. Thus it is not yet settled whether coated vesicles are required for the removal of synaptic vesicles from the axolemma. Possibly all of the processes (discussed above) occur to some extent and the process that predominants at any given time may depend on the rate at which membrane is added and on factors in the axoplasm that determine rates of recovery. A meaningful choice among the various possibilities probably cannot be made until unambiguous markers for the vesicle membrane have been identifed" (quote from p. 425 of Ceccarelli & Hurlbut, 1980). In this endeavor, the scientists who trained with Ceccarelli and who are determined to carry on in his absence are continuing to make rapid progress (cf. chapters by Grohovaz et al. and Valtorta et al. in this Volume).

ACKNOWLEDGEMENTS

Current work supported by NIH grant #GM29647; earlier work was largely supported by the Muscular Dystrophy Association of America.

REFERENCES

Birks, R., H.E. Huxley and B. Katz. (1960) The fine structure of the neuromuscular junction of the frog. J. Physiol. 150: 134-144.

Ceccarelli, B., W.P. Hurlbut and A. Mauro. (1972) Depletion of vesicles from frog neuromuscular junctions by prolonged tetanic stimulation. J. Cell Biol. 54: 30-38.

Ceccarelli, B., W.P. Hurlbut and A. Mauro. (1973) Turnover of transmitter and synaptic vesicles at the frog neuromuscular junctions. J. Cell Biol. 57: 499-524.

Ceccarelli, B., F. Grohovaz, W.P. Hurlbut and N. Iezzi. (1979a) Freeze fracture studies of frog neuromuscular junctions during intense release of neurotransmitter. I. Effects of black widow spider venom and Ca^{++}-free solutions on the structure of the active zone. J. Cell Biol. 81: 163-177.

Ceccarelli, B., F. Grohovaz, W.P. Hurlbut and N. Iezzi (1979b) Freeze-fracture studies of frog neuromuscular junctions during intense release of neurotransmitter. II. Effects of electrical stimulation and high potassium. J. Cell Biol. 81: 178-192.

Ceccarelli, B. and W.P. Hurlbut. (1980) Ca^{2+}-dependent recycling of synaptic vesicles at the frog neuromuscular junction. J. Cell Biol. 87: 297-303.

Ceccarelli, B. and W.P. Hurlbut. (1980) Vesicle hypothesis of the release of quanta of acetylcholine. Physiol. Rev. 60: 396-441.

Ceccarelli, B., R. Fesce, F. Grohovaz and C. Haimann. (1988) The effect of potassium on exocytosis of transmitter at the frog neuromuscular junction. J. Physiol. 401: 163-183.

Ceccarelli, B., P.C. Molenaar, B.S. Oen, R.L. Polak, F. Torri-Tarelli and G.Th.H. Van Kempen. (1989) The effect of anions on bound acetylcholine in frog sartorius muscle. J. Physiol. 408: 233-249.

Couteaux R. and M. Pecot-Dechavassine. (1970) Vesicles synaptiques et poches au niveau des "zones actives" de la jonction neuromusculaire. Comptes Rend. Acad. Sci. (Paris) Ser D 271: 2346-2349.

Couteaux, R. and M. Pecot-Dechavassine. (1974) Les zones specialisees des membranes presynaptique. Comptes Rend. Acad. Sci. (Paris) Ser D 280: 299-301.

Davoust, J., J. Gruenberg and K.E. Howell. (1987) Two threshold values of low pH block endocytosis at different stages. Eur. Mol. Biol. Organ. J. 6: 3601-3609.

Dreyer, F., K. Peper, K. Akert, L. Sandri and H. Moor. (1973) Ultrastructure of the "active zone" in the frog neuromuscular junction. Brain Res. 62: 373-380.

Fesce, R., J.R. Segal, B. Ceccarelli and W.P. Hurlbut. (1986) Effects of black widow spider venom and Ca^{2+} on quantal secretion at the frog neuromuscular junction. J. Gen. Physiol. 88: 59-81.

Haimann, C., F. Torri-Tarelli, R. Fesce and B. Ceccarelli. (1985) Measurement of quantal secretion induced by ouabain and its correlation with depletion of synaptic vesicles. J. Cell Biol. 101: 1953-1965.

Heuser, J.E. and R. Miledi. (1971) Effect of lanthanum ions on function and structure of frog neuromuscular junctions. Proc. Roy. Soc. Lond. B 179: 247-278.

Heuser, J.E. and T.S. Reese. (1973) Evidence for recycling of synaptic vesicle membrane during transmitter release at the frog neuromuscular junction. J. Cell Biol. 57: 315-344.

Heuser, J.E., T.S. Reese and D.M.D. Landis. (1974) Functional changes in frog neuromuscular junctions studied with freeze-fracture. J. Neurocytol. 3: 109-131.

Heuser, J.E. (1976) Morphology of synaptic vesicle discharge and reformation at the frog neuromuscular junction. In: Motor Innervation of Muscle. S. Thesleff, editor. Academic Press, Lond, pp. 51-115.

Heuser, J.E. (1977) Synaptic vesicle exocytosis revealed in quick-frozen frog neuromuscular junctions treated with 4-aminopyridine and given a single electrical shock. In: Neuroscience Symposia, Vol. 2. W.M. Cowan and J.A. Ferrendelli, editors. Society for Neuroscience. Bethesda, MD, pp. 215-239.

Heuser, J.E., T.S. Reese, L.Y. Jan, Y.N. Jan, M.J. Dennis and L. Evans. (1979) Synaptic vesicle exocytosis captured by quick-freezing and correlated with quantal transmitter release. J. Cell Biol. 81: 275-300.

Heuser, J.E. and T.S. Reese. (1981) Structural changes after transmitter release at the frog neuromuscular junction. J. Cell Biol. 88: 564-580.

Heuser, J. (1989a). Effects of cytoplasmic acidification on clathrin lattice morphology. J. Cell Biol. 108: 401-411.

Heuser, J.E. (1989b) Changes in lysosome shape and distribution correlated with changes in cytoplasmic pH. J. Cell Biol. 108: 855-864.

Miller, T.M. and J.E. Heuser. (1984) Endocytosis of synaptic vesicle membrane at the frog neuromuscular junction. J. Cell Biol. 98: 685-698.

Peper, K., F. Dreyer, C. Sandri, K. Akert and H. Moor. (1974) Structure and ultrastructure of the frog motor endplate. A freeze-etching study. Cell Tissue Res. 149: 437-455.

Roos, A. and W.F. Boron. (1981) Intracellular pH. Physiol. Rev. 61: 296-434.

Roth, T.F. and K.R. Porter. (1964) Yolk protein uptake in the oocyte of the mosquito Aedes aegypti L. J. Cell Biol. 20: 313-332.

Sandvig, K., S. Olsnes, O.W. Peterson and B. van Deurs. (1987) Acidification of the cytosol inhibits endocytosis from coated pits. J. Cell Biol. 106: 679-689.

Segal, J.R., B. Ceccarelli, R. Fesce and W.P. Hurlbut. (1985) Miniature endplate potential frequency and amplitude determined by an extension of Campbell's therum. Biophys. J. 47: 183-202.

Torri-Tarelli, F., F. Grohavaz, R. Fesce and B. Ceccarelli. (1985) Temporal coincidence between synaptic vesicle fusion and quantal secretion of acetylcholine. J. Cell Biol. 101: 1386-1399.

Torri-Tarelli, F., C. Haimann and B. Ceccarelli. (1987) Coated pits and coated vesicles during enhanced quantal release of acetylcholine at the neuromuscular junction. J. Neurocytol. 16: 205-214.

Valtorta, F., A. Villa, R. Jahn, P. De Camilli, P. Greengard and B. Ceccarelli. (1988a) Localization of synapsin I at the frog neuromuscular junction. Neurosci. 24: 593-603.

Valtorta, F., R. Jahn, R. Fesce, P. Greengard and B. Ceccarelli. (1988b) Synaptophysin (p38) at the frog neuromuscular junction: I incorporation into the axolemma and recycling after intense quanta secretion. J. Cell Biol. 107: 2717-2727.

Willingham, M.C. and I. Pastan. (1980) The receptosome: an intermediate organelle of receptor-mediated endocytosis in culture fibroblasts. Cell 21: 67-77.

ACETYLCHOLINE COMPARTMENTS IN SKELETAL MUSCLE

Peter C. Molenaar
Department of Pharmacology, Sylvius Laboratory,
Wassenaarseweg 72, 2333 AL Leiden, The Netherlands

ABSTRACT:

I studied acetylcholine compartments in skeletal muscle with the aim to find their anatomical origin, and, in addition, their correlation with functional compartments, i.e. the pools in which synthesis, storage and release take place.

INTRODUCTION:

For about forty years the neuromuscular junction (NMJ) has served the role of a model system for electrophysiology and electron microscopy. Unfortunately, the NMJ is not a particularly suitable system for chemical measurements of acetylcholine (ACh) because it contains very little of this substance. For example, a typical skeletal muscle, such as the frog sartorius which has been very popular for electrophysiological studies, contains about one million times less ACh than the electric organ of the electric ray, which has been a biochemical model system for the last two decades (fig. 1). Nevertheless there is a need for ACh measurements in the NMJ because the electrophysiologist cannot look into the nerve terminal and the electron microscopist cannot see where the ACh is located.

In collaboration mostly with Rob Polak of the Medical Biological Laboratory-TNO at Rijswijk and Ricardo Miledi of University College London, I have studied ACh in skeletal muscle. In this article I review our work on ACh compartments.

RESULTS AND DISCUSSION:

Measurement of ACh

It is clear that anyone who wishes to measure such small amounts of ACh must use a powerful analytical technique. At the time when Polak and I started biochemical measurements of ACh in muscle there was only one type of apparatus that was suitable for this purpose, a GCMS system in which the separating power of gas chromatography is combined with the high sensitivity of the mass spectrometer. Thus, the mass spectrometer is used as a selective detector of ions. The principle is as follows. Since ACh is a non-volatile quaternary nitrogen salt it is not suitable for chromatography in the gas phase. The ACh can be transformed into a volatile compound by demethylation either with a chemical procedure (Jenden et al., 1973) or by heating (Szilagyi et al., 1968). We developed 'slow' pyrolysis, a simple method which produces the demethylated ACh with a high yield (Polak and Molenaar, 1979). A bonus of the GC-MS method is that using variants containing deuterium as a label we can apply deuterated internal standards and incorporated precursors, all of which can be analyzed at the same time. However, the usage of deut-

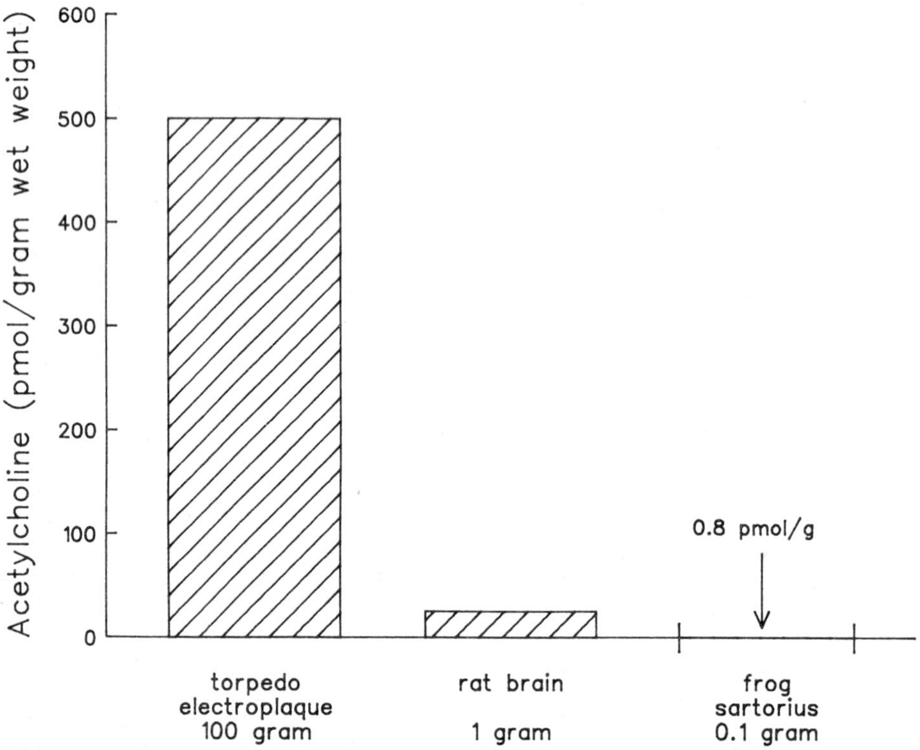

Fig.1. ACh content of model systems for ACh (electric organ of the ray), for synaptosomes (from brain) and for electrophysiology and morphology (skeletal muscle of the frog).

erium in combination with the demethylation step involves the risk of deuterium exchange, via the free choline (Polak and Molenaar, 1974) so that we eliminate the choline extracted from the tissue during the purification procedure. The sensitivity of the method, roughly between 0.1 and 0.2 pmol, is more than enough for measuring ACh from muscle.

Neural and non-neural ACh

It has been known for some time that cutting the motor nerve causes degeneration which begins at the nerve terminals and then crawls back along the distal part of the severed motor nerve. In frog muscle the motor nerve terminals desintegrate after a delay of about five days, whereas the axons degenerate much later (Birks et al., 1960a, 1960b). Thus denervation is an appropiate technique to find out how much ACh is located in the nerve terminals. When we tested this (Miledi et al., 1977), we found that no more than 70 % of the ACh disappeared between 4 and 8 days after denervation and that the remaining ACh stayed in the muscle for at least 25 days. Also in denervated mammalian muscle we found some ACh with mass spectrometry (Miledi et al., 1982b). In the early sixties there already had been a hint that some post-denervation ACh persisted in mammalian muscle (Bhatnagar and MacIntosh, 1960; Hebb, 1962), but since these measurements had been made with bioassay methods there was some doubt about the identity of the ACh-response.

As the next step we divided the muscles into segments containing the endplates and segments that were free of them in order to find out whether the ACh which remains shortly after denervation is located in the intramuscular branches of the motor nerve. (As a matter of fact the endplate segment in the frog sartorius has to be quite large because its fibres have a multiple innervation, Katz and Kuffler, 1941.) However, it appeared that endplate-free segments of the muscle contained substantial amounts of ACh which could not be decreased by denervation. On the other hand, denervation caused a decrease of ACh in the endplate segment and after denervation the concentrations of ACh (in pmoles per gram of wet tissue) became exactly the same as in the endplate-free segments. These experiments (Miledi et al., 1977, 1982b) indicated that ACh is located in the muscle fibres themselves and the question arose whether they also contain choline acetyltransferase (ChAT). In fact, enzymatic analysis indicated that muscle fibres are free of ChAT (Molenaar and Polak, 1980; Miledi et al., 1982b). Instead, we suggested that non-neural ACh is synthesized by carnitine acetyltransferase which may accept choline as a substrate (Molenaar and Polak, 1980; Tucek, 1982).

The Schwann cells which cover the nerve terminals make contact with the postsynaptic membrane after denervation and release quanta of ACh upon stimulation (Dennis and Miledi, 1974). Apparently, these cells synthesize and contain some ACh. However, this ACh is negligible compared to the amounts of ACh contained in nerve terminals and muscle fibres.

Surplus ACh

When a diaphragm muscle is incubated in the presence of a cholinesterase inhibitor, the level of ACh starts to rise (Molenaar et al., 1987), a paradoxical effect in view of the fact that cholinesterase in located extracellularly. This is called surplus ACh in analogy to the surplus ACh first discovered in the ganglion by Birks and MacIntosh (1961). However, in the frog sartorius no formation of surplus takes place (Miledi et al., 1977; Molenaar et al., 1987). Consequently, there is no reason to believe that surplus ACh is an essential aspect of transmitter metabolism at the NMJ.

Bound and free ACh

The background of our approach is that the ACh in synaptic vesicles is supposed to be protected against the action of cholinesterase (Marchbanks and Israël, 1971). So when the tissue is homogenized, the soluble ACh is destroyed by the enzyme whereas the vesicular ACh is protected. Our method (Miledi et al., 1982a) is similar to that originally developed for the Torpedo by Israël and Dunant (Dunant et al., 1972). The principle of the method is as follows (fig. 2). The muscle is homogenized in Ringer; one part is extracted with trichloro acetic acid (TCA): this gives the <u>total</u> ACh of the tissue. The other part is treated with a large amount of cholinesterase from

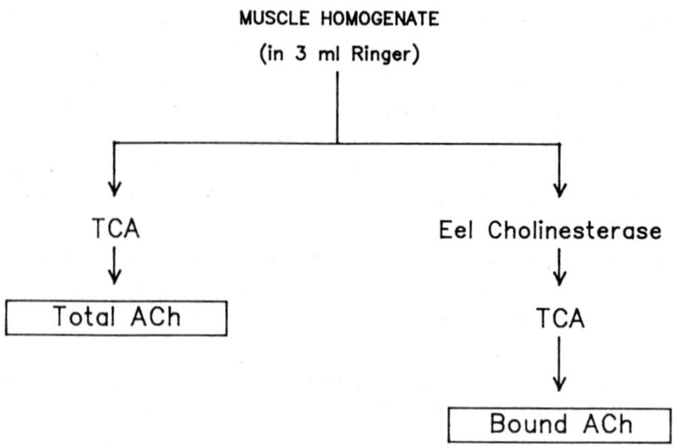

Fig. 2. Scheme of preparation of total and bound ACh. Free ACh is the difference between total and bound ACh.

electric eel to destroy any freely dissolved ACh. (This is necessary because frog muscle by itself does not contain enough enzyme for this purpose.) The ACh surviving this step is then extracted with TCA and this gives the bound ACh.

In a typical frog sartorius (R. temporaria) 50 pmol total and 25 pmol bound ACh are measured (in R. esculenta these values are somewhat higher). Thus 25 pmol is hydrolysed, corresponding to the free ACh fraction. Using again denervation as a technique for probing the fraction of ACh in nerve terminals, we found that 18 pmol bound ACh was lost by denervation.

It is important to bear in mind that bound and free ACh are biochemically defined fractions. Whether or not these fractions are derived from synaptic vesicles and cytoplasmic ACh remains to be seen. (For instance it has been suggested that some vesicular ACh may turn up in the free fraction because of 'exocytosis' of ACh during homogenization, Heuser and Lennon, 1973; Miledi et al., 1982a.)

Effect of stimulation on ACh compartments

Here I focuss on the effect of stimulation on ACh in the tissue, rather than on the release itself. In principle some deductions can be made on (sub)compartments of the releasable store (Gorio et al., 1978; Molenaar and Oen, 1988).

We tested the effect of three stimulation methods on ACh levels in the tissue. 1. Lanthanum as a stimulating agent is of interest because it causes an outburst of ACh quanta leading to an irreversible depletion of synaptic vesicles (Heuser and Miledi, 1971). 2. Potassium propionate gives also an outburst of quanta but this is associated with a reversible depletion of vesicles (Ceccarelli et al., 1989). 3. Electric stimulation (in the absence or presence of propionate ion).

For release studies we found that ordinary inhibitors such as neostigmine and DFP are useless, especially in frog muscle, and that very potent nerve gases must be applied to prevent destruction of the released ACh (Miledi et al., 1984). First, when we tested the effect of lanthanum on ACh release (Miledi et al., 1980), we found that lanthanum failed to cause ACh release from denervated muscle, whereas lanthanum caused much ACh release from a normal, innervated muscle. High potassium similarly failed to evoke ACh release from denervated muscle. We concluded, therefore, that the non-neural ACh in the tissue is an inert store. Furthermore, labelling studies indicated that non-neural ACh had a small turnover rate (Molenaar and Polak, 1983).

We then made an unexpected finding. It might have been anticipated that a full length treatment with lanthanum would cause a thorough depletion of ACh in the tissue, simply because of the morphological evidence that this causes a total depletion of synaptic vesicles. In fact, we found that after an initial trough in the content coinciding with the maximal rate of ACh release, the ACh content increased and at the time of vesicle depletion at 5 h, the tissue contained even more ACh than in the beginning of the experiment. Apparently, this ACh must have had a cytoplasmic localization. It was therefore of interest to investigate the effect of lanthanum on bound and free ACh (Miledi et al., 1982a; Molenaar and Polak, 1989). We found that lanthanum reduced the bound ACh to a low level, about the same low level as found after denervation. Apparently, lanthanum depletes nearly all the bound ACh from the nerve terminals. In contrast, lanthanum does not deplete the free ACh.

Subsequently, we wanted to know whether or not the free ACh after lanthanum was available for transmitter release under the influence of a calcium ionophore (A 23187), a second dose of lanthanum and high potassium (Miledi et al., 1983). However, none of these substances increased the transmitter release from lanthanum treated muscles. This was the first indication that bound, but not the free ACh is important for transmitter release.

In another type of experiment we stimulated frog sartorius muscles for 5 min in high potassium propionate (Molenaar and Polak, 1989), a treatment leading to a marked reduction of synaptic vesicles (Gennaro et al., 1978). We found that after 5 min there was a profound reduction of bound ACh whereas the free ACh remained unchanged. This was another indication that bound rather than free ACh is important for transmitter release.

Recovery of ACh and synaptic vesicles after stimulation

In these experiments (Ceccarelli et al., 1989) we used a 30 min stimulation period in potassium propionate in order to obtain a practically complete depletion of bound ACh. We then allowed the muscles to recover for 3 h in normal low potassium medium with either chloride or propionate ions. We found that total ACh recovered in 3 h, regardless whether chloride or propionate had been present during the recovery period. On the other hand, bound ACh did not recover in a propionate medium whereas it did recover fairly well in a chloride medium. Apparently, the revovery of bound ACh required the presence of chloride ions. There was an increase of the free ACh, which was most marked in a propionate medium. Subsequently, we found that synaptic vesicles, which were thoroughly depleted during the 30 min stimulation period, recovered within 1 h in a chloride medium. However, in propionate medium the vesicles did not reappear

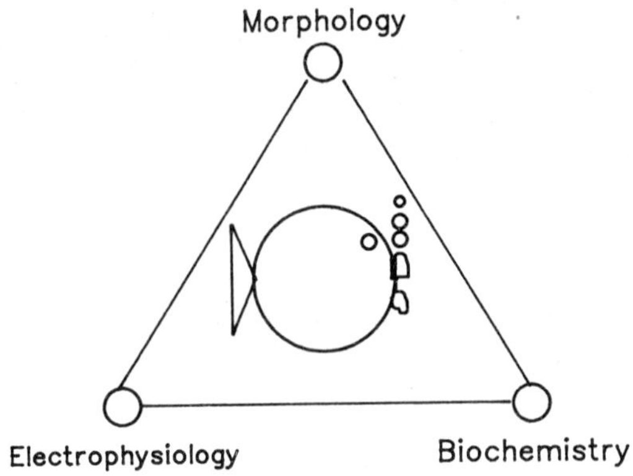

Fig. 3. A triangular net as a symbolic representation how the ACh release mechanism may be caught.

except for a few vesicles clustered at the active zones. After 3 h recovery in propionate there were still very few vesicles in the terminals. Apparently, both vesicle recycling and the recovery of bound ACh are both inhibited in a propionate medium. (It was the lack of chloride rather than the presence of propionate which was responsible for the effect, because bound ACh did recover when chloride ions had been added to the propionate medium).

Labelling experiments

When the tissue was exposed to deuterated choline during the recovery period the labelled ACh first appeared in the free fraction: after one hour the labelling ratio in the free was about two times higher than that of the bound fraction (Molenaar and Polak, 1989) In resting muscle the ACh was practically not labelled at all.

In recent experiments (unpublished) we labelled the ACh either in the absence or the presence of AH 5183 (a blocker of the vesicular uptake of ACh, Parsons et al., 1987). We found that AH 5183 completely prevented the formation of bound deuterium-labelled ACh, although there was an abundant formation of labelled ACh in the free fraction. In addition AH 5183 prevented the release of labelled ACh during a second stimulation period. In the absence of AH 5183, however, there was formation of labeled bound ACh and stimulation then evoked the release of labelled ACh. Apparently, the labelled ACh in the free fraction was unavailable for ACh release.

Conclusion

Free and bound ACh are different fractions, apparently with a different subcellular origin. It appears that bound ACh is more important than free ACh for transmitter release, since we could evoke ACh release in the presence of bound ACh. But it was not the other way round: the presence of free ACh alone was not sufficient for ACh release.

It is clear that so far with electrophysiology or electron microscopy alone it has been impossible to pin point the release mechanism of ACh. Nor is this possible on the basis of the present results, nothwithstanding their suggestive power. As illustrated symbolically in the cartoon of fig. 3 results from electrophysiology, electron microscopy and biochemical measurements of ACh may be thought to form together a sort of triangular net. The optimistic idea is that eventually the fish, that is the release mechanism for ACh, can be caught in this net and its form distinguished when the ropes are pulled.

ACKNOWLEDEGEMENT:

Financial support by MEDIGON/ZWO is gratefully acknowledged.

REFERENCES:

Bhatnagar, S.P. and MacIntosh, F.C. (1960) Acetylcholine content of striated muscle. Proc. Can. Fed. Biol. Soc. 3, 12-13.

Birks, R., Huxley, H.E. and Katz, B. (1960) The fine structure of the neuromuscular junction of the frog. J. Physiol., Lond. 150, 134-144.

Birks, R., Katz, B. and Miledi, R. (1960) Physiological and structural changes at the amphibian myoneural junction in the course of nerve degeneration. J. Physiol., Lond. 150, 145-168.

Birks, R. and MacIntosh, F.C. (1961) Acetylcholine metabolism in a sympathetic ganglion. Canad. J. Biochem. Physiol. 39, 787-827.

Ceccarelli, B., Molenaar P.C., Oen, B.S., Polak, R.L. Torri-Tarelli, F. and Van Kempen G.Th.H. (1989) The effect of anions on bound acetylcholine in frog sartorius muscle. J. Physiol., Lond. 408, 233-249.

Dennis, M.J. and Miledi, R. (1974) Electrically induced release of acetylcholine from denervated Schwann cells. J. Physiol., Lond. 237, 431-452.

Dunant, Y., Gautron, J., Israël, M., Lesbats, B. and Manaranche, R. (1972) Les compartiments d'acétylcholine de l'organe électrique de la Torpille et leurs modifications par la stimulation. J. Neurochem. 19, 1987-2002.

Gennaro, J.F., Nastuk W.L. and Rutherford, D.T. (1978) Reversible depletion of synaptic vesicles induced by application of high external potassium to the frog neuromuscular junction. J. Physiol. Lond. 280, 237-247.

Gorio, A., Hurlbut, W.P. and Ceccarelli, B.(1978) Acetylcholine compartments in mouse diaphragm: comparison of the effects of black widow spider venom, electrical stimulation and high concentrations of potassium. J. Cell Biol. 78, 716-733.

Hebb, C.O. (1962) Acetylcholine content of rabbit plantaris muscle after denervation. J. Physiol., Lond. 163, 294-306.

Heuser, J. and Lennon, A.M. (1973) Morphological evidence for exocytosis of acetylcholine during the formation of synaptosomes from Torpedo electric organ. J. Physiol., Lond. 223, 39-41P.

Heuser, J. and Miledi, R (1971) Effect of lanthanum ions on function and structure of frog neuromuscular junctions. Proc. R. Soc. Lond. B. 192, 475-480.

Jenden, D.J., Roch, M. and Booth, R.A. (1973) Simultaneous measurement of endogenous and deuterium-labelled tracer variants of choline and acetylcholine in sub-picomole quantities by gas chromatography/mass spectrometry. Analyt. Biochem. 55, 438-448.

Katz, B. and Kuffler, S.W. (1941) Multiple motor innervation of the frog's sartorius muscle. J. Neurophysiol. 6, 99-110.

Marchbanks, R.M. and Israël, M. (1971) The heterogeneity of bound acetylcholine and synaptic vesicles. Biochem. J. 129, 1049-1061.

Miledi, R., Molenaar, P.C. and Polak, R.L. (1977) An analysis of acetylcholine in frog muscle by mass fragmentography. Proc. R. Soc. B. 197, 285-297.

Miledi, R., Molenaar, P.C. and Polak, R.L. (1980) The effect of lanthanum ions on acetylcholine in frog muscle. J. Physiol., Lond. 309, 199-214.

Miledi, R., Molenaar, P.C. and Polak, R.L. (1982a) Free and bound acetylcholine in frog muscle. J. Physiol., Lond. 333, 189-199.

Miledi, R., Molenaar, P.C. and Polak, R.L. (1983) Electrophysiological and chemical determination of acetylcholine release at the frog neuromuscular junction. J. Physiol. Lond. 334, 245-254.

Miledi, R., Molenaar, P.C. and Polak, R.L. (1984) Acetylcholinesterase activity in intact and homogenized skeletal muscle of the frog. With an appendix by P.C. Molenaar. J. Physiol., Lond. 349, 663-686.

Miledi, R., Molenaar P.C., Polak, R.L., Tas J.W.M. and Van der Laaken, T. (1982b) Neural and non-neural acetylcholine in the rat diaphragm. Proc. R. Soc. Lond. B. 214, 153-168.

Molenaar, P.C. and Oen, B.S. (1988) Analysis of quantal acetylcholine noise at end-plates of frog muscle during rapid transmitter secretion. J. Physiol., Lond. 400, 335-348.

Molenaar, P.C., Oen, B.S., Polak, R.L. and Van der Laaken, A.L. (1987) Surplus acetylcholine and acetylcholine release in the rat diaphragm. J. Physiol., Lond. 385, 147-167.

Molenaar, P.C. and Polak, R.L. (1980) Acetylcholine synthesizing enzymes in frog skeletal muscle. J. Neurochem. 35, 1021-1025.

Molenaar, P.C. and Polak, R.L. (1983) Potassium propionate causes preferential loss of 'bound' acetylcholine in frog muscle. Neuroscience Letters 43, 209-213.

Molenaar, P.C. and Polak, R.L. (1989) Effect of potassium propionate on free and bound acetylcholine in frog muscle. Brain Res. 477, 109-117.

Parsons, S.M., Bahr, B.A., Gracz, L.M., Kaufman, R., Kornreich,W.D., Nilsson, L. and Rogers, G.A. (1987) ACh transport: fundamental properties and effects of pharmacologic agents. Ann. N.Y. Acad. Sci. 493, 220-223.

Polak, R.L. and Molenaar, P.C. (1974) Pitfalls in determination of acetylcholine from brain by pyrolysis-gas chromatography/ mass spectrometry. J. Neurochem. 23, 1295-1297.

Polak, R.L. and Molenaar, P.C. (1979) A method for determination of acetylcholine by slow pyrolysis combined with mass fragmentography on a packed capillary column. J. Neurochem. 32, 407-412.

Szilagyi, P.I.A., Schmidt, D.E. and Green, J.P. (1968) Microanalytical determination of acetylcholine, other choline esters, and choline by pyrolysis-gas chromatography. Anal.Chem. 40, 2009-2013.

Tucek, S. (1982) The synthesis of acetylcholine in skeletal muscles of the rat. J. Physiol., Lond. 322, 53-69.

DUAL EFFECT OF POTASSIUM ON TRANSMITTER EXOCYTOSIS.

F. Grohovaz, R. Fesce and C. Haimann.

C.N.R. Center of Cytopharmacology and "Bruno Ceccarelli" Center, Department of Pharmacology, University of Milano, Italy.

The time course of exocytosis of quanta of acetylcholine induced by 20 mM K^+ was studied at the frog neuromuscular junction. Images of vesicle fusion on freeze-fracture replicas were mostly localized at the active zones in resting preparations fixed in 20 mM K^+. Fusions appreared also outside the active zones in preparations fixed after 1 min exposure to 20 mM K^+ and were evenly distributed over the presynaptic membrane after 5 min in 20 mM K^+ (even though secretion was prevented by withdrawing Ca^{2+} until 30 s before fixation). The mean densities of vesicle fusions were comparable in all conditions, as were the total number of quanta released during the fixation period. This indicates that fusions outside active zones represent ectopic exocytosis, slowly activated by potassium. Partial inactivation of K^+-induced quantal release (time and concentration-dependent) was observed electrophysiologically; this may be related to the observed decrease in density of vesicle fusions along the active zones, with time. Consistently, after 5 min in 15 mM K^+ fusion density at the active zones remained high. It is concluded that active zone-associated and ectopic fusions are two exocytotic processes activated with differential time courses and concentration-dependence by K^+.

INTRODUCTION.

With the lead of Bruno Ceccarelli our group has worked in the last few years on a series of projects aimed at clarifying the cellular processes involved in quantal turnover of ACh at the neuromuscular junction. In particular, using as a working hypothesis the concept that release of quanta is sustained by the exocytotic fusion of synaptic vesicles with the presynaptic axolemma (vesicle hypothesis), the mechanisms of exocytosis and endocytotic retrieval of vesicle membrane have been investigated. The freeze-fracture technique, which provides the unique opportunity of visualizing large portions of cell membrane surface, has been employed by our group to study the interactions between vesicle membrane and axolemma that accompany active quantal secretion. The main result was that under most experimental conditions vesicles fused with the axolemma along the so called active zones (Plate 1A), as previously reported (Heuser et al., 1974), whereas prolonged (15-60 min) exposure to elevated concentrations of K^+ led to a uniform distribution of vesicle openings all over the presynaptic membrane (Ceccarelli et al., 1979 a & b). This observation was of particular interest since elevated concentrations of potassium are widely used as a substitute for the physiological stimulus to induce secretion in a variety of excitable cells. Isolated frog nerve muscle preparations exposed to solutions containing high K^+ show increased frequencies of miniature end plate potentials (MEPPs), that were originally attributed to the depolarizing effect of the elevated concentration of the ion (Liley, 1956). However, though electrical depolarization can similarly activate spontaneous secretion, electrophysiological evidence has accumulated indicating an action of K^+ distinct from simple depolarization (Gage & Quastel, 1965; Parsons et al., 1965). In particular, it appears that the time course of the activation of quantal release induced by K^+ differs from that induced by equivalent electrical depolarizations of the nerve terminal, in that MEPP frequency rises faster due to an initial "specific effect" of potassium (Cooke & Quastel, 1973). As K^+ induces also a peculiar pattern of exocytosis, it seemed appropriate to study in detail K^+-induced exocytosis at earlier times (Fesce et al., 1982; Pecot-Dechavassine, 1982).

We investigated (i) the changes in the distribution of images of vesicle fusion on freeze fracture replicas of presynaptic membranes from junctions fixed in 20 mM K^+ after several different times of exposure to 20 mM K^+, and (ii) the relation between density of vesicle fusion and total quantal secretion from the same preparation, as measured by fluctuation analysis of intracellular recordings during fixation (Ceccarelli et al., 1988).

EXOCYTOSIS INDUCED BY POTASSIUM AT EARLY TIMES.

On freeze-fracture replicas of P-faces of the presynaptic membrane, the active zones appear as gentle ridges running perpendicular to the major axis of the nerve terminal and, at higher magnification, display two parallel double rows of large particles. No images of vesicle fusions are evident on the presynaptic membrane of resting terminals fixed with a control fixative containing 20 mM Na^+. Instead, with 20 mM K^+-containing fixative, the presynaptic membranes are marked by a large number of vesicle fusions, that appear as dimples, confined to the region immediately adjacent to the active zones (Plate 1B). When extracellular K^+ is raised to 20 mM 1 min before fixation (in 20 mM K^+), more than 50% of dimples are locat- ed near the active zones (Plate 1C). After 5' in 20 mM K^+ fusions appear evenly distributed on the axolemma (Plate 1D), as was previously reported for later times (Ceccarelli et al., 1979 b), although no infoldings of the membrane could be seen at the shorter times investigated here.

The distributions of vesicle fusions in the three conditions are illustrated in Fig.1, where the points

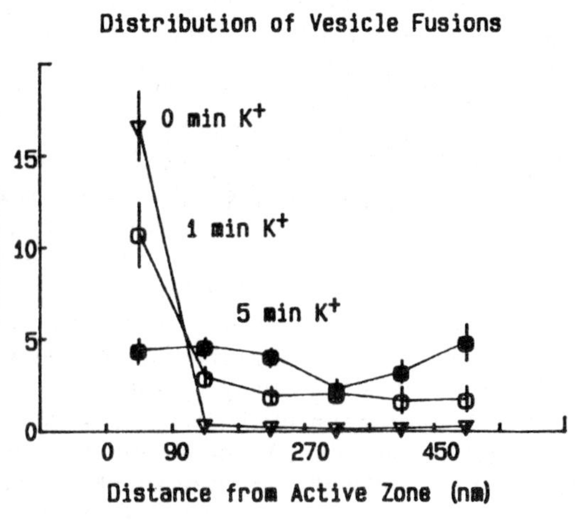

1

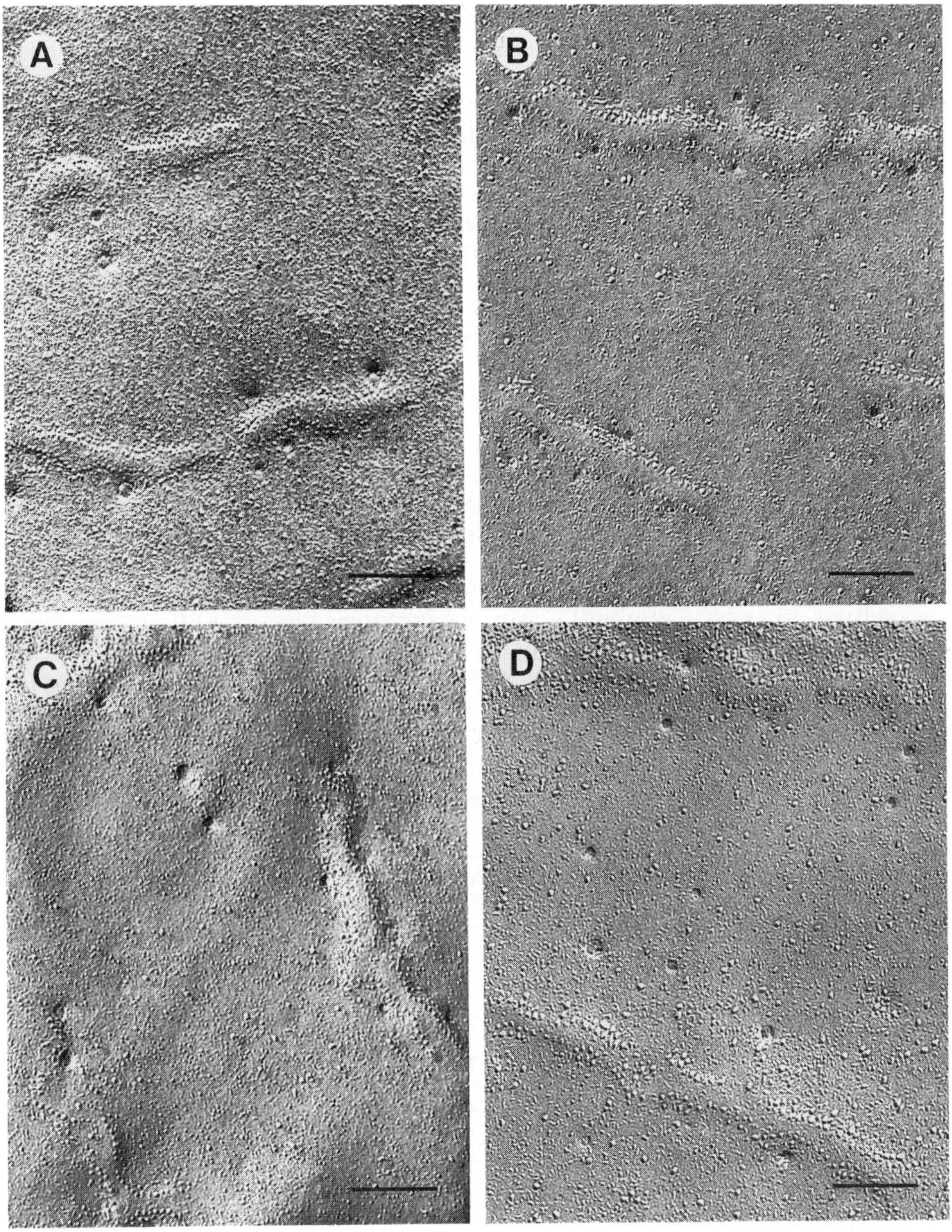

Plate 1. Cutaneous pectoris muscles from frogs were fixed with aldehydes, glicerinated and frozen in propane-isopenthane mixture before being freeze-fractured and shadowed. Freeze-fracture replicas of P-faces of presynaptic axolemma are illustrated.
A: Terminal electrically stimulated for 20 min at 10 Hz;
B, C, D: terminals fixed in 20 mM K^+-containing fixative after 0, 1 and 5 min exposure to 20 mM K^+ (Calibration bar = 0.2 μm).

represent the average density within successive regions extending from the border of an active zone to a point half-way to the next active zone. As can be seen in the figure, fusions outside the active zones are virtually absent at 0 min K^+, begin to appear at 1 min K^+ and reach by 5 min their maximum density.

CORRELATION BETWEEN THE DENSITY OF VESICLE FUSIONS AND THE NUMBER OF QUANTA SECRETED.

Fusions outside the active zones, ectopic fusions, might represent delayed endocytotic events which follow the collapse of vesicle membrane and the translocation of its components in the axolemma (Heuser & Reese, 1973; Miller & Heuser, 1984). This interpretation was already challenged by the extreme paucity of ectopic fusions observed under different conditions of intense recycling (Ceccarelli et al., 1979). The issue can be clarified, in principle, by studying the correlation between the number of quanta secreted during fixation and the density of vesicle fusions on the presynaptic axolemma. This was not performed at that time because MEPP rate increased to such an extent that it was not possible to obtain a precise estimate. A specific fluctuation analysis procedure is now available for measuring high MEPP rates from endplate recordings (Segal et al, 1985; Fesce et al., 1986). We therefore attempted such a correlation.

We checked the reliability of the fluctuation analysis procedure under our experimental conditions, by simulating a typical time course of MEPP rate during fixation. The measured rates (Fig. 2, O) and cumulative quantal secretion (*) are in good agreement with the actual MEPP rates and cumulative MEPP number in the artificial record (continuous and dashed lines), although the rate rapidly changes from zero to a peak >5000/s within about 2 s (1 s time constant) and falls back to zero within 30 s (5 s time constant).

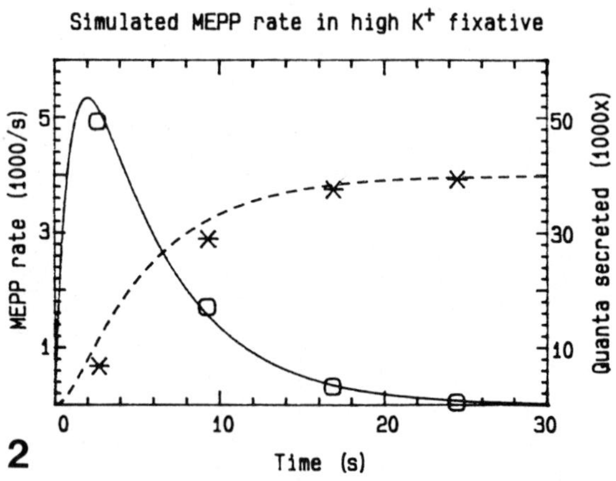

2

Following the application of a fixative containing 20 mM Na^+, MEPP rate barely increased. On the contrary when a fixative containing K^+ was applied to resting preparations (0 min K^+) MEPP rate rapidly increased to such high levels that fluctuation analysis was necessary to measure it. Single MEPPs could be clearly recognized 1 to 2 min after addition of fixative, indicating that the secretory machinery is impaired and blocked by the fixative, before the sensitivity of the acetylcholine receptor is abolished.

The power spectra of endplate noise retain, even during fixation, the shape corresponding to the typical time course of the

MEPP (the difference between two exponentials), thus permitting the application of fluctuation analysis.

When fixative containing 20 mM K^+ was applied to a resting preparation MEPP rate rose to a peak within about 30 s and declined to zero whithin about 1.5 min. Marked increases in MEPP rate were observed upon fixation also in preparations exposed to 20 mM K^+ for either 1 or 5 min. The membrane potential rapidly decreased after the fixative was added reaching its minimum at the peak of MEPP rate. MEPP height usually increased with time notwithstanding the marked depolarization, which suggests an early inhibitory effect of the fixative on cholinesterase activity.

A one to one correlation between vesicle fusions and quantal secretion cannot be obtained directly because images of chemically fixed preparations show an integration of the events occurring during the fixation process (Heuser et al., 1974; Ceccarelli et al., 1979 b; Smith & Reese, 1980), and the limits of the integration period (the time during which vesicle openings are captured) are not known. Still, it is possible to perform significant comparisons between the numbers of quanta and fusions, if we assume that fixation of the nerve terminal begins when MEPP rate starts to decline and it is complete by the time MEPPs disappear from electrophysiological recordings. The numbers measured this way are reported in Fig.3 (*), together with the corresponding densities of vesicle fusions (●), for the three different times; the relative contribution of fusions near the active zones is also shown (O). The average numbers of fusions/μm^2 of nerve terminal axolemma are not significantly different in the three conditions; in fact the decrease with time in the density of fusions near the active zones is paralleled by the increase outside the zones.

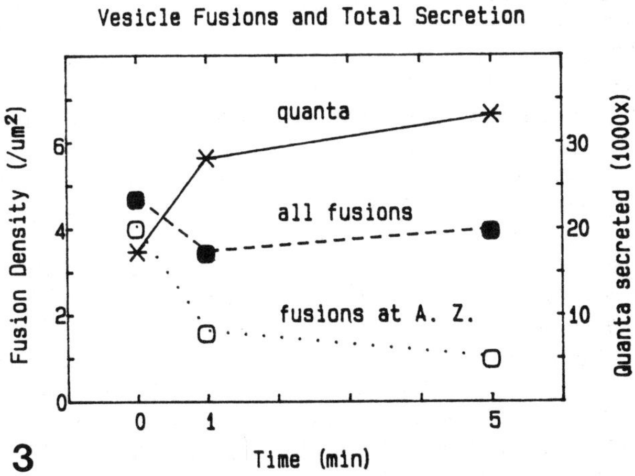

3

If the occurrence of ectopic vesicle openings were due to the delayed onset of endocytosis, then the density of fusions along the active zones should remain comparable at the different times, as it is the case for the number of quanta secreted during fixation. The observation that the <u>total</u> density of fusions remains relatively constant, while active zone-associated events decrese, indicates instead that both active zone-associated and ectopic fusions represent exocytotic events (Ceccarelli et al., 1988). This result is consistent with the idea that exo- and endocytosis are immediately subsequent steps of a single process (Ceccarelli et al., 1973), at least under non-exhaustive stimulation, the vesicles being immediately interiorized after a transient opening to the synaptic cleft (Ceccarelli & Hurlbut, 1980; Torri-Tarelli et al., 1987). This hypothesis is corroborated by the findings that (i) no signs of vesicle-membrane collapse into the axolemma are evident in preparations quick frozen up to 10 ms after single electrical shock to the nerve, in 4-aminopyridine (Torri- Tarelli et al., 1985), and (ii) the vesicle-associated protein, synaptophysin, becomes incorporated on the axolemma after intense secretion in the presence of block of endocytosis, but not when vesicle recycling is active (Valtorta et al. 1988, see also this volume).

THE MECHANISM RESPONSIBLE FOR THE REDISTRIBUTION OF EXOCYTOSIS.

The time dependent redistribution of vesicle fusions might be due to the prolonged exposure to K^+ as well as to the previous secretory activity.

No redistribution was observed when secretion was similarly activated by other means of stimulation (Ceccarelli et al, 1979). We studied exocytosis in preparations exposed for 5 min to hypertonic Ringer's (150 mM added sucrose), which induces asynchronous quantal secretion (Furshpan, 1956) comparable to that elicited by 20 mM K^+, and found that vesicle fusions predominate (55%) along the active zones.

This suggests that prolonged exposure to potassium, rather than previous activity, is responsible for the relocation of exocytosis. We therefore investigated the possible effect of predepolarization without secretion. The K^+ concentration was raised, for 5 min, in the absence of Ca^{2+}; as expected, MEPP rate did not increase. The fixative was added 30 s after readmitting Ca^{2+}, when MEPP rate had reached its peak value. In replicas of presynaptic membranes from these preparations many vesicle fusions were observed, uniformly distributed over the membrane, which supports the view that relocation of exocytosis is dependent on the duration of exposure to K^+ but not on the number of quanta previously secreted.

It is possible that the specific effect of K^+ described elecrophysiologically (see above, Cooke and Quastel, 1973) is responsible for relocation of exocytosis. Alternatively, time-dependent changes in cytosolic distributions of Ca^{2+} may be responsible. It has been suggested that calcium dependent exocytosis is generally localized at the active zones because calcium channels are selectively localized at the active zones (Pumplin et al., 1981). Prolonged depolarization would then induce an initially localized Ca^{2+} influx, followed by a slow rise in cytosolic Ca^{2+} concentration. This interpretation for the delayed ectopic fusions, however, is highly unlikely, since ectopic openings occur even after a very brief exposure to Ca^{2+} (see above) and, on the contrary, fusions still predominate near the active zones in hypertonic solutions, a condition where quantal secretion is thought to be activated by cytosolic Ca^{2+} increase following intracellular redistribution (Kita & Van der Kloot, 1977; Shimoni et al., 1977). It is still possible that different populations of Ca^{2+} channels are present in different regions of the presynaptic axolemma, and that they are activated with different time courses.

A DUAL EXOCYTOTIC MECHANISM.

One interesting point is that, as density of ectopic vesicle fusions rises, the density along the active zones declines. Depletion of vesicles would not account for this phenomenon, which is independent of the amount of previous secretion and is not observed with means of stimulation other than 20 mM K^+. This suggests that either some factor involved in exocytosis migrates during the effect of potassium, or two distinct processes are activated with differential time courses, the faster one becoming inactivated as the slower one ensues. If this were the case, then electrophysiological measurement of quantal secretion might also evidentiate some kind of inactivation. In order to investigate this possibility we studied the kinetics of quantal secretion induced by various K^+ concentrations at single neuromuscular junctions. In particular, peak and steady-state rates of secretion were measured. A steady-state rate is achieved when the rate of quantal secretion equals the rate of recycling. Therefore, a higher steady state rate is expected if either secretion or recycling or both are activated more intensely, and a stronger stimulus must produce a higher MEPP rate. If not so, inactivation of some step of the synaptic transmission machinery must be assumed.

In particular, if a nerve terminal is endowed with a population of releasable quanta, Q, equal to the sum of free vesicles and vesicles with their membrane fused with the axolemma, then the steady-state MEPP rate sustained by this terminal is Q/T, where T is the "recycling time", i.e. the average time necessary to fuse with and be recovered from the axolemma. If either secretion or recycling are more activated, then T must decrease and the steady-state rate must increase. Conversely, lower steady state rates indicate lower activation of secretion (or recycling).

In this series of experiments, at least two concentrations (between 15-25 mM K^+) were tested at each junction, with a period of rest of about 30 min in Ringer solution between successive treatments. MEPP rates were measured only when it was possible to apply a final treatment equal to the first one which produced a superimposable time course, indicating that neither irreversible depletion nor relevant fatigue in synaptic transmission had occurred (viz Q, as above defined, had remained constant). The MEPP rate time course in one of these experiments is illustrated in Fig.4. The maximum MEPP rate attained was always higher in the higher concentration of K^+, as expected. Conversely much higher steady-state rates (even more than twofold) were often obtained at the lower K^+ concentrations. This indicates that either secretion or

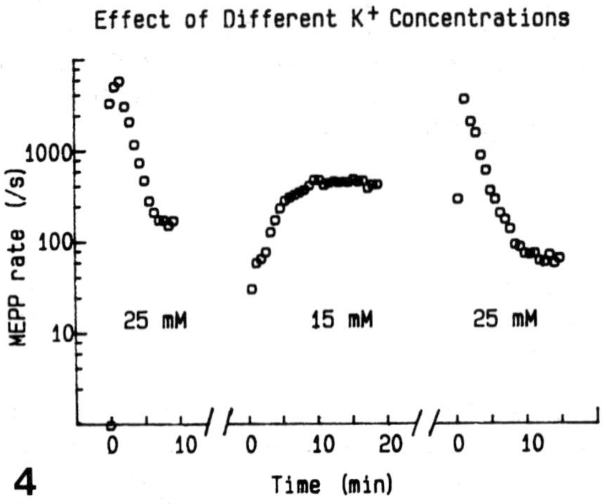

4

Modified from Ceccarelli et al. 1988

recycling or both are impared by the prolonged exposure to high K^+ to such an extent that the relation between steady-state MEPP rate and K^+ concentration becomes inverted in the range between 15 and 25 mM.

These kinetic data indicate that some concentration dependent inactivation occurs in K^+-treated terminals. It seemed therefore interesting to examine whether the decline in fusion density along the active zones were also concentration dependent. This appears to be the case, as in preparations exposed for 15' to 15 mM K^+, we observed fusions predominantly concentrated along the active zones.

Alhough a direct connection cannot be demonstrated, it is tempting to see a relation between the time and concentration dependent decline in vesicle fusions along the active zones and the time and concentration-dependent partial inactivation of quantal release induced by potassium.

CONCLUSION.

Our data suggest that two populations of fusion sites can be identified, which are activated by high K^+ with differential time courses. In particular, fusion sites at the active zones, traditionally implied in the physiological exocytosis, appear to undergo partial inactivation with time. It is tempting to hypothesize that the two populations of exocytosis sites might reflect different types of calcium channels or, alternatively, that activation of ectopic fusions may depend on some slow intracellular process, like biochemical pathways involving second messengers.

The complex mechanism of activation of secretion by elevated concentrations of extracellular K^+ can be relevant in the physiology of the synapse. It is well known that K^+ accumulates in the intercellular space as a result of neuronal activity. The changes in extracellular K^+ concentration depend on neuronal activity (Sykova, 1981); accumulation of K^+ up to possibly 20 mM has been reported in CNS synapses following tetanic stimulation. Evidence is available (Sykova, 1981) that an increase of K^+ up to 6 mM induces an increase in spontaneous as well as evoked activity, whilst larger increase in K^+ concentration inhibits transmission in the spinal cord because of unknown alterations in synaptic function.

REFERENCES.

Ceccarelli, B., Fesce, R., Grohovaz, F. & Haimann, C. (1988). The effect of potassium on exocytosis of transmitter at the frog neuromuscular junction. J. Physiol. **401**: 163-183.

Ceccarelli, B., Grohovaz, F. & Hurlbut W.P. (1979, a). Freeze-fracture studies of frog neuromuscular junctions during intense release of neurotransmitter. I. Effects of black widow spider venom and Ca^{2+}-free solutions on the structure of the active zone. J. Cell Biol. **81**: 163-177.

Ceccarelli, B., Grohovaz, F. & Hurlbut, W.P. (1979, b). Freeze-fracture studies of frog neuromuscular junctions during intense release of neurotransmitter. II. Effects of electrical stimulation and high potassium. J. Cell Biol. **81**: 178-192.

Ceccarelli, B., Hurlbut, W.P. & Mauro, A. (1973). Turnover of transmitter and synaptic vesicles at the frog neuromuscular junction. J. Cell Biol. **57**: 499-524.

Ceccarelli, B. & Hurlbut, W.P. (1980). The vesicle hypothesis of the release of quanta of acetylcholine. Physiol. Rev. **60**: 396-441.

Cooke, J.D. & Quastel, D.M.J. (1973). The specific effect of potassium on transmitter release by motor nerve terminals and its inhibition by calcium. J. Physiol. **228**: 435-458.

Fesce, R., Grohovaz., F., Haimann, C. & Ceccarelli, B. (1982). Different patterns of vesicle fusion during quantal release of acetylcholine at the frog neuromuscular junction. Caryol. **35**: 122.

Fesce, R., Segal, J.R. & Hurlbut, W.P. (1986). Fluctuation analysis of nonideal shot noise. Application to the neuromuscular junction. J. Gen. Physiol. **88**: 25-58.

Furshpan, E.J. (1956). The effects of osmotic pressure changes on the spontaneous activity at motor nerve endings. J. Physiol. **134**: 689-697.

Gage, P.W. & Quastel, D.M.J. (1965). Dual effect of potassium on transmitter release. Nature **206**: 625-626.

Heuser, J.E. & Reese, T.S. (1973). Evidence for recycling of synaptic vesicle membrane during transmitter release at the frog neuromuscular junction. J. Cell Biol. **57**: 315-344.

Heuser, J.E., Reese, T.S. & Landis, D.M.D. (1974). Functional changes in frog neuromuscular junctions studied with freeze-fracture. J. Neurocytol. **3**: 109-131.

Kita, H. & Van der Kloot, W. (1977). Time course and magnitude of effects of changes in tonicity on acetylcholine release at frog neuromuscular junction. J. Neurophysiol. **40**: 212-224.

Liley, A.W. (1956). The effects of presynaptic polarization on the spontaneous activity at the mammalian neuromuscular junction. J. Neurophysiol. **16**: 509-527.

Miller, T.M. & Heuser, J.E. (1984). Endocytosis of synaptic vesicle membrane at the frog neuromuscular junctions. J. Cell Biol. **98**: 685-698.

Parsons, R.L., Hoffmann, W.W. & Feigen, G.A. (1965). Presynaptic effects of potassium ion on the mammalian neuromuscular junction. Nature **208**: 590-591.

Pecot-Dechavassine, M. (1982). Synaptic vesicle openings captured by cooling and related to transmitter release at the frog neuromuscular junction. Biol. of The Cell **46**: 43-50.

Pumplin, D.W., Reese, T.S. & Llinas, R. (1981). Are the presynaptic membrane particles the calcium channels? Proc. Nat. Acad. Sci. USA **78**: 7210-7213.

Segal, J.R., Ceccarelli, B., Fesce, R. & Hurlbut, W.P. (1985). Miniature endplate potential frequency and amplitude determined by an extension of campbell's theorem. Biophys. J. **47**: 183-202.

Shimoni, Y., Alnaes, E. & Rahamimoff R. (1977). Is hyperosmotic neurosecretion from motor nerve endings a calcium dependent process? Nature **267**: 170-172.

Smith, J.E & Reese, T.S. (1980). Use of aldehyde fixatives to determine the rate of synaptic transmitter release. J. Exp. Biol. **89**: 19-29.

Syková, E. (1981). K^+ changes in the extracellular space of the spinal chord and their physiological role. J. Exp. Biol. **95**: 93-110.

Torri Tarelli, F., Grohovaz, F., Fesce, R. & Ceccarelli, B. (1985). Temporal coincidence between synaptic vesicle fusion and quantal secretion of acetylcholine. J. Cell Biol. **101**: 1386-1399.

Torri Tarelli, F., Haimann, C. & Ceccarelli, B. (1987). Coated vesicles and pits during enhanced quantal release of acetylcholine at the neuromuscular junction. J. Neurocytol. **16**: 205-214.

Torri Tarelli, F., Villa, A., Valtorta, F., De Camilli, P., Greengard, P. & Ceccarelli, B. (1989). Redistribution of synaptophysin and synapsin I during alpha-latrotoxin induced release of neurotransmitter at the neuromuscular junction. J. Cell Biol. **in press**.

Valtorta, F., Jahn, R., Fesce, R., Greengard, P. & Ceccarelli, B. (1988). Synaptophysin (p-38) at the frog neuromuscular junction: its incorporation into the axolemma and recycling after intense quantal secretion. J. Cell Biol. **107**: 2717-2727.

CHARACTERIZATION OF A POLYCLONAL ANTISERUM RAISED AGAINST MEDIATOPHORE, A PROTEIN THAT TRANSLOCATES ACETYLCHOLINE.

ISRAEL, M, LESBATS, B. and *SUZUKI, A.
Laboratoire de Neurobiologie Cellulaire et Moléculaire, CNRS, 91198 Gif sur Yvette Cedex (France)
*Laboratoire du Métabolisme de la Nutrition des Plantes, CNRA, 78026 Versailles Cedex (France)

ABSTRACT.

A protein (the mediatophore) purified from Torpedo electric organ nerve terminals was identified by its ability to translocate acetylcholine upon calcium action. The recent large scale production of this protein led us to prepare a polyclonal antibody that was used to study the localization of the protein.

INTRODUCTION.

The release of acetylcholine (ACh) from synaptosomal suspensions may be triggered by a variety of depolarizing agents that lead to an increase of calcium within the nerve terminal. In order to induce release in a more direct way it is necessary to bypass the natural calcium channel. Neurotoxins or calcium ionophores have proved to be good tools for activation of the release mechanism itself. Until recently, the most convenient way to measure the efflux of the transmitter was to label, with radioactive precursors, the ACh pools and to separate from the perfusion fluid the released radioactive transmitter. The choline oxidase procedure for measuring ACh has the advantage of being applicable to suspensions of synaptosomes, allowing monitoring in real time of the efflux of the transmitter. The principle of the procedure is simple. Synaptosomes are kept in a physiological solution, a reaction mixture containing choline oxidase is then added, this oxidizes all external choline. Stimulation of synaptosomes induces the release of the transmitter which will be hydrolyzed by acetylcholinesterase, the resulting choline is oxidized to betaine and hydrogen peroxide. Several reactions may be used to measure the hydrogen peroxide. We have obtained good results with the luminol-peroxidase system that gives a blue chemiluminescence which can be continuously recorded. In a series of preliminary experiments we have studied several aspects of the release process from synaptosomal suspensions. We have also analysed their metabolism, ACh compartmentation, and the action of drugs (Israël and Lesbats 1981a,b; 1982,1985,1986). Our main concern was, however, to identify the final steps of the release mechanism, the step that allows the transmitter to cross the presynaptic membrane. From the very first formulation of the quantal theory (Fatt and Katz 1952; Katz 1959) until more recent work on exocytosis, a mysterious "little dot" was placed between the synaptic vesicle and the nerve terminal membrane. This point of impact forms a transient channel through which release takes place and may be the first step of a fusion process (Brenckenridge and Almers 1987). This view is not necessarily true, and a direct release of transmitter from the cytoplasmic pool might take place if a membrane channel establishes a communication between the cytoplasm and the cleft. Whatever will be the final answer, the pool of transmitter might be released through a classical exocytotic process (Heuser et al. 1979) or a more transient exocytotic event (Ceccarelli and Hurlbut 1980; Torri-Tarelli et al. 1985; Zimmermann 1979) or through a structure having mixed vesicular and gate properties, the vesigate (Tauc 1982). The necessary presence of a presynaptic membrane element that would either be a docking protein for vesicles or an independent channel appears as a logical necessity. A concensus on that point may thus certainly be reached (see also reviews by Dunant 1986, Dunant and Israël 1985). We isolated from the nerve terminal membrane a protein called mediatophore (Birman et al. 1986; Israël et al. 1986) that endows artificial membranes with a calcium dependent release mechanism and we know that integral membrane proteins are involved in the final step of the transmitter translocation. This has been found in many laboratories (Venzin et al. 1977; Takano and Kamiya 1979, Israël et al. 1980, 1987; Muller et al. 1987; Egea et al. 1987). If the mediatophore protein is shown to be a constituent of such particles that become more numerous when the transmitter is tanslocated, then the final step of the release mechanism would no longer be a mysterious dot but become an identified protein with an essential physiological function.

RESULTS

Synaptosomal acetylcholine release: its reconstitution in artificial membranes.

The synaptosomes isolated from Torpedo electric organ have been prepared in sucrose-saline solutions in order to preserve their physiological and metabolic properties (Israël et al. 1976; Morel et al. 1977). Figure 1A shows a synaptosomal fraction and a typical ACh release experiment (1B). Transmitter efflux was monitored with the choline oxidase procedure, release was induced by generating a calcium influx with the ionophore A23187 in the presence of calcium. Release may also be triggered by KCl depolarization or by a variety of agents producing a calcium entry. Figure 1C shows a fraction of membranes derived from nerve terminal plasma membranes. These membranes have been used as the starting material to prepare proteoliposomes. Reconstitution was performed by mixing them to lipids in the presence of organic solvents or detergents (Israël et al. 1984, 1988).

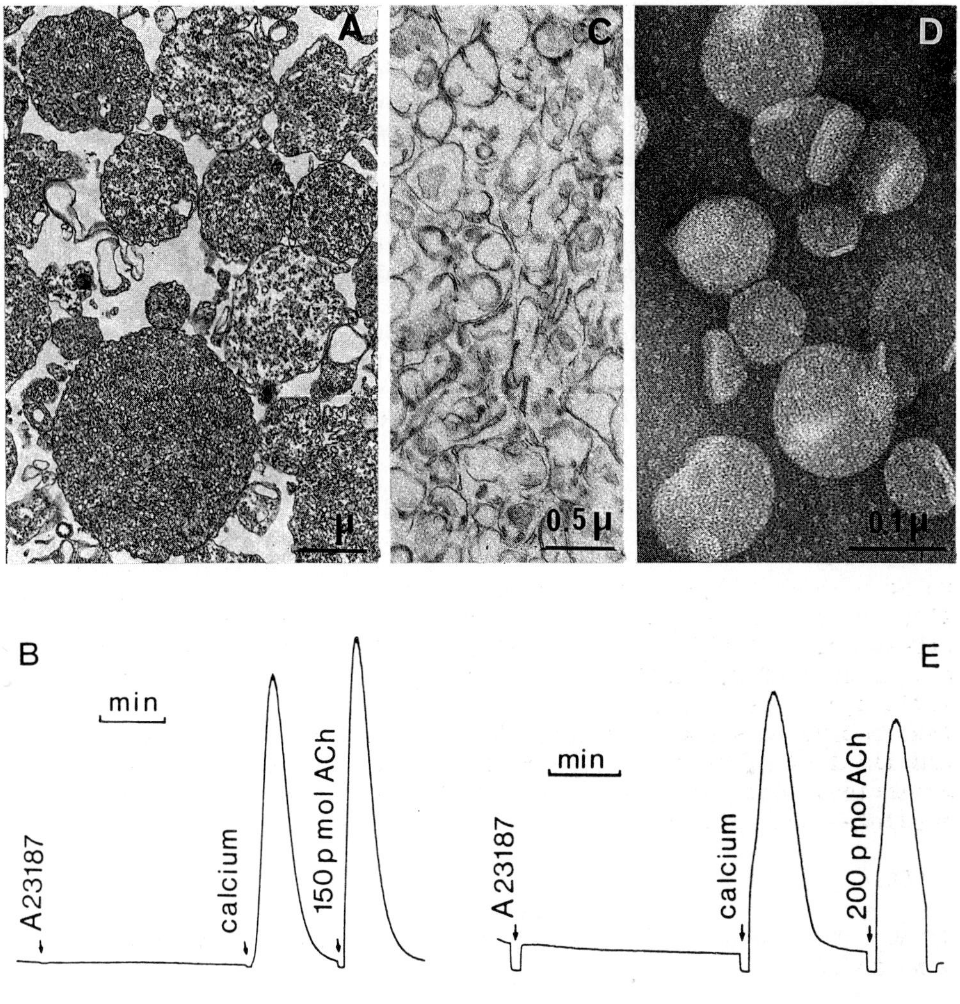

Figure 1. Reconstitution of the synaptosomal release mechanism in liposomal membranes

A - Synaptosomal fraction prepared from Torpedo electric organ.

B - Acetylcholine release by synaptosomes in response to a calcium influx. Release was monitored with the choline oxidase-chemiluminescent procedure, and calibrated with a 150 pmol standard.

C - Presynaptic plasma membranes which serve for starting material for reconstitution experiments.

D - Proteoliposomes formed from the presynaptic membrane material.

E - Calcium induced acetylcholine release from proteoliposomes filled with acetylcholine. They have inherited, from the synaptosomal membrane, a calcium dependent release mechanism.

Figure 1D shows the fraction of proteoliposomes. When these were filled with ACh in controlled ionic conditions they were able to release Ach in response to a calcium influx (Fig. 1E). These proteoliposomes are the minimal organized structure in which one may recover the calcium dependent ACh release event.
When the totality of the synaptosomal membrane is incorporated into the liposomal membrane, ACh release may be triggered by Glycera neurotonin or by the calcium ionophore. After several purification steps of synaptosomal membrane constituents, the meurotoxins receptor is no longer associated with the nerve terminal membrane protein that translocates ACh. We showed that a single protein, associated to some endogenous lipids, was sufficient to endowe artificial membranes with a calcium dependent ACh release mechanism. This protein was purified and named the mediatophore. Figure 2A shows an electron micrograph of a negatively stained preparation of mediatophore. The molecule (7 to 8 nm) seems pentameric with a

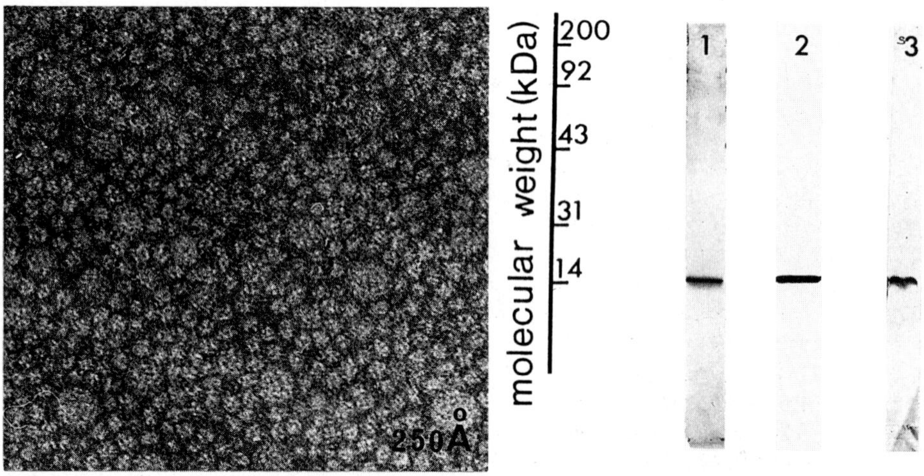

Figure 2. The mediatophore protein. Electron micrograph of a negatively stained preparation of mediatophore, the protein that endowes artificial membranes with a calcium dependent release mechanism.

Acrylamide gels of mediatophore and synaptosomal membranes.

Lane 1, SDS-PAGE of the mediatophore. A single 15 Kda subunit is found - Coomassie blue staining.

Lane 2, Western blot. Staining of the 15 Kda subunit with the rabbit antiserum and peroxydase labelled antirabbit immunoglobulin.

Lane 3, Western blot of total synaptosomal membranes proteins. The serum stained specifically the 15 Kda subunit at a dilution 1/4000.

central hole, its apparent molecular weight is of about 200 Kda. When submitted to acrylamide gel electrophoresis after solubilization in sodium dodecyl sulfate, a single subunit at 15 Kda was found to be the major mediatophore constituent, Fig. 2B. It is not our intention to explain the whole release process with a single protein activated by calcium, as would be the case with an ordinary channel. In contrast we are probably dealing with the final step of a more complex process. The over-simplified view that may emerge comes from the fact that only a single event is considered here i.e. the translocation of the transmitter through the presynaptic membrane.

Preparation of a antimediatophore antibody

The preparation of mediatophore was recently scaled up (Israël et al. 1988). A polyclonal antiserum was raised by injecting a rabbit with about 1.5 mg protein. The two first injections were made with the 15 Kda band cut from the acrylamide gel and powdered in liquid nitrogen. The third injection was made directly with the native protein which was injected half intravenously and half sub-cutaneously. The serum obtained had antibodies that bound to the 15 Kda band of the purified mediatophore, Fig. 2C. When the western blot was done with total synaptosomal membranes the 15 Kda mediatophore subunit was specifically recognized among the other synaptosomal proteins at a serum dilution of $1/_{4000}$. For more concentrated serum, some higher molecular weight bands (200 and 100 Kda) were faintly stained. The mediatophore activity was immunoprecipitated from a mediatophore solution in the detergent Chaps (10 mM). The antimediatophore antiserum was added to the mediatophore solution together with goat antirabbit antiserum. The complex was sedimented with protein A linked to sepharose beads. When gold labelled goat antiserum is used, sedimentation of the immunocomplex is visualized by the mauve color covering the beads.

The Figure 3 compares the mediatophore activity of a sample treated with non immune or immune rabbit sera, in both cases goat antirabbit and sepharose protein A beads were added. The activity remained in the supernatant in the "non immune" treated sample but markedly decreased in the "immune" treated sample. The activity was measured as described earlier by incorporating the protein into ACh containing liposomes, release was induced by the influx of calcium (Israël et al. 1984). The detergent Chaps was removed from the sample by gel filtration. A western-blot analysis showed that the 15 Kda band decreased in the sample treated with the immune serum. When the sepharose beads were treated with sodium dodecyl sulfate, the immune complex was dissociated and a 15 Kda band recovered from the pellet showing that it had been removed from the supernatant together with the mediatophore activity (Fig. 3).

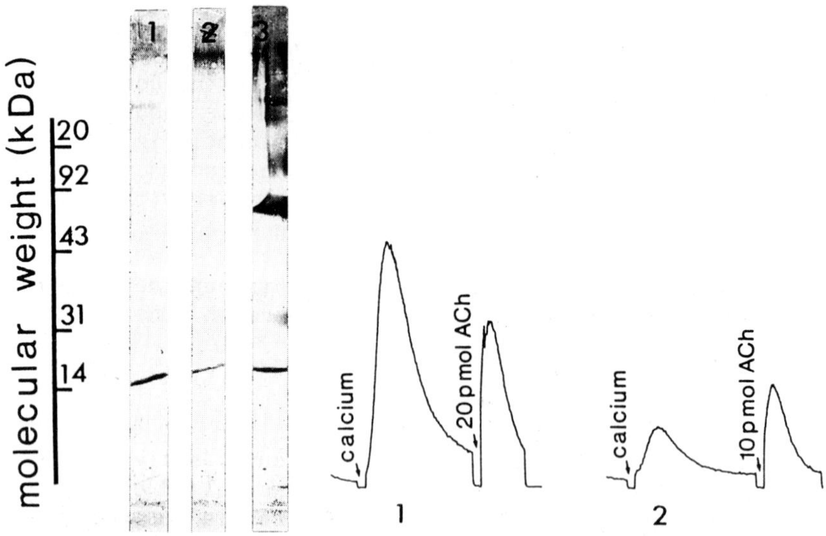

Figure 3. Immuno-precipitation of mediatophore activity
The mediatophore was disolved in a detergent (10 mM Chaps) and the sample split into two halves. One batch received rabbit non immune serum, the other the anti-mediatophore rabbit serum. In both cases goat antirabbit and sepharose protein A beads were added. Lane 1 shows that the mediatophore is not sedimented in the case of non immunoserum while in lane 2 a marked decrease of the 15 Kda band is observed with the immune serum. The precipitated 15 Kda band is detached from the beads with sodium dodecylsylfate and recovered in lane 3 together with the rabbit immunoglobulins. The samples before (1) and (2) after immunoprecipitation were tested for their mediatophore activity, a clear decrease of ACh release is observed in the immuno precipitated sample. Release from proteoliposomes was tested as for Figure 1.

Localization of the mediatophore

We were tempted to use the polyclonal antiserum to localize the mediatophore in tissues (see Morel et al. 1988, 1989). Torpedo muscles were fixed in formalin-buffer, bundles of muscle fibers were dissociated and incubated with the first antibody. They were washed and incubated with an antirabbit second antibody labelled with fluorescein. The fibers were observed with a fluorescence microscope. The motor end-plates were found to fluoresce, the reaction being localized at the level of nerve terminals but also on the terminal parts of axons.

When electroplaques were treated in a similar way, the fluorescence was found in the nerve endings as bright spots and also in the fine nerve branches (Fig. 4). These results suggest that the mediatophore is indeed localized in nerve endings but the localization was not exclusively in the terminal region of the nerve. It is difficult to know if the localization observed reflects the fact that the protein is synthesized in the cell body and migrates to the nerve terminal or if the antibody stains in the nerve, proteins that are not mediatophore. This is always a danger with a polyclonal antiserum.

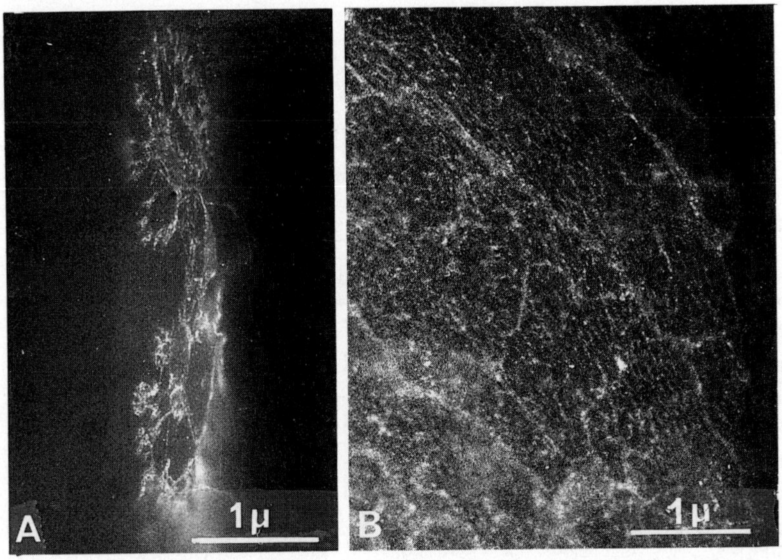

Figure 4. Immunochemical staining of structures with the antimediatophore antiserum

A - Torpedo motor end-plate.

B - Torpedo electroplaque.

The tissues were incubated with the antiserum at a dilution 1/1000 after washing, a second antirabbit antibody fluorescein labelled was added and washed. Observation was carried in an ultra-violet light microscope.

In order to demonstrate at least, the presence of the antigen in the nerve terminal membrane, we treated synaptosomes with the antimediatophore antiserum. A light fixation (01% permanganate) stabilized the synaptosomes. A goat anti-rabbit antibody labelled with 5 nm gold particles was then added. The unreacted antibody was separated from the synaptosomes by sedimenting the latter through a 0.5 M sucrose layer. The unreacted antibody remains in the supernatant.

Figure 5 shows at a low magnification, that the synaptosomes were preserved by the fixation used, which was compatible with the immunogold method. At a higher magnification, we show a control synaptosome treated with non-immune serum and a synaptosome treated with the antimediatophore serum. In this case the structure is decorated with numerous gold particles showing the nerve terminal

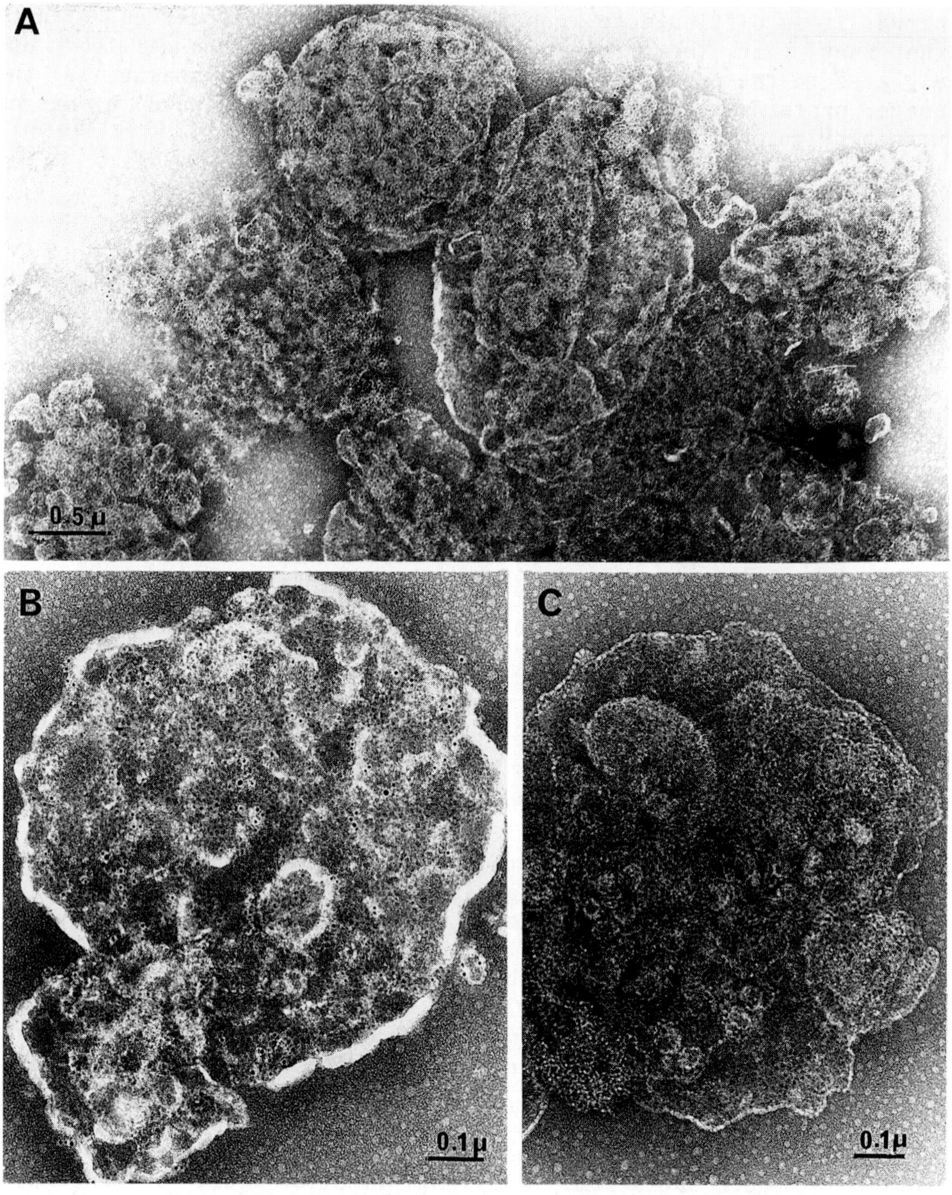

Figure 5. Electron microscopic localization of the antigen in synaptosomes permeabilized with 0.1 % saponin

A - Low magnification view of synaptosomes negatively stained (2% neutral phosphotungstic acid).

B - Synaptosome reacted with the antimediatophore antiserum. The whole surface of the synaptosomes is decorated with 5 nm gold particles.

C - Control synaptosomes treated with non immune rabbit antiserum.

localization of the antigen, probably the mediatophore. About 20% to 30% of the synaptosomes were decorated with gold particles showing that either we did not add enough antibody or that the pinched-off nerve terminals are not equally rich in mediatophore, the protein being more concentrated in some areas of the terminal network.

CONCLUSION

The localization of mediatophore in nerve terminals has been established in previous studies with a first generation of polyclonal antibodies that stained the 15 Kda subunit but also labelled some other bands (see Morel et al. 1989). The present antibody appeared to be more specific but far from the ideal tool studying localization. In parallel work (Morel et al., in preparation) monoclonal antibodies have been prepared in order to study the protein and we hope that some of them will be suitable for morphological localization studies at the electron microscopic level.

References

Birman, S., Israël, M., Lesbats, B. and Morel, N. (1986) Solubilisation and partial purification of a presynaptic membrane protein ensuring calcium-dependent acetylcholine releasae from proteoliposomes. J. Neurochem., 47, 433-444.

Breckenridge, L.J. and Almers, W. (1987) Currents through the fusion pore that forms during exocytoses of a secretory vesicle. Nature, 328, 814-817.

Ceccarelli, B. and Hurlbut, W.P. (1980) The vesicle hypothesis of the release of quanta of acetylcholine. Physiolog. Rev., 60, 396-441.

Dunant, Y. (1986) On a mechanism of acetylcholine release. Progress in Neurobiol., 26, 55-92.

Dunant, Y. and Israël, M. (1985) The release of acetylcholine. Scientific American, 252, 58-66.

Egea, G., Esquerda, JE., Calvet, R, Solsona, C. and Marsal, J. (1987) Structural changes at pure cholinergic synaptosomes during the transmitter release induced by A 23187 in Torpedo marmorata. A freeze-fracture study. Cell Tissue Res., 248, 207-214.

Fatt, P. and Katz, B. (1952) Spontaneous subthreshold activity at motor nerve endings. J. Physiol. (London), 117, 109-128.

Heuser, J.E., Reese, T.S., Dennis, M.J., Jan, Y., Jan, L. and Evans, L. (1979) Synaptic vesicle exocytosis captured by quick-freezing and correlated with quantal transmitter release. J. Cell Biol., 81, 275-300.

Israël, M., Manaranche, R, Mastour, P. and Morel, N. (1976) Isolation of pure cholinergic nerve endings from ther electric organ of Torpedo marmorata. Biochem. J., 160, 113-115.

Israël, M. and Lesbats, B. (1981a) Chemiluminescent determination of acetylcholine and continuous detection of its release from Torpedo electric organ synapses and synaptosomes. Neurochem. Int., 3, 81-90.

Israël, M. and Lesbats, B. (1981b) Continuous determination by a chemiluminescent method of acetylcholine release and compartmentation in Torpedo electric organ synaptosomes. J. Neurochem., 37, 1475-1483.

Israël, M. and Lesbats, B. (1982) Application to mammalian tissues of the chemiluminescent method of acetylcholine. J. Neurochem., 39, 248-250.

Israël, M, Lesbats, B., Morel, N., Manaranche, R., Gulik-Krzywicki, T., and Dedieu, J.C. (1984) Reconstitution of a functional synaptosomal membrane possessing the protein constituents involved in acetylcholine translocation. Proc. Natl. Acad. Sci. USA, 81, 277-281.

Israël, M. and Lesbats, B. (1985) Chemiluminescent determination of acetylcholine and continuous detection of its release from tissues. In Bioluminescence and Chemiluminescence. Instruments and Applications, Vol. 2, CRC Press, Boca Raton, Florida, pp. 1-12.

Israël, M. and Lesbats, B. (1986) The use of bioluminescence techniques in neurobiology, with emphasis on the cholinergic system. In Neurochemistry, A Practical Approach, IRL Press, Oxford, pp. 113-135.

Israël, M., Manaranche, R., Morel, N., Dedieu, J.C., Gulik-Krzywicki, T. and Lesbats, B. (1980) Redistribution of intramembrane particles related to acetylcholine release by cholinergic synaptosomes. J. Ultrasctruct. Res., 75, 162-178.

Israël, M., Morel, N., Lesbats, B., Birman, S. and Manaranche, R. (1986) Purification of a presynaptic membrane protein which mediates a calcium-dependent translocation of acetylcholine. Proc. Natl. Acad. Sci. USA, 83, 9226-9230.

Israël, M., Manaranche, R, Morot Gaudry-Talarmain, Y., Lesbats, B., Gulik-Krzywicki, T. and Dedieu, J.C. (1987) Effect of cetiedil on acetylcholine release and intramembrane particles in cholinergic synaptosomes. Biol. Cell, 61, 59-63.

Israël, M., Lesbats, B., Morel, N., Manaranche, R. and Birman, S. (1988) The lipid requirements of mediatophore for acetylcholine release activity. Large scale purification of this protein in a reactive form. Neurochem. Int., 13, 199-205.

Katz, B. (1969) The release of neuronal transmitter substanaces. The Sherrington Lectures, Liverpool University Press.

Morel, N., Israël, M., Manaranche, R. and Mastour, P. (1977) Isolation of pure cholinergic nerve endings from Torpedo electric organ. Evaluation of their metabolic properties. J. Cell Biol., 75, 43-55.

Morel, N., Manaranche, R. and Israël, M. (1988) Immunological detection of mediatophore in motor end-plates and electric organ subcellular fractions of Torpedo marmorata. Neurochem. Int., 13, 207-215.

Morel, N., Israël, M. Synguelakis, M. and Le Gal La Salle, G. (1989) Identification of two proteolipid antigens with different localization at Torpedo neuromuscular synapses. Neurochem. Int., 15,169-177.

Muller, D., Garcia-Segura, L.M., Parducz, A. and Dunant, Y. (1987) Brief occurence of a population of presynaptic intramembrane particles coincides with transmission of a nerve impulse. Proc. Natl. Acad. Sci. USA, 84, 590-594.

Tauc, L. (1982) Non vesicular release of neurotransmitter. Physiol. Rev., 62, 857-892.

Takano, Y. and Kamiya, H. (1979) Effect of ionic environment on densities of membrane-associated pârticles in presynaptic membranes observed in freeze-fractured synaptosomes. Experientia, 35, 1076-1078.

Torri-Tarelli, Grohovaz, F., Fesce, R. and Ceccarelli, B. (1985) Temporal coincidence between synaptic vesicles fusion and quantal secretion of acetylcholine. J. Cell Biol., 101, 1386-1399.

Venzin, M., Sandri, C., Akert, K. and Wyss, U.R. (1977) Membrane-associated particles of the presynaptic active zone in rat spinal cord. A morphometric analysis. Brain Res., 130, 393-404.

Zimmermann, H. (1979) Commentary: Vesicle recycling and transmitter release. Neuroscience 4, 1773-1803.

PRESYNAPTIC REGULATION OF ACETYLCHOLINE RELEASE IN THE CNS

Maurizio Raiteri, Mario Marchi, Guido Maura and Giambattista Bonanno
Istituto di Farmacologia e Farmacognosia, Università degli Studi di Genova, Viale Cembrano 4, 16148 Genova, Italy

The release of ACh appears to be under the control of autoreceptors localized on cholinergic nerve terminals. Moreover, the process can be regulated by transmitters other than ACh or by modulators either through receptor-mediated or carrier-mediated mechanisms. In this chapter we report on our recent results concerning the regulation of the release of ACh by ACh itself, 5-HT and GABA in the rat hippocampus. In particular it will be shown: 1) that the release of the cholinergic transmitter can be inhibited through muscarinic receptors of the M_3 subtype; 2) that 5-HT can interact with ACh by depressing ACh release through the activation of receptors of the 5-HT_{1B} subtype; 3) that the release of ACh can be enhanced by GABA by a novel mechanism involving a selective penetration of the amino acid into the cholinergic terminals.

Introduction

Acetylcholine release in the CNS can be studied by various in vivo and in vitro techniques. Although the in vivo techniques, such as the microdialysis and the "push-pull cannula" possess the advantage of being performed in the living animal, brain slices or synaptosomes are more commonly used since they provide more easily quantitative information on the release process as well as on the mechanisms by which release is modulated.

Brain slices and synaptosomes are complementary systems, both possessing advantages and pitfalls. The major advantage of slices is their integrity which allows, for example, to study release-regulating receptors which are sited on cell bodies or dendrites. On the other hand, synaptosomes allow to determine the exact location of those receptors (presynaptic receptors) which, being sited on the releasing terminals themselves, represent the last controllers of the release process.

As it is known, the exocytotic release of a given transmitter can be regulated by the transmitter itself, through the activation of the so called presynaptic autoreceptors located on the releasing terminal; the same terminal may also possess other receptors (presynaptic heteroreceptors) regulating the release of the same transmitter once activated by various modulating compounds (for reviews see Starke, 1981; Langer, 1981; Chesselet, 1984; Raiteri et al., 1984). It has been also shown that, in selective areas of the rat brain, the release of a neurotransmitter from nerve endings can be regulated through a mechanism which involves the membrane transport system (Bonanno and Raiteri 1987a,b).

In the present chapter we discuss some aspects concerning the presynaptic regulation of the release of ACh in the rat hippocampus. The release of ACh in this area can be modulated by ACh itself through an autoreceptor-mediated mechanism, by 5-HT through a heteroreceptor-mediated system and by GABA which causes release of ACh following penetration into cholinergic nerve terminals through a transport system selective for the aminoacid.

Cholinergic regulation of ACh release

The existence of an inhibitory feed-back regulation of the release of ACh has been proposed on the basis of experiments with brain slices (Molenaar and Polak, 1970; Szerb and Somogyi, 1973; Hadhàzy and Szerb, 1977) and synaptosomes (Nordström and Bartfai, 1980; Marchi et al., 1981). The results obtained with nerve endings isolated from rat hippocampus clearly indicate that this inhibitory mechanism occurs through the activation of muscarinic receptors located on cholinergic nerve terminals.

It is well known that, on the basis of their affinity for pirenzepine, muscarinic receptors were originally subdivided into M_1 (high-affinity for pirenzepine) and M_2 (low affinity

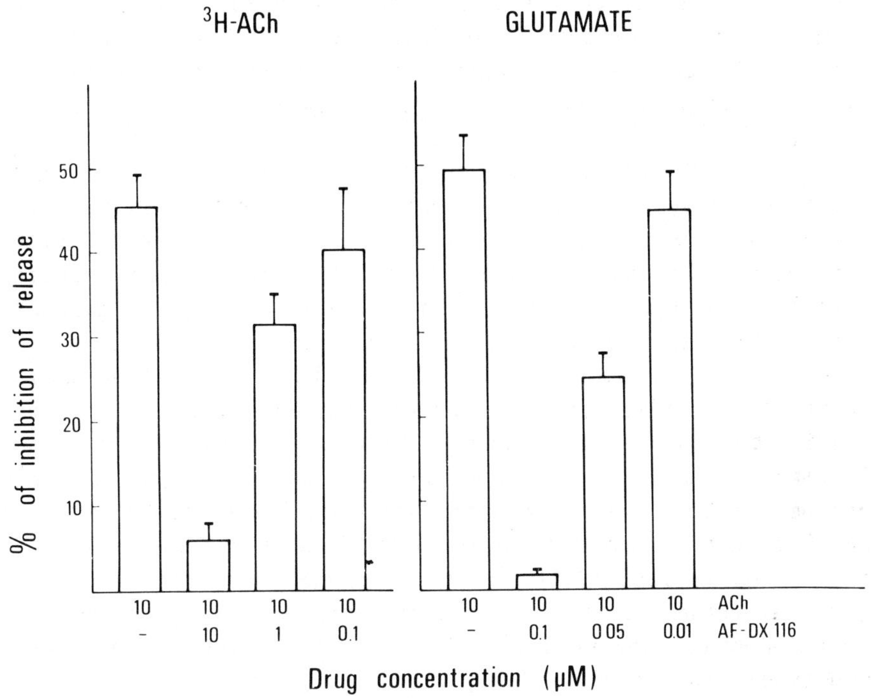

Fig. 1. Antagonism by AF-DX 116 of the effect of exogenous ACh (10 μM) on the release of ^{3}H-ACh and glutamate

for pirenzepine) (Hirschowitz et al., 1984). The lipophilic drug dicyclomine was subsequently found to be at least as useful as pirenzepine to discriminate between M_1 and M_2 receptor subtypes (Potter et al., 1984; Raiteri et al., 1984; Giachetti et al., 1986).

In previous reports it was found that the muscarinic autoreceptors regulating ACh release displayed relatively low sensitivity to pirenzepine or dicyclomine (Raiteri et al., 1984; Meyer and Otero, 1985). It has been therefore proposed that these receptors belong to the M_2 subtype. For the same reason we proposed that the muscarinic receptors recently found to regulate glutamate release in rat hippocampus could be classified as M_2 (Marchi and Raiteri, 1989). However, recent data have suggested that also the receptors having low affinity for pirenzepine are heterogeneous. In fact, the selective M_2 muscarinic antagonists (11-[[2-[diethylamino) methyl]-1-piperidinyl] acetyl] -5-11-dihydro-6H-pyrido-[2-3-b][1,4]benzodiazepine-6-one) (AF-DX 116) or methoctramine discriminate between "cardiac" and "glandular" receptors (Doods et al., 1987; Duckles et al., 1987; Hammer et al., 1987; Micheletti et al., 1987; Giraldo et al., 1987). On the basis of this heterogeneity of the pirenzepine-insensitive receptors, it was proposed to term M_2 the cardiac receptors (relatively high affinity for AF-DX 116) and M_3 the glandular receptors (Doods et al., 1987). The availability of the selective M_2 antagonist AF-DX 116, offered the opportunity to compare the muscarinic receptors located on ACh with those sited on GLU nerve endings. The results of figure 1 show clearly that the effectiveness of AF-DX 116 as an antagonist of ACh at the M_2 autoreceptors was much lower than that at the M_2 heteroreceptors regulating GLU release.

These data suggest that the presynaptic autoreceptors are more similar to the M_3 muscarinic receptors whereas the receptors located on GLU nerve endings resemble most the M_2 subtype (Marchi and Raiteri, 1989).

Serotonergic modulation of ^{3}H-ACh release from hippocampus

The possible interaction between serotonin and ACh has been investigated by studying the effects of 5-HT and of various serotonergic agents on the release of ^{3}H-ACh from rat hippocampal synaptosomes (depolarized with 15 mM KCl) and slices (stimulated electrically).

In both systems the Ca^{2+}-dependent release of ^{3}H-ACh was concentration-dependently inhibited by 5-HT; this effect was antagonized by methiothepin, but not by ketanserin. The $5\text{-}HT_2$ agonist (±)DOI did not mimic 5-HT. The release of ^{3}H-ACh was however reduced, both in synaptosomes and in slices, by the $5\text{-}HT_1$ agonist RU 24969, but not by the $5\text{-}HT_{1A}$ agonist 8-OH-DPAT. In synaptosomes the purported $5\text{-}HT_{1B}$ agonist CGS 12066B was effective as an inhibitor of ^{3}H-ACh release . (-)Propranolol, used as a $5\text{-}HT_{1A}/5\text{-}HT_{1B}$ blocker, antagonized 5-HT in synaptosomes, whereas mesulergine, spiperone, MDL 72222 and ICS 205930 did not counteract 5-HT. In slices the electrically-evoked release of ^{3}H-ACh was increased by methiothepin, but not by ketanserin; fenfluramine (a releaser of 5-HT) and 6-nitroquipazine (a 5-HT uptake blocker) inhibited ^{3}H-ACh release, their effect being reverted by methiothepin.

It can be concluded that hippocampal cholinergic terminals are endowed with a tonically activated inhibitory 5-HT heteroreceptor which appears to belong to the 5-HT_{1B} subtype (see Table I and Table II).

Table I. Pharmacological characterization of 5-HT presynaptic heteroreceptors regulating hippocampal ^{3}H-ACh

Drugs	used as		^{3}H-ACh release synaptosomes	^{3}H-ACh release slices
RU 24969	5-$HT_{1A/B/D}$	agonist	active	active
mCPP	5-$HT_{1A/B}$	agonist	active	-
TFMPP	5-$HT_{1A/B}$	agonist	active	-
8-OH-DPAT	5-HT_{1A}	agonist	inactive	inactive
Ipsapirone	5-HT_{1A}	agonist	inactive	-
CGS 12066B	5-HT_{1B}	agonist	active	-
(±)DOI	5-HT_{2}	agonist	inactive	-
Methiothepin	5-HT_{1}/5-HT_{2}	antagonist	active	active
Cinanserin	5-HT_{2}	antagonist	-	-
Ketanserin	5-HT_{2}	antagonist	inactive	inactive
Methysergide	5-HT_{2}/5-$HT_{1C/D}$	antagonist	inactive	-
Mesulergine	5-HT_{2}/5-HT_{1C}	antagonist	inactive	-
Spiperone	5-HT_{2}/5-HT_{1A}	antagonist	inactive	-
(-)Propranolol	5-$HT_{1A/B}$	antagonist	active	-
MDL 72222	5-HT_{3}	antagonist	inactive	-
ICS 205-930	5-HT_{3}	antagonist	inactive	-

TABLE II. Effects of methiothepin, ketanserin, 6-nitroquipazine and d-fenfluramine on the release of ^{3}H-ACh from hippocampal and cerebellar slices, respectively

Drugs	^{3}H-ACh (hippocampus)
Methiothepin	increase
Ketanserin	no effect
6-Nitroquipazine	decrease
d-Fenfluramine	decrease

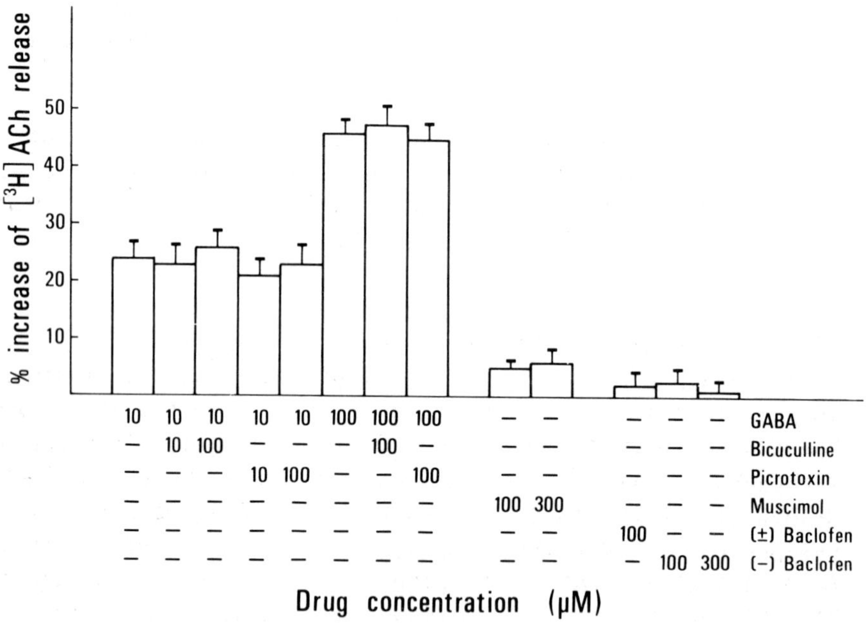

Fig. 2. Effects of $GABA_A$ and $GABA_B$ drugs on the GABA-induced release of ^{3}H-ACh

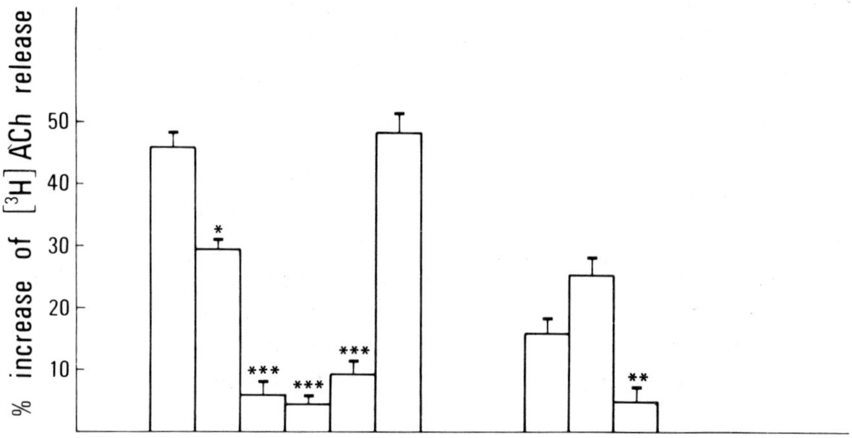

100	100	100	100	100	100	—	—	—	GABA
—	1	10	—	—	—	—	—	10	SKF 89976 A
—	—	—	10	—	—	—	—	—	SKF 100561
—	—	—	—	10	—	—	—	—	SKF 100330 A
—	—	—	—	—	10	—	—	—	Hemicholinium-3
—	—	—	—	—	—	100	300	300	Nipecotic acid

Drug concentration (μM)

Fig. 3. Inhibition by GABA uptake inhibitors but not by hemicholinium-3 of the enhancement of ^{3}H-ACh release induced by GABA or by nipecotic acid. * $P < 0.05$; ** $P < 0.005$; *** $P < 0.001$.

GABAergic regulation of ACh release

The effects of GABA on the release of ^{3}H-ACh were studied in synaptosomes prepared from rat hippocampus. When hippocampal synaptosomes prelabelled with ^{3}H-Ch were exposed to GABA in superfusion a dose-dependent increase of ^{3}H-ACh release could be observed. The effect of GABA was not mimicked by the $GABA_A$ agonist muscimol or by the $GABA_B$ agonist (-)baclofen and was not antagonized by the $GABA_A$ antagonists bicuculline or picrotoxin (Fig. 2). These results seem to exclude a possible involvement of the two known GABA receptor subtypes in the effects observed. Unexpectedly, the GABA-induced ^{3}H-ACh release was strongly counteracted by the new and potent GABA uptake inhibitors, SK&F 89976A, SK&F 100330A, SK&F 100561 (Yunger et al., 1984; Bonanno and

Raiteri, 1987a) (Fig. 3). Fig. 3 also shows that nipecotic acid, an inhibitor-substrate for the GABA transport system (Martin, 1976), increased although less potently than GABA, the basal release of ^{3}H-ACh and that its effect was prevented by SK&F 89976A.

A similar pattern was observed when the effect of GABA was studied using synaptosomes prepared from other rat brain areas: GABA increased in a dose-dependent way the spontaneous outflow of ^{3}H-ACh in cortex and hypothalamus while its effect was negligible in the corpus striatum. Also the GABA-induced ^{3}H-ACh release observed in the cortex and hypothalamus was insensitive to $GABA_A$ and $GABA_B$ drugs but was abolished by SK&F 89976A (Bonanno and Raiteri, 1987b).

On the basis of the above results it seems justified to propose that GABA penetrates into the cholinergic terminals, in selective areas of the rat brain, through a transport system selective for the aminoacid and through such a mechanism stimulates the release of ^{3}H-ACh.

This work was supported by grants from the Italian Ministry of Education and from the Italian C.N.R.

References

- Bonanno, G. and Raiteri, M. (1987a) Coexistence of carriers for dopamine and GABA uptake on a same nerve terminal in the rat brain. Br. J. Pharmacol. **91**: 237-243.
- Bonanno, G. and Raiteri, M. (1987b) Regional selectivity of a GABA-induced [^{3}H]ACh release sensitive to inhibitors of GABA uptake. J. Neurochem. **48**: 1454-1458.
- Chesselet, M.F. (1984) Presynaptic regulation of neurotransmitter release in the brain: Facts and hypothesis. Neurosci. **12**: 347-375.
- Doods, H.N., Mathy, M.J., Davidesko, D., van Charldorp, K.J., de Jonge, A. and van Zwieten, P.A. (1987) Selectivity of muscarinic antagonists in radioligand and in vivo experiments for the putative M_1, M_2 and M_3 receptors. J. Pharmacol. Exp. Ther. **242**: 257-262.
- Duckles, S.P., Yamamura, H.I. and Lee, V. (1987) AF-DX 116 discriminates between muscarinic M_2 receptors of the heart and vasculature. Life Sci. **40**: 1507-1511.

- Giachetti, A., Giraldo, E., Ladinsky, H. and Montagna, E. (1986) Binding and functional profiles of the selective M_1 muscarinic receptor antagonists trihexyphenidyl and dicyclomine. Br. J. Pharmacol. **89**: 83-90.
- Giraldo, E., Hammer, R. and Ladinsky, H. (1987) Distribution of muscarinic receptor subtypes in rat brain as determined in binding studies with AF-DX 116 and pirenzepine. Life Sci. **40**: 833-840.
- Hadhàzy, P. and Szerb, J.C. (1977) The effect of cholinergic drugs on ^{3}H-acetylcholine release from slices of rat hippocampus, striatum and cortex. Brain Res. **123**: 311-322.
- Hammer, R., Monferini, E., Deconti, L., Giraldo, E., Schiavi, G.B. and Ladinsky, H. (1987) Distinct muscarinic receptor subtypes in the heart and in exocrine glands, in Dowdall, M.J. and Hawthorne, J.N. (eds.) Cellular and Molecular Basis of Cholinergic Function. Chichester, England: Ellis Horwood, pp. 56-63.
- Hirschowitz, B.I., Hammer, R., Giachetti, A., Keirns, J.J. and Levine, R.R. (eds.) (1984) Subtypes of Muscarinic Receptors. North Holland: Elsevier.
- Langer, S.Z. (1981) Presynaptic regulation of the release of catecholamines. Pharmacol. Rev. **32**: 337-362.
- Marchi, M., Paudice, P. and Raiteri, M. (1981) Autoregulation of acetylcholine release in isolated hippocampal nerve endings. Eur. J. Pharmacol. **73**: 75-79.
- Marchi, M. and Raiteri, M. (1989) Interaction ACh-GLU in rat hippocampus: involvement of two subtypes of M-2 muscarinic receptors. J. Pharmacol. Exp. Ther. **248**: 1255-1260.
- Martin, D.L. (1976) Carrier-mediated transport and removal of GABA from synaptic regions, in Roberts, E., Chase, T.N. and Tower, D.B. (eds.). GABA in Nervous System Function. New York: Raven Press, pp. 347-386.
- Meyer, E.M. and Otero, D.H. (1985) Pharmacological and ionic characterizations of the muscarinic receptors modulating ^{3}H-acetylcholine release from rat cortical synaptosomes. J. Neurosci. **5**: 1202-1207.
- Micheletti, R., Montagna, E. and Giachetti A. (1987) AF-DX 116, a cardioselective muscarinic antagonist. J. Pharmacol. Exp. Ther. **241**: 628-634.
- Molenaar, P.C. and Polak, R.L. (1970) Stimulation by

atropine of acetylcholine release and synthesis in cortical slices from rat brain. Br. J. Pharmacol. **40**: 406-417.
- Nordström, O. and Bartfai, T. (1980) Muscarinic autoreceptors regulate acetylcholine release in the rat hippocampus: in vitro evidence. Acta Physiol. Scand. **108**: 347-353.
- Potter, L.T., Flynn, D.D., Hanchett, H.E., Kalinoski, D.L., Luber-Narod, J. and Mash, D.C. (1984) Independent M_1 and M_2 receptors: Ligands, autoradiography and function. Trends Pharmacol. Sci. **4** (Suppl.): 22-31.
- Raiteri, M., Marchi, M. and Maura, G. (1984) Release of catecholamines, serotonin, and acetylcholine from isolated brain tissues. In: Lajtha, A. (ed.) Handbook of Neurochemistry, vol. 6, New York: Plenum Publishing Co., pp. 431-462.
- Starke, K. (1981) Presynaptic receptors. Ann. Rev. Pharmacol. Toxicol. **21**: 7-30.
- Szerb, J.C. and Somogyi, G.T. (1973) Depression of acetylcholine release from cortical slices by cholinesterase inhibition and by oxotremorine. Nature (London) **241**: 121-123.
- Yunger, L.M., Fowler, P.J., Zarevics, P. and Setler, P.E. (1984) Novel inhibitors of γ-aminobutyric acid (GABA) uptake: anticonvulsant actions in rats and mice. J. Pharmacol. Exp. Ther. **228**: 109-115.

SPONTANEOUS AND NERVE-EVOKED QUANTAL TRANSMISSION IN REGENERATED MOTOR TERMINALS

F. Di Gregorio, R. Fesce*, S. Cereser, G. Favaro and M.G. Fiori

Department of Peripheral Nervous System Research, Fidia Research Laboratories, Abano Terme (PD), Italy and *"Bruno Ceccarelli" Center for the Study of Peripheral Neuropathies and Neuromuscular Diseases, Department of Pharmacology, University of Milano, Milano, Italy

ABSTRACT

Quantal acetylcholine release was studied in sciatic nerve - extensor digitorum longus muscle preparations from normal rats and in reinnervated muscles at different times following peroneus nerve crush. The efficiency of nerve-evoked transmission was regained almost completely at a time (20 days after crush) when the secretory response to increased extracellular K^+ was very weak. This suggests that K^+-induced secretion might be activated through mechanisms at least partially different from those involved in the response to nerve stimulation.

INTRODUCTION

The present study has its origins in the collaborative work we were fortunate to undertake with Bruno Ceccarelli shortly before his untimely and sudden death. His expertise in probing the molecular and cellular biology of the phenomena underlying neurotransmission at the endplate level has attracted generations of neurobiologists to the fascinating topic of the interactions between nerve and muscle.

The biological mechanisms that lead to nerve regeneration and muscle reinnervation after a lesion to a peripheral nerve have been extensively investigated in the last decades. Particular attention has been paid to the role of the extracellular matrix, Schwann cells and trophic factors in promoting the formation and elongation of axonal sprouts (Sanes and Covault, 1985; Taniuchi et al., 1988). Within this framework, one of the most intriguing issues is the nature of the intra- and extracellular signals that induce the differentiation of motor axons from pathfinding growth cones into transmitter-releasing nerve terminals. It has been demonstrated that reinnervation commonly occurs at pre-existing endplate sites, and that the endplate basal lamina is capable of inducing synaptogenesis even in the absence of viable muscle fibers. The actual contact between the two components of the neuromuscular junction triggers the formation of specialized release structures, the so-called active zones, in the presynaptic terminal (Sanes et al., 1978; Herrera and Wernig, 1987). In contrast, little information is available on the functional performance of the regenerated motor terminal and on the factors involved in the maintenance and maturation of either newly formed or reformed endplates.

The process of neurotransmitter release requires a complex secretory machinery, involving acetylcholine (ACh) synthesis and storage, quantal ACh release by Ca^{++}-dependent exocytosis, vesicle mobilization and recycling during sustained activity. Using in-vitro electrophysiologic techniques we analyzed different features of quantal transmission in normal and regenerating neuromuscular junctions, in an attempt to assess the degree and time course of the functional recovery that follows mammalian skeletal muscle reinnervation.

NEW TOOLS FOR STUDYING EVOKED RELEASE UNDER PHYSIOLOGICAL CONDITIONS

One of the major problems in neuromuscular junction electrophysiology derives from the peculiar properties of the endplate potential (EPP), which is generally high enough in the normal junction to induce an action potential (AP) in the postsynaptic membrane, followed by mechanical activation of the muscle fiber. In order to avoid muscle contraction and to separate EPP from the all-or-none AP, the EPP must be decreased to subthreshold levels. This may be achieved by reducing either ACh output or postsynaptic sensitivity. However, by artificially reducing transmitter output, information about the physiological release capacity of the system is lost. When cholinergic antagonists are used, miniature end-plate potentials (MEPPs) can rarely be recorded. In addition, the block of presynaptic autoreceptors may result in modification of ACh release (Magleby et al., 1981; Wilson, 1982). Hence, the need arises for new tools that allow the study of evoked release under conditions as similar to those occurring in vivo as possible.

Recently, a 22-aminoacid peptide capable of blocking voltage-gated Na^+ channels in the sarcolemma, but not in nervous tissue, was isolated from the venom of the fish-eating snail Conus geographus (Cruz et al., 1985). This peptide, known as CGIIIA μ-conotoxin, allowed us to perform a series of experiments on nerve-evoked quantal transmission at the extensor digitorum longus (EDL) neuromuscular junction of the rat, in the presence of normal concentrations of Ca^{++} and Mg^{++} (2 and 1 mM, respectively). Application of 1 μM CGIIIA abolished AP generation in the muscle, while EPPs with an amplitude of up to 50 mV could be recorded. The mean EPP amplitude during low-rate (0.3 Hz) sciatic nerve stimulation was 32.8 ± 1.3 mV (results expressed as mean ± SEM over the group of fibers studied). To perform quantal analysis, EPPs were corrected for non-linearity between conductance and potential, according to the modified Martin's correction (McLachlan and

Martin, 1981):

$$V_c = V[1 - fV/(RMP - RP)]^{-1}$$

where V is the peak EPP amplitude, V_c its corrected value, RMP the resting membrane potential, RP the reversal potential of the activated endplate. RP was assumed equal to 0, and the correction coefficient f was set at 0.8.

The mean quantal content, calculated in individual fibers as the ratio between the mean of corrected EPPs and the mean MEPP amplitude, averaged 134.0 ± 7.4 in the sampled group. The distribution of the corrected EPP amplitudes, analyzed in each fiber according to the binomial model of synaptic transmission (McLachlan, 1978), gave average p values (the mean probability of activation of the release units) of 0.87 ± 0.02. In normal EDL, 46% of the endplates had $0.9 < p < 1$ and 35% had $0.8 < p < 0.9$. Consequently, the quantal content approached the estimated number of release units per nerve terminal (n), which averaged 155.2 ± 8.0.

Repetitive stimulation of the sciatic nerve at 50 Hz induced only a very slight facilitation of evoked release (2.1 ± 1.3% increase of EPP amplitude at the second pulse of the series). The subsequent rundown of the synaptic signal is illustrated in Fig. 1 (open circles).

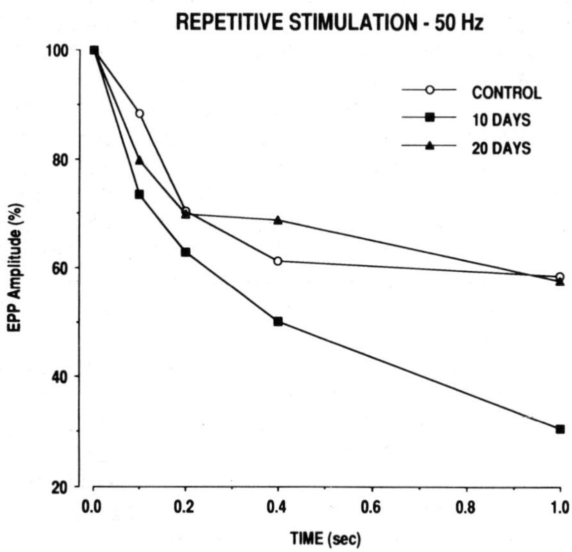

Fig. 1. EPP rundown during trains of repetitive stimulation at 50 Hz for 1 sec. EPPs were corrected for non-linearity and expressed as percent of the first evoked response in any given fiber. The percent residual amplitude was then averaged over the number of tested fibers. Standard errors ranged between 1.9 and 5.1.

ASYNCHRONOUS QUANTAL RELEASE

Spontaneous quantal transmission, resulting in the occurrence of MEPPs at the postsynaptic membrane, may be accelerated by several means such as α-latrotoxin, ouabain, hypertonic media, or depolarizing agents (Haimann et al., 1985; Fesce et al., 1986a). Although this kind of stimulation is certainly not physiological, it offers the advantage of inducing massive ACh release, that can be followed-up for an extended period of time. Statistical analysis of the fluctuations in postsynaptic potential produced by ACh quanta allows for an accurate determination of the rate of secretion even under conditions of intense asynchronous release. Mean waveform parameters of the MEPPs constituting the postsynaptic noise can be derived from the power spectrum of membrane potential; MEPP rate and amplitude can be calculated from the semiinvariants of the probability density function of membrane potential by an extension of Campbell's theorem (Segal et al., 1985; Fesce et al., 1986b). We followed this method to estimate motor terminal secretory response during Ca^{++}-dependent release activation induced by Krebs solution containing 25 mM K^+ at the mammalian EDL endplate. Resting MEPP frequency in 5 mM K^+ Krebs solution was 3.7 ± 0.6 MEPPs/sec; in 25 mM K^+ the frequency rose to a peak of 2403 ± 659 MEPPs/sec, increasing 623-fold (± 110). After 20 min of stimulation, MEPP frequency decreased to 37% (± 7.0%) of the peak value. The secretion rate remained virtually constant from 15 to 20 min after K^+ addition; this steady state (about 900 MEPPs/sec) presumably represents the level of release that can be counterbalanced by the active process of vesicle recycling, which allows the maintenance of a constant pool of releasable quanta.

SYNAPTIC FUNCTION IN REGENERATED MOTOR TERMINALS

The efficiency of the release system after muscle reinnervation was investigated with respect to both nerve-evoked and K^+-induced secretion. EDL denervation was achieved by crushing the peroneal nerve. One week after nerve crush, subthreshold EPPs could already be recorded from superficial EDL fibers, demonstrating that muscle reinnervation had begun. After 10 days, most of the endplates showed overthreshold EPPs, which resulted in AP generation and muscle twitch. Nerve stimulation at 0.3 Hz in the presence of 1 μM CGIIIA produced EPPs in the 3.4 - 39.1 mV range. Although polyinnervated fibers were numerous, quantal analysis was limited to monoinnervated endplates. Since resting MEPP frequency was very low at this stage of reinnervation (few events per minute in most fibers), MEPP amplitude was measured during nerve stimulation at 10 Hz. The induced facilitation of MEPP occurrence made it possible to calculate the mean MEPP amplitude over a suitable number of events. The mean quantal content, at 0.3 Hz stimulation, averaged 57.9 ± 6.0 in the sampled fibers. Simple binomial statistics could not always be applied to describe ACh release at these early stages; the calculated p were spread over the whole possible range (0 - 1), and attained negative values in 20% of the tested fibers. Unexpectedly low or negative p values are generally considered an expression of non-stationarity of the binomial parameters n or p (McLachlan, 1978). In this case, only a complex binomial model would fit the distribution of EPP amplitudes. As a consequence, the number of release units per nerve terminal could not be reliably defined in recently reinnervated EDL. Twenty days after crush, p, derived from the simple binomial model, ranged between 0.4 and 1, averaging 0.80 ± 0.04. The quantal content increased to 96.4 ± 5.9, the estimated number of release units being 120.1 ± 8.0.

The capacity to sustain high-frequency repetitive activity was tested by comparing EPP rundown during 50 Hz stimulation in normal and regenerated junctions (Fig. 1). Ten days after crush, regenerated terminals fatigued more quickly than normal, and EPP amplitude was greatly reduced within 1 sec (Fig. 2). Very often, failures of transmission occurred after a few seconds of repetitive activity. In contrast, twenty days after nerve crush, EPP rundown during repetitive stimulation was quite similar to that of control endplates (Fig. 1, triangles). After 10 sec of stimulation at 50 Hz, the mean residual amplitude of EPP, corrected for non-linear summation, was 32.6% (± 2.2) and 34.4% (± 2.4) of the first EPP of the train in normal and regenerated junctions, respectively.

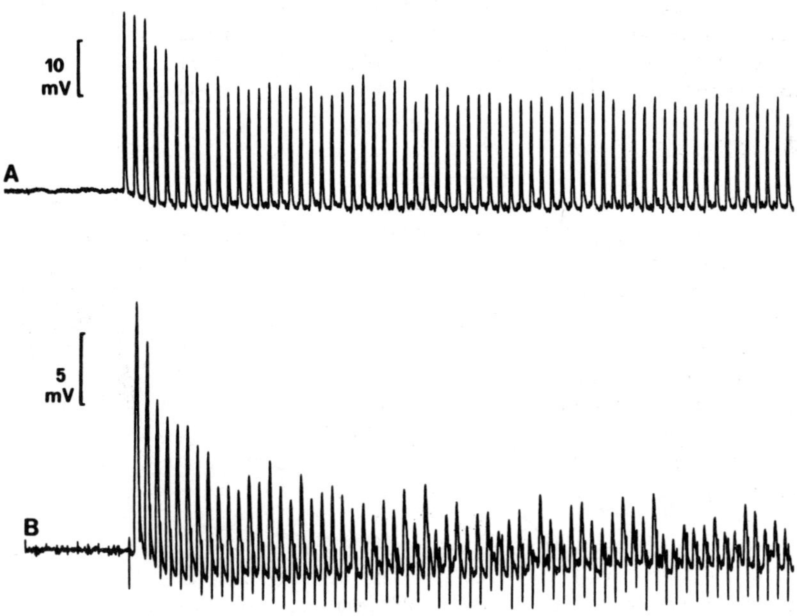

Fig. 2. Repetitive stimulation of sciatic nerve at 50 Hz. Typical recordings of EPP trains from a normal endplate (A) and a reinnervated fiber, 10 days after nerve crush (B).

The response to K^+ application was studied starting twenty days after crush, in order to by-pass the polyinnervation phase. Only junctions showing a unimodal distribution of MEPP amplitude were included in the analysis. The mean MEPP frequency in the presence of normal K^+ (5 mM) was 1.2 ± 0.2 MEPPs/sec, i.e., 33% of the frequency detected in normal EDL endplates. Exposure to 25 mM K^+ increased MEPP frequency 162-fold (± 29), leading to a peak response of 174 ± 22 MEPPs/sec, that is only 7% of the frequency reached at normal junctions. The typical response to K^+ was restored 30 days after nerve crush, with a 607-fold (± 92) increase of MEPP frequency. The time course of MEPP frequency changes during 20 min exposure to 25 mM K^+, and the total number of quanta secreted as a function of time, are illustrated in Fig. 3, A and B, in controls and in reinnervated muscles, 20, 25, and 30 days after crush.

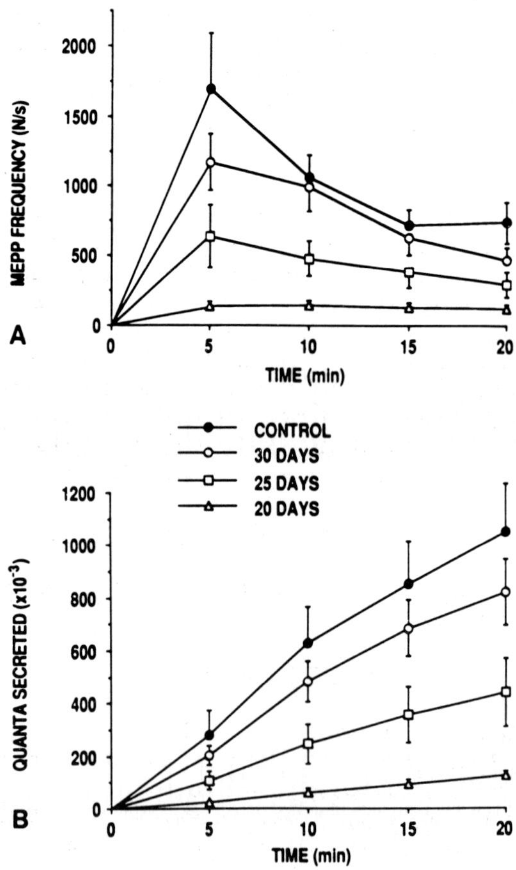

Fig. 3. MEPP frequency (A) and total number of quanta secreted (B) during exposure to 25 mM K^+-Krebs solution. Mean values ± SEM. Control: n=7; 20-day reinnervated: n=14, 25-day reinnervated: n=11; 30-day reinnervated: n=10.

DISCUSSION

In accordance with previously reported evidence (Carmignoto et al., 1983), the present study demonstrates that synaptic transmission is already efficient enough to produce overthreshold EPPs at very early stages of EDL reinnervation. However, the quantal content is low and the variance of EPP amplitude is quite large even in the presence of normal Ca^{++} concentration, many endplates show negative or very small p values, and nerve terminals tend to fatigue rapidly during repetitive stimulation. The mechanisms underlying nerve-evoked transmission mature quickly: by twenty days after crush, quantal content, binomial parameters, and performance during high frequency release approach normal levels. In contrast, spontaneous quantal release recovers more slowly. This might reflect the persistence of small nerve endings since MEPP frequency has been related to the size of the presynaptic terminal (Kuno et al., 1971). Actually, twenty days after nerve crush MEPP frequency is only 33% of the control value, whereas the number of release units involved in nerve-evoked transmission, which depends on the number of sites where ACh release can take place, is 77% of normal. In spite of the large number of release sites and the virtually normal capacity to sustain repetitive activity, the response to K^+ is weak.

This observation is complementary to previous reports by Ceccarelli et al. (1988), who demonstrated that, in the frog, vesicle exocytosis during exposure to high K^+ concentrations occurs initially along the active zones, but unlike nerve-evoked release, within few minutes it spreads over the whole presynaptic membrane. The different time courses of recovery after muscle reinnervation displayed by synchronous, nerve-evoked, and asynchronous, K^+-induced, quantal release, support the suggestion that these two Ca^{++}-dependent processes could be mediated by partially different mechanisms and subcellular structures.

ACKNOWLEDGMENTS

We thank Dr. Mei Satake for kindly supplying μ-conotoxin, and B. Corey for editorial assistance.

REFERENCES

Carmignoto, G., Finesso, M., Siliprandi, R. and Gorio, A. (1983) Muscle reinnervation-1. Restoration of transmitter release mechanisms. Neuroscience 8(3), 393-401.

Ceccarelli, B., Fesce, R., Grohovaz, F. and Haimann, C. (1988) The effect of potassium on exocytosis of transmitter at the frog neuromuscular junction. J. Physiol. (London) 401, 163-183.

Cruz, L.J., Gray, W.R., Olivera, B.M., Zeikus, R.D., Kerr, L., Yoshikami, D. and Moczydlowski, E. (1985) Conus geographus toxins that discriminate between neuronal and muscle sodium channels. J. Biol. Chem. 260, 9280-9283.

Fesce, R., Segal, J.R., Ceccarelli, B. and Hurlbut, W.P.

(1986a) Effects of black widow spider venom and Ca^{2+} on quantal secretion at the frog neuromuscular junction. J. Gen. Physiol., 88, 59-81.

Fesce, R., Segal, J.R. and Hurlbut, W.P. (1986b) Fluctuation analysis of nonideal shot noise. Application to the neuromuscular junction. J. Gen. Physiol. 88, 25-57.

Haimann C., Torri-Tarelli, F., Fesce, R. and Ceccarelli, B. (1985) Measurement of quantal secretion induced by ouabain and its correlation with depletion of synaptic vesicles. J. Cell Biol. 101, 1953-1965.

Kuno, M., Turkanis, S.A. and Weakly, J.R. (1971) Correlation between nerve terminal size and transmitter release at the neuromuscular junction of the frog. J. Physiol. (London) 213, 545-556.

Magleby, K.L., Pallotta, B.S. and Terrar, D.A. (1981) The effect of (+)tubocurarine on neuromuscular transmission during repetitive stimulation in the rat, mouse and frog. J. Physiol. (London) 312, 97-113.

McLachlan, E.M. (1978) The statistics of transmitter release at chemical synapses. Int. Rev. Physiol. Neurophysiol. III 17, 49-117.

McLachlan, E.M. and Martin, A.R. (1981) Non-linear summation of end-plate potentials in the frog and mouse. J. Physiol. (London) 311, 307-324.

Sanes, J.R. and Covault, J. (1985) Axon guidance during reinnervation of skeletal muscle. Trends NeuroSci. 8, 523-528.

Sanes, J.R., Marshall, L.M. and McMahan, U.J. (1978) Reinnervation of muscle fiber basal lamina after removal of myofibers. Differentiation of regenerating axons at original synaptic sites. J. Cell Biol. 78, 176-198.

Segal, J.R., Ceccarelli, B., Fesce, R. and Hurlbut, W.P. (1985) Miniature endplate potential frequency and amplitude determined by an extension of Campbell's theorem. Biophys. J. 47, 183-202.

Taniuchi, M., Clark, H.B., Schweitzer, J.B. and Johnson, E.M. Jr (1988) Expression of nerve growth factor receptors by Schwann cells of axotomized peripheral nerves: ultrastructural location, suppression by axonal contact, and binding properties. J. Neurosci. 8, 664-681.

Wernig, A. and Herrera, A.A. (1986) Sprouting and remodelling at the nerve-muscle junction. Prog. Neurobiol. 27, 251-291.

Wilson, D.F. (1982) Influence of presynaptic receptors on neuromuscular transmission in rat. Am. J. Physiol. 242, C366-C372.

THE GENETICS OF TYPE A POTASSIUM CHANNELS IN *DROSOPHILA MELANOGASTER*.

A. Mallart.
Unité de Physiologie Neuromusculaire, Laboratoire de Neurobiologie Cellulaire et Moléculaire, C.N.R.S., F-91198 Gif sur Yvette, France.

The A-current (I_A), first described in the somata of molluscan neurones (Connor and Stevens, 1971), is a voltage dependent, fast transient K current whose main action is to repolarize the action potential. Type-A K-channel block causes action potential widening and/or membrane re-excitation; transmitter release by pre-synaptic terminals is thereby enhanced. I_A has been subsequently described throughout the animal kingdom from insect muscle to mammalian brain.

A family of *Drosophila melanogaster* mutants showing absence (or defectiveness) of I_A were called *Shaker* (*Sh*) because of their abnormal leg shaking behaviour on recovery from ether anesthesia, caused by anomalous action potential electrogenesis (Jan, Jan and Dennis, 1977; Salkoff and Wyman, 1981; Wu and Haugland, 1986). Using chromosomal rearrangements, these *Shaker* mutations have been mapped to polytene chromosomal position 16F on the X chromosome (map units 57.7 and 58.2 for Sh^{KS133} and Sh^{5} respectively). Thanks to the availability of a DNA fragment that hybridized nearby, Baumann et al. (1987), Papazian et al. (1987) and Pongs et al. (1988) started a chromosomal walk through the *Shaker* locus using overlapping clones from genomic libraries until over 200 kb of genomic DNA had been isolated. The *Shaker* gene complex was located in the genomic DNA using as landmarks several chromosomal breakpoints giving a *Shaker* phenotype. Probes obtained from the genomic DNA were used to screen *Drosophila* cDNA libraries to isolate different cDNA clones. The aminoacid composition of the *Shaker* protein was deduced from the base sequence of these cDNAs. It turned out that the A-channel is a 616 aminoacid protein of about 70 kDa showing, in hydropathy tests, six putative transmembrane helices, one of which contains the S4 region which is thought to be the voltage sensor present also in Na and Ca voltage sensitive channels. The type-A K-channel thus resembles one of the four domains forming the α subunit of Na and Ca channels (Pongs et al. 1988; Jan and Jan, 1989).

The question now arises of how a protein of one fourth the size of the other voltage sensitive channels can form a transmembrane channel? The possibility that the A-channel is formed by a multimeric assembly of subunits was considered following the results of gene dosage tests using null *Shaker* mutants (e.g. Sh^{KS133} or Sh^{102}): I_A in heterozygous (Sh/Sh^+) was smaller than the expected value of 50%. The interpretation was that, in these crosses, the mutated *Shaker* gene produced abnormal subunits which formed multimeric assemblies with their normal counterparts to give non-functionnal type-A K-channels (Ganetzky and Wu, 1986).

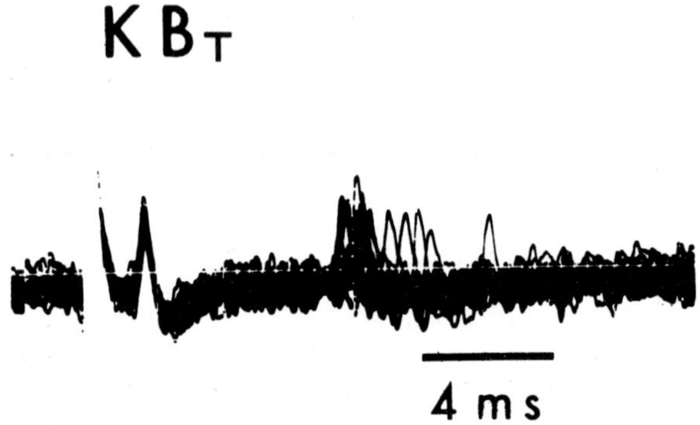

Figure. Backfiring of a presynaptic terminal recorded by an external electrode from a transgenic larval neuromuscular preparation (see Gisselmann et al. 1989).

We examined the hypothesis of abnormal subunits being generated at the Shaker gene of null mutants such as Sh^{102} (Gisselmann et al. 1989). We found by cloning and sequencing the appropriate part of the Sh^{102} DNA that the mutation caused a base exchange giving a termination codon thereby generating truncated A-channel subunits lacking the 6th presumed transmembrane helix and the entire carboxy terminus. The capability of these abnormal subunits to assemble with normal A-channel proteins was tested by constructing transgenic flies carrying a heat-inducible gene encoding truncated A-type K-channel subunits together with the normal dose of wild type *Sh* gene. The heat-induced expression of the altered gene at larval, pupal or adult stages lead to the transformation of wild type into *Shaker* flies as shown by a 30% reduction in larval muscle potassium current, backfiring of motor axons (see the Figure), increased transmitter release in neuromuscular junctions and leg shaking behaviour in adult flies (Gisselmann et al., 1989).

The next question to be asked concerns the number of constitutive subunits of the A-channel and whether it is composed of identical (homomultimer) or different (heteromultimer) subunits. Since the protein sequence of the type-A K-channel shows a striking similarity with each one of the four homologous domains of the protein that forms Na and Ca channels, it is conceivable that a multimeric assembly of four *Shaker* gene products forms a type A channel (Pongs et al. 1988). Since several clones differing by their amino and carboxy termini, but conserving a common central core, have been obtained from the *Shaker* locus by alternative splicing of a primary transcript (Kamb et al. 1988; Schwarz et al. 1988; Pongs et al. 1988), one possibility is that the channel is formed by an heteromultimeric assembly of different gene products from the *Shaker* locus.

Another possibility is that other regions of the genome contribute subunits to form, together with the *Shaker* gene, the type-A K-channel in *Drosophila*. In fact, several other mutations such as *V7*, located on the X chromosome centrally relative to the *Shaker* complex (Tanouye et al., 1981), *ether á gogo* (*eag*), also on the X chromosome at position 50.0 and *hyperkinetic* (*Hk*) on the same chromosome at position 30.9 cause a reduction of I_A and/or nerve hyperexcitability and enhanced trans-

PHENOTYPIC EXPRESSION OF MUTATIONS IN THE

SHAKER GENE SUPERFAMILY

	Neuron	Nerve	Nerve endings	Muscle
Shaker	o	+	+	+
V7	--	+	+	o
eag	--	--	+	+
Hk	+	--	--	+

\+ mutant phenotype
o normal "
-- no data

mitter release (Ganetzky and Wu, 1986). As shown in the Table, these different genes are expressed preferentially in a tissue specific way. For instance, the protein coded at *V7* has been shown to contribute to express I_A in nerves rather than in muscles while the *Shaker* product goes preferentially to muscle and peripheral nerves but not to neuronal somata (Solc, Zagotta and Aldrich, 1987). Furthermore, by using a *Shaker* cDNA probe Butler et al. (1989) have isolated three genes, *Shab*, *Shaw* and *Shal*, in different chromosomes whose deduced proteins have a high homology with the *Shaker* protein, but whose physiological significance has not yet been established.

One may now ask how a point mutation affecting only one of the genes coding for subunits of the type-A K-channel in *Drosophila* can cause a *Shaker* phenotype in spite of the continued production of normal subunits elsewhere in the genome? If the A-channel was formed by a single molecule (like Na and Ca channels) one would expect only a moderate reduction in I_A, if any. But, if the A-channel is formed by the assembly of several subunits, as I have shown above, the production of relatively few abnormal subunits which can assemble with normal ones, will interfere with the function of a large number of channels. The severity of the *Shaker* phenotype will, thus, depend on the ability of the normal or abnormal gene products from different members of the *Shaker* superfamily to assemble with each other to form type-A K-channels.

This work was supported by the Association des Myopathes de France.

REFERENCES

Baumann, A., Krah-Jentgens, I., Müller, R., Müller-Holtkamp, F., Seidel, R., Kecskmethy, N., Casal, J., Ferrús, A. and Pongs, O. (1987). Molecular organization of the maternal effect region of the *Shaker* complex of *Drosophila*: characterization of an I_A channel transcript with homology to vertebrate Na^+ channel. EMBO J. **6**: 3419-3429.

Butler, A., Wei, A., Baker, K. and Salkoff, L. (1989) A family of putative potassium channel genes in *Drosophila*. Science **243**: 943-947.

Connor, J. A. and Stevens, C. F. (1971). Voltage clamp studies of a transient outward membrane current in gastropod neural somata. J. Physiol. (Lond.) **213**: 21-30.

Ganetzky, B. and Wu, C.-F. (1986). Neurogenetics of membrane excitability in *Drosophila*. Ann. Rev. Genet. **20**: 13-44.

Gisselmann, G., Sewing, G., Madsen, W. B., Mallart, A., Angaut-Petit, D. Müller-Holtkamp, F., Ferrús, A. and Pongs, O. (1989). The interference of truncated with normal potassium channel subunits leads to abnormal behaviour in transgenic *Drosophila melanogaster*. EMBO J. **8**: 2359-2364.

Jan, L. Y. and Jan, Y. N. (1989). Voltage-sensitive ion channels. Cell **56**: 13-25.

Jan, L. Y., Jan, Y. N. and Dennis, M. J. (1977). Two mutations of synaptic transmission in *Drosophila*. Proc. Roy. Soc. Lond. B **198**: 87-108.

Kamb, A., Iverson, L. E. and Tanouye M. A. (1987). Molecular characterization of *Shaker*, a Drosophila gene that encodes a potassium channel. Cell **50**: 405-413.

Papazian, D. M., Schwarz, T. L., Tempel, B. L., Jan, Y. N. and Jan, L. Y. (1987). Cloning of complementary DNA from *Shaker*, a putative potassium channel gene from *Drosophila*. Science **237**: 749-753.

Pongs, O., Kecskemethy, N., Muller, R., Krah-Jentgens, I., Baumann, A., Kiltz, H. H., Canal, I., Llamazares, S. and Ferrús, A. (1988). Shaker encodes a family of putative potassium channel proteins in the nervous system of *Drosophila*. EMBO J. **7**: 1087-1096.

Salkoff, L. and Wyman, R. (1981). Genetic modification of potassium channels in *Drosophila Shaker* mutants. Nature **293**: 228-230.

Schwarz, T. L., Tempel, B. L., Papazian, D. M., Jan, Y. N. and Jan, L. Y. (1988). Multiple potassium-channel components are produced by alternative splicing at the *Shaker* locus in *Drosophila*. Nature **331**: 137-142.

Solc, C. K., Zagotta, W. N. and Aldrich, R. W. (1987). Single-channel and genetic analyses reveal two distinct A-type potassium channels in *Drosophila*. Science **236**: 1094-1098.

Tanouye, M. A., Ferrús, A. and Fujita, S. C. (1981). Abnormal action potentials associated with the *Shaker* complex locus of *Drosophila*. Proc. Nat. Acad. Sci. U.S.A. **78**: 6548-6552.

Wu, C.-F. and Haugland, F. N. (1985). Voltage-clamp analysis of membrane currents in larval muscle fibers of *Drosophila*: alteration of potassium currents in *Shaker* mutants. J. Neurosci. **5**: 2626-2640.

SODIUM-ACTIVATED POTASSIUM CHANNEL IN AVIAN SENSORY NEURONS

C. Haimann* and C.R. Bader §

Département de Physiologie, Centre Médical Universitaire, Genève, *CNR Center of Cytopharmacology and "B. Ceccarelli" Center for the Study of Peripheral Neuropathies and Neuromuscular Diseases, Department of Pharmacology, University of Milano, Italy, § Division de Neurophysiologie Clinique, Hôpital Cantonal, Genève, Switzerland.

Potassium currents contribute to the control of neuronal excitability through their effects on the resting membrane potential and on the firing pattern of neurons. Several types of potassium currents are involved in these various tasks (see Rudy, 1988). Recently, a new type of potassium current characterized by its sensitivity to the concentration of intracellular sodium has been described. This sodium-activated potassium current (KNa) has been observed in cardiac cells (Kameyama et al., 1984), in vertebrate (Bader et al., 1985; Dryer et al., 1989; Haimann et al., 1990; Schwindt et al., 1989) and in invertebrate neurons (Hartung, 1985). In this report, we review results of single-channel recordings of KNa which suggest the existence of at least two distinct types of channels in neurons and in cardiac cells. A full account of the results obtained so far is given elsewhere (Haimann et al., 1990).

THE ELEMENTARY PROPERTIES OF KNa IN NEURONS

KNa was identified in vertebrate sensory and parasympathetic neurons (Bader et al., 1985) by comparing whole-cell current recordings obtained in the absence and in the presence of tetrodotoxin (TTX) during step depolarizations in voltage clamp. The membrane current suppressed by TTX consisted of an early inward sodium current followed by a potassium current. Similar results were also reported in invertebrate neurons (Hartung, 1985) and in chick mesencephalic neurons (Dryer et al., 1989). The interpretation of these surprising results was that the potassium current suppressed by TTX was activated by a transient accumulation of sodium underneath the membrane. Whole-cell recordings in trigeminal neurons also indicated that the presence of a high intracellular sodium concentration could steadily activate KNa at potentials where voltage-dependent potassium currents (delayed rectifier, A-current) were not activated (Bader et al., 1985).

---

* to whom correspondence should be addressed
§ This work was supported by grants from the Swiss National Science Foundation n. 3.651.0.84 and n. 3.594.0.87.

0309–1651/89/121133–7/$03.00/0

Single-channel activity of KNa was studied by applying sodium to the cytoplasmic face of inside-out patches (Hamill et al., 1981) from cultured trigeminal neurons of the quail (Haimann et al., 1990). The single-channel activity induced by sodium could not be evoked when sodium was substituted by choline or lithium. Also, KNa was not suppressed by the calcium chelator EGTA and the presence of 5 uM calcium failed to activate this channel; this indicated that the KNa channel is distinct from the calcium-activated K channels.

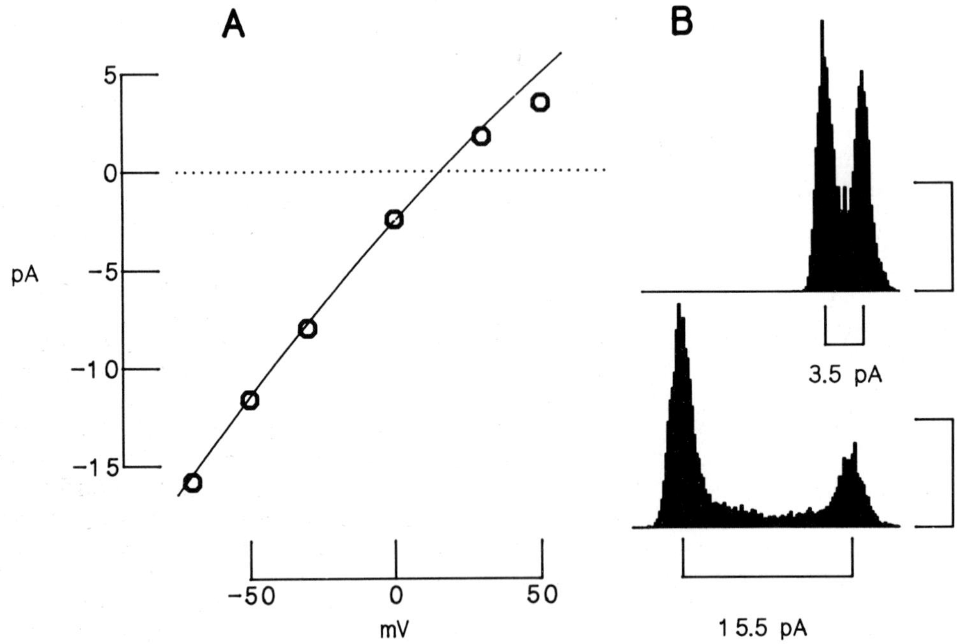

Fig. 1. Voltage-dependence of KNa single-channel activity. A. Current-voltage relationship measured in an inside-out patch exposed to 100 mM sodium. The voltage was changed stepwise and the amplitude of the current measured at each voltage. The continuous line is the Goldman-Hodgkin-Katz equation. The permeability was 4×10^{-13} cm^3/s. B. Amplitude histograms of 20 current traces, each lasting 600 ms recorded from the same patch as in A at +50 mV (top) and -70 mV (bottom). The value of the calibration bar for the number of events is 250. Methods: inside-out patches were excised from dissociated quail trigeminal ganglion neurons cultured for 12-48 hours. The ganglia were dissected at embryonic day 7. Methods for preparing dissociated neurons and for recording have been described previously (Bader et. al., 1987). Acquisition, analysis, and graphical representation of data were performed with the program DATAC (Bertrand and Bader, 1986). The solution inside the pipette was (mM): KCl (140), KF (10), NaCl (5), HEPES (5), EGTA (5) and TTX 1 μM. The superfusion solution was (mM): NaCl (100), KF (75), HEPES (5), EGTA (20).

The current-voltage relationship for one inside-out patch superfused at the cytoplasmic face with a solution containing 100 mM sodium is shown in Fig. 1A. It can be seen that between -70 mV and +50 mV the elementary conductance has no clear voltage dependence. The chord conductance measured at -50 mV was 180 pS (150 mM Ko and 75 mM Ki). In 5 patches the mean slope conductance was 174 ± 24 pS. The fitting of the data with a Goldman-Hodgkin-Katz equation (Goldman, 1943; Hodgkin and Katz, 1949) suggests that potassium ions are the major charge carriers of KNa. The selective permeability for potassium ions was confirmed by experiments which demonstrated that the reversal potential of KNa shifted during potassium substitutions as predicted by the Nernst equation (Haimann et al., 1990).

The elementary conductance of KNa depends upon the extracellular potassium concentration and it decreases, as predicted by the constant-field theory, to 50 pS in the presence of a physiological potassium gradient (Haimann et al., 1990). A sodium-activated potassium current with similar single-channel properties has been described in avian brainstem neurons (Dryer et al., 1989).

Fig. 1B shows the amplitude histograms of the single-channel currents at membrane potentials of -70 mV (bottom) and +50 mV (top). In both histograms, the peaks at the left represent the background noise distribution and the peaks at the right represent the distribution of the current sizes when the channel is in the maximally conducting state. The area of the peak at the right divided by the total area of an histogram gives an estimate of the probability for the KNa channel to be in the maximally conducting state. This probability was found to be increased at depolarized voltages with an e-fold increase for a depolarization of 108 mV. This voltage sensitivity increased in the presence of lower sodium concentrations (Haimann et al., 1990). There were no additional peaks to the right of the largest current peak in the amplitude histograms. Therefore, we believe that the smaller current levels, which can be clearly observed between the "noise peak" and the largest current peak at -70 mV (see Fig. 1B), represent substates of the KNa channel (Haimann et al., 1990).

KNa SENSITIVITY TO SODIUM

An important issue was to determine whether the sodium sensitivity of KNa was compatible with the cytoplasmic concentrations of sodium during neuronal activity. By various techniques, the sodium concentration in the neuronal cytoplasm has been estimated to be approximately 5 mM in mammalian sympathetic neurons (Galvan et al., 1984) and between 4 and 50 mM in frog motoneurons (Grafe et al., 1982; Bührle and Sonnhof, 1983). The relationship between the sodium concentration and the probability for KNa to be open has now been examined. Figure 2 illustrates examples of recordings obtained from an inside-out patch exposed to solutions containing sodium concentrations in the physiological range. At 12.5 mM internal sodium KNa was already active (top panel) and when the concentration was increased to 50 mM, the channel activity increased markedly (bottom panel). The dose-response relationship for patches exposed to intracellular sodium concentrations between 12 and 100 mM indicated that the probability for the KNa channel to be open increased approximately three-fold between 12 and 50 mM sodium. Beyond this concentration, saturation occurred. The

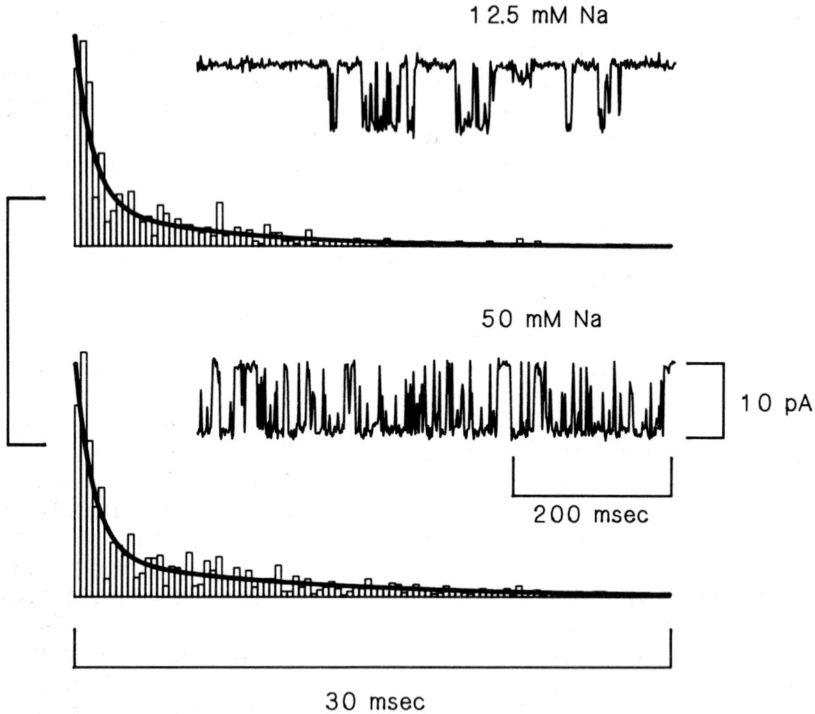

Fig. 2. Sodium-dependence of KNa single-channel activity. An inside-out patch was exposed to 12.5 mM (top panel) and 50 mM sodium (bottom panel). The open time distribution and one typical current trace recording of KNa are shown for each sodium concentration. The holding potential was -50 mV. Data were acquired at 3.3 kHz and filtered at 1.6 KHz. Open times were measured automatically at an amplitude corresponding to 20% of the maximum single-channel current amplitude, in order to include all identified substates. At both sodium concentrations, a sum of two exponentials gave the best fit to the data. The time constants of the exponentials were: at 12.5 mM, t_1 = 0.88 ms and t_2 = 7.1 ms; at 50 mM, t_1 = 0.93 ms and t_2 = 10.7 ms. The total time over which open times were measured was 12 s at 12.5 mM and 15 s at 50 mM. The value of the calibration bar for the number of events is 90 at 12.5 mM and 180 at 50 mM. The pipette solution was as described in Fig. 1. The superfusion solution contained (mM): KF (75), EGTA (20), HEPES (5) and either NaCl (12.5) and choline (87.5) or NaCl (50) and choline (50).

dose-response relationship could be fitted by a Hill equation with a Hill coefficient greater than 2 (Haimann et al., 1990). Such a power relationship suggested that more than one sodium ion has to bind to the channel before the channel opens. Another possibility would be that when a channel is opened by the interaction with one single sodium ion, the sodium concentration affects the channel open time. The latter possibility seems however unlikely in view of the open time distributions illustrated in Fig. 2: at both sodium concentrations the time constants were in the vicinity of 0.9 ms and 9 ms. Also, the relationship between the brief and longer open times was not significantly modified by the increase in sodium concentration.

In brainstem neurons, Dryer et al. (1989) investigated the effect of intracellular sodium in patches containing many KNa channels. They found that the overall current induced by sodium increased between 20 and 150 mM, with no sign of saturation. This difference with our results could be due to the existence of subpopulations of less sensitive KNa channels that we did not observe in our single-channel recordings.

THE ROLE OF KNa IN NEURONS AND IN HEART CELLS

The functional role of KNa will remain a matter of speculation until specific blockers or positive modulators are found. In heart, the elementary conductance of KNa is high (207 pS with Ki 49 mM and Ko 150 mM) and shows marked inward rectification. No conductance substates were reported. The gating of the channel appears to be regulated exclusively by intracellular sodium and the opening probability begins to increase at concentrations of approximately 30 mM (Kameyana et al., 1984). Because the cytoplasmic sodium concentration of cardiac cells has been reported to be less than 10 mM (Lee and Fozzard, 1975), Kameyana et al. (1984) concluded that KNa played a functional role only under pathological conditions: KNa might promote membrane repolarization when, for example, a limited oxygen supply and the associated decrease of sodium extrusion lead to marked intracellular sodium accumulation.

In neurons, KNa can be activated under physiological conditions and recently, Schwindt et al. (1989) identified a potassium current activated by the persistent sodium current which exists in neocortical neurons. This sodium-activated potassium current provides a tonic repolarizing effect, complementary to that of the calcium-activated potassium currents. It has not yet been demonstrated whether this particular current is due to the activation of the KNa channel described here.

KNa in neurons has a high elementary conductance, between 105 pS (Dryer et al., 1989) and 174 pS (Haimann et al., 1990), but it does not show any significant rectification and possesses several conductance levels. The gating of the channel is primarily sodium-dependent but the probability for the channel to be open increases at depolarized voltages in the presence of sodium (Haimann et al., 1990). Finally, physiological intracellular sodium concentrations can activate KNa at a membrane potential corresponding to the resting potential of trigeminal neurons. Thus, neuronal KNa probably contributes to the resting membrane potential of neurons. In addition, during an action potential, the sodium influx combined with the voltage-dependence of the probability for the channel to be open could accelerate the repolarizing phase of the action potential and, as a consequence, contribute to the control of the firing pattern of a neuron. Indeed, the hyperpolarization triggered by an increase in the cytosolic sodium concentration could facilitate the reactivation of those currents which are inactivated by a depolarization, such as the sodium current, the A current (Connor and Stevens, 1971), and the low-threshold calcium current (Carbone and Lux, 1984; Nowicky et al., 1985). It is possible that, depending upon the time course of the sodium influx, the sodium-activated potassium current would participate in distinct phases of the electrical signal in different types of neurons.

REFERENCES

Bader, C.R., Bernheim, L. and Bertrand, D. (1985) Sodium-activated potassium current in cultured avian neurons. Nature 317:540-542

Bader, C.R., Bertrand, D. and Schlichter, R. (1987) Calcium-activated chloride current in cultured sensory and parasympathetic quail neurons. J. Physiol. 394:125-148

Bertrand, D. and Bader, C.R. (1986) DATAC, a multipurpose biological data analysis program based on a mathematical interpreter. Int. J Biomed. Comp. 18:193-202

Bührle, C. P. and Sonnhof, U. (1983) Intracellular ion activities and equilibrium potentials in motoneurons and glia cells of the frog spinal cord. Pflüg. Archiv. 396:144-153.

Carbone, E. and Lux, H. (1984) A low-voltage-activated, fully inactivating Ca channel in vertebrate sensory neurons. Nature 310:501-502

Connor, J.A. and Stevens, C. F. (1971) Voltage clamp studies of a transient outward membrane current in gasteropod neural somata. J. Physiol. 213:21-30

Dryer, S.E., Fujii, J.T., and Martin, A. R. (1989) A Na+-activated K+ current in cultured brainstem neurons from chicks. J. Physiol. 410:283-296

Galvan, M., Dörge, A. Beck, F. and Rick, R. (1984) Intracellular electrolyte concentrations in rat sympathetic neurones measured with an electron microprobe. Pflüg. Arch. 400:274-279

Goldman, D.E. (1943). Potential, impedance, and rectification in membranes. J. Gen. Physiol. 27:37-60.

Grafe, P., Rimpel, J., Reddy, M.M. and Ten Bruggencate, G. (1982) Changes of intracellular sodium and potassium ion concentrations in frog spinal motoneurons induced by repetitive synaptic stimulation. Neuroscience 7:3212-3220

Haimann, C., Bernheim, L., Bertrand, D. and Bader, C. R. (1990) Potassium current activated by intracellular sodium in quail trigeminal ganglion neurons. J. Gen. Physiol. in press

Hamill, O. P., Marty, A., Neher, E., Sakmann, B. and Sigworth, F.J. (1981). Improved patch clamp techniques for high resolution current recording from cells and cell-free membrane patches. Pflüg. Archiv. 391:85-100.

Hartung, K. (1985). Potentiation of a transient outward current by Na+ influx in crayfish neurons. Pflüg. Archiv. 404:41-44.

Hodgkin, A.L. and Katz, B. (1949). The effect of sodium ions on the electrical activity of the giant axon of the squid. J. Physiol. 108:37-77.

Kameyama, M., Kakei, M., Sato, R., Shibasaki, T., Matsuda, H. and Irisawa, H. (1984). Intracellular Na+ activates a K+ channel in mammalian cardiac cells. Nature 309:394-356.

Lee, C. O. and Fozzard, H. A. (1975). Activities of potassium and sodium ions in rabbit heart muscle. J. Gen. Physiol. 65:695-708.

Nowycky, M. C., Fox, A.P. and Tsien, R.W. (1985). Three types of neuronal calcium channels with different calcium agonist sensitivity. Nature 316:440-443.

Rudy, B. (1988). Diversity and ubiquity of K channels. Neuroscience 25:729-749.

Schwindt, P. C., Spain, W. J. and Crill, W. E. (1989). Long-lasting reduction of excitability by a sodium-dependent potassium current in cat neocortical neurons. J. Neurophysiol. 61:233-244.

INTRACELLULAR MECHANISM OF NEUROTRANSMITTER-INDUCED MODULATIONS OF VOLTAGE-DEPENDENT Ca CURRENT IN SNAIL NEURONS

H.M. Gerschenfeld, Danièle Paupardin-Tritsch, Constance Hammond and R. Harris-Warrick*
Laboratoire de Neurobiologie, Ecole Normale Supérieure, 46, rue d'Ulm, 75230 Paris cedex 05, France

ABSTRACT

This paper reviews our work on the modulation of voltage-dependent Ca currents in identified snail neurons. Ca currents of snail neurones are enhanced or decreased by neurotransmitters. Serotonin and acetylcholine enhance the Ca current of identified neurons, the effect of serotonin being mediated by cGMP and cGMP-dependent protein kinase. Cholecystokinin (CCK8) and dopamine both decrease the Ca current of identified neurons. The effect of CCK8 is irreversible and involves the activation of protein kinase C. The dopamine-induced decrease in Ca current is reversible and involves an α_{40} subunit of a snail G protein immunologically and functionally related to α_o of mammalian brain.

Second messengers and protein kinases play a key role in synaptic actions involving the regulation of voltage-dependent ionic channels by neurotransmitters and, in particular, in the modulation of voltage-dependent Ca channels (see Greengard, 1978; Levitan, 1988; Hosey and Lazdunski, 1988; Bean, 1989). These Ca channels play an important role in the regulation of neuronal excitability and the release of synaptic transmitters.

Neurotransmitters have been reported to either enhance or reduce the voltage-dependent Ca current through different intracellular mechanisms. The mechanism of a neurotransmitter-induced increase in voltage-dependent Ca current was first described in vertebrate cardiac muscle fibres in which β-adrenergic agonists by stimulating adenylate cyclase evoke an increase in intracellular cAMP (Brum et al., 1983) that activates the cAMP-dependent protein kinase (protein kinase A, PKA, Osterrieder et al., 1982; Brum et al. 1983; Reuter et al., 1983) which, in turn, phosphorylates the Ca channels or some associated protein/s. Phosphorylation would increase the number of open Ca channels (Reuter et al., 1983; Brum et al., 1984) and may alter the kinetics of Ca channel activation and inactivation (Bean et al., 1984; Brum et al., 1984).

A neurotransmitter-induced reduction of the voltage-dependent Ca current was first found in neurons. Noradrenaline (NA) decreases the duration of the Ca-dependent spike recorded in the soma of both chick embryo dorsal root sensory ganglion (DRG) neurons in culture and rat sympathetic ganglion neurons and these NA-induced effects are due to a decrease in voltage-dependent Ca currents (Dunlap and Fischbach, 1980; Horn and McAffee 1980; Galvan and Adams, 1982). The mechanism of the different neurotransmitter-induced decreases in Ca current has not been yet completely elucidated. It has been shown that the NA- and GABA-induced decreases in Ca current of chick embryo DRG neurons in culture, involve a G protein which is ADP-ribosylated by the toxin of *Bordetella pertussis* (PTX) since PTX

* Section of Neurobiology and Behavior, Seeley Mudd Hall, Cornell University, Ithaca N.Y. 14583, USA.

blocks these neurotransmitter-induced reductions of Ca current in DRG neurons (Holz et al., 1986; Dolphin and Scott, 1987). Hescheler et al. (1987) have also shown that PTX blocks the decrease in Ca current induced by opiate peptides in a neuroblastoma x glioma hybrid cell line, the NG 108-15 cells. The PTX effect on these cells could be reversed by the intracellular perfusion of two different G proteins, Gi and Go, Go being ten times more potent than Gi in reversing the effect of PTX. The use of patch-clamp whole cell recording in these experiments, which involves a wash-out of the phosphorylation substrates from the cytoplasm could suggest that Go acts by coupling directly the opiate receptors to the voltage-dependent Ca channels. Nevertheless, in DRG neurons, the extracellular application of a diacylglycerol analog, oleylacetylglycerol (OAG), evokes a decrease in Ca current (Rane and Dunlap, 1986) and inhibitors of the Ca/ diacylglycerol-dependent protein kinase (protein kinase C, PKC) blocked the NA-induced decrease in Ca current (Rane et al., 1989). These results strongly suggest that PKC is involved in the mechanism of the NA-induced modulation of the Ca current.

In this paper, we will review our own results concerning the neurotransmitter-induced modulation of voltage-dependent Ca current in identified neurons of the snail *Helix aspersa* . The soma of these neurons discharge Ca-dependent action potentials resulting from the activation of voltage-dependent Ca channels. The Ca-dependent plateau component of the somatic action potential can be revealed by bathing the neurons in a saline containing 30 mM tetraethylammonium (TEA) chloride. The voltage-dependent Ca current was analyzed by voltage-clamping with two microelectrodes, the snail neurons bathed in a saline containing 30 mM TEA, and in which Ca was replaced by Ba that is known to permeate the Ca channels and to block outward K currents. The voltage-dependent current of snail neurons is largely due to the activation of a predominant class of Ca channels which resemble the high voltage-activated Ca channels (L-type channels) of Vertebrates (see Hoffmann et al., 1987; Tsien et al. 1988; Bean, 1989). To confirm that the neurotransmitters specifically affected the voltage-dependent Ca current of the snail neurons we established current-voltage curves both in the presence and the absence of the neurotransmitters. Moreover, a modulation of the inward Na current was ruled out by monitoring the inward current amplitude 40 msec after the onset of the depolarizing pulse, when the Na current was already inactivated. Finally, all possible contaminations of the inward current recordings by hidden outward K currents was ruled out by suppressing the K currents of the snail neurons by loading them with Cs using the ionophore nystatin (see Tillotson, 1979).

I. NEUROTRANSMITTER-INDUCED ENHANCEMENTS OF VOLTAGE DEPENDENT Ca CURRENT IN SNAIL NEURONS

Serotonin (5-HT) enhances the voltage-dependent Ca current in identified snail neurons. Role of cGMP and cGMP-dependent protein kinase

In a group of identified neurons located in the ventral face of the parietal ganglion of *Helix* bathed in a saline containing 30 mM TEA, 5-HT (1 mM) induces an increase of the duration of the somatic Ca-dependent action potential. This effect shows a latency of seconds and is rapidly reversed by washing-out of the neurotransmitter. When 5-HT is continuously applied for 15 minutes or more, no desensitization is observed. In these identified neurons

5-HT (1-5) mM does not affect any TEA-insensitive, Ca-independent outward current component, but induces a 25-30 % increase of the amplitude of the Ca current (Paupardin-Tritsch et al., 1986).

Cyclic AMP was not involved in this 5-HT response since neither its intracellular injection nor the extracellular application of forskolin, an adenylate cyclase activator, alter the current of the ventral neurons or its modulation by 5-HT. An involvement of cytosolic Ca in this 5-HT-induced response was also ruled out since prolonged and repetitive intracellular injections of EGTA in the identified neurons had no effect on the 5-HT induced increase in Ca current.

In contrast, the intracellular injection of cGMP in the identified ventral neurons mimicked the effect of 5-HT increasing both the duration of the Ca-dependent action potential and the amplitude of the voltage-dependent Ca current. That 5-HT and cGMP act on the same population of Ca channels is suggested by the observation that when 5-HT application evoked a maximal increase in Ca current amplitude, the intracellular injection of cGMP became ineffective and vice-versa. Moreover, when the intracellular concentration of cGMP was increased by the extracellular application of zaprinast, a specific inhibitor of the cGMP-dependent phosphodiesterase zaprinast (see Windquist et al., 1984), the Ca current amplitude of the ventral neurons was increased.

Therefore, the 5-HT-induced increase in Ca current in the identified ventral neurons of Helix was mediated by cGMP (Paupardin-Trisch et al. 1986). How does 5-HT induce the increase in intracellular cGMP? Is it by stimulating a membrane-bound guanylate cyclase (see Waldman and Murad, 1987) or does 5-HT stimulate the cGMP synthesis via the arachidonic acid pathway (see Goldberg and Haddox, 1977)? We attempted to answer these questions experimentally. Our results show that 4-bromophenacyl bromide, a blocker of phospholipase AII, did not affect the 5-HT response, and that the extracellular application of arachidonic acid (50-100 mM) to the identified ventral neurons affected neither the Ca current nor its modulation by 5-HT. Moreover, no G-protein appears to be involved in the 5-HT-induced enhancement of Ca current since the intracellular injection of GTPγS neither increases the Ca current in the identified neurons nor alters the 5-HT-induced response (Paupardin-Tritsch and Gerschenfeld, unpublished results).

Another important point that required clarification was how cGMP modulated the voltage-dependent Ca channels. Did cGMP act directly on the Ca channels from the inner surface of the cell in the same way as it activates the "light-sensitive" cationic channels of vertebrate phoreceptors (Fesenko et al., 1985; Hayne and Yau, 1985)? Or did cGMP regulate the Ca current of snail neurons by activating a cGMP-dependent protein kinase (PKG)? To understand how cGMP modulates the Ca current we studied, in collaboration with P. Greengard and A.C. Nairn (Paupardin-Tritsch et al., 1987), the effect of the intracellular injection of PKG in the identified ventral neurons. Since both the regulatory and the catalytic sites of PKG are located on the same peptide chain it was not possible, as in the case of PKA, to dissociate the catalytic subunit from the regulatory subunit of PKG. Therefore, we used two different procedures to activate the enzyme. In some experiments, we first injected PKG in the identified neuron and then activated it by inducing an increase in intracellular cGMP by applying low concentrations of either 5-HT or zaprinast. Using this protocol, we observed that the Ca-current increase elicited by these agents was markedly potentiated when their application was preceded by the intracellular injection of PKG. This was an indication that the exogenous PKG injected into the cell became activated by the intracellular increase in cGMP induced by 5-HT and zaprinast. In other experiments, we preactivated PKG by adding to it a low concentration of cGMP (1 mM) prior to its intracellular injection. When this pre-activated PKG was injected in the cells, we observed a small but consistent increase in Ca current (Fig. 1, a). Moreover, when pre-activated PKG was released into the cytoplasm of the identified ventral neurons from a "leaky" intracellular micropipette, the amplitude of the Ca current of the ventral neurons became increased by 200-300% (Fig. 1, b), thus showing that the activated enzyme had a similar effect to those of 5-HT and cGMP. The effects of the PKG disappeared when the enzyme was inactivated bvy heating prior to its injection.

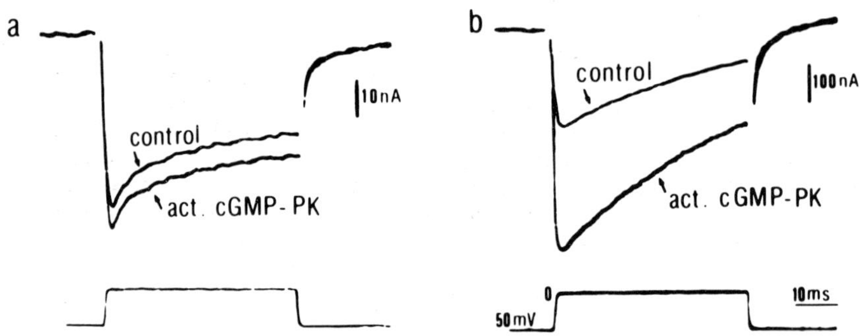

Fig. 1. Effect of the intracellular injection of cGMP-PK on the Ca current of identified snail ventral neurons bathed in a Ba/TEA saline. In **a** the cell has been impaled with two recording KCl-filled micropipettes and a third normal tip micropipette was filled with cGMP-PK pre-activated by addition of 1 μM cGMP. After recording the control Ca current, the intracellular pressure-injection of cGMP-PK (10 pulses of 40 ms duration pressure 3 bars) evoked an increase in the amplitude of the Ca current. In **b**, a control recording of the Ca current was obtained from another identified ventral neuron impaled with two recording KCl micropipettes. The neuron was then bathed again in normal saline and impaled with a third "leaky" micropipette containing cGMP-PK activated by cGMP (1 μM). When the cell was bathed again with a Ba/TEA saline it could be observed that the activated cGMP-PK released inside the cell from the "leaky" micropipette had induced a large increase in the amplitude of the Ca current. From Paupardin-Tritsch et al. (1987).

These results (Paupardin-Tritsch et al., 1987) confirm that the increase in Ca current evoked by 5-HT in the identified ventral snail neurons is mediated by cGMP which activates PKG, which in turn phosphorylates the Ca channels.

Cholinergic agonists also enhance voltage-dependent Ca current in a single identified snail neuron

Acetylcholine (ACh) is the chemical transmitter of many identified excitatory and inhibitory synapses of molluscan nervous systems where its action involves three different receptors, each of them associated either to a Cl, K channel or cation-selective channel (Tauc and Gerschenfeld, 1961, Kehoe, 1972)

To analyze whether cholinergic agonists regulate voltage-dependent Ca channels, TEA ions were excluded from the snail saline because they block ACh receptors. Therefore our experiments (Gerschenfeld and Paupardin-Tritsch 1988) were performed in a saline containing 4-aminopyridine (1 mM) and in which Ca was replaced by Ba and K by Cs. After prolonged (30-45 min) bathing in this medium, the Ca current of F1 could be almost totally blocked by nifedipene or nitrendipene (Fig. 1). In all the experiments on the cholinergic modulation of the Ca current, d-tubocurarine (10 mM) and hexamethonium (10-20 mM) were also added to the saline to block both the cationic-dependent and the Cl-dependent responses to cholinergic agonists.

When carbamylcholine (CCh, 5-25 mM), which is not inactivated by acetylcholinesterase, was applied to snail neuron F1 it evoked an increase in the amplitude in the voltage-dependent Ca current (Fig.2). This effect was reversed by wash-out. When the CCh application was prolonged, the response became desensitized. The effect of CCh persisted after prolonged intracellular injection of Cs ions (Fig. 2) or after loading the neurons with Cs using nystatin (see above).

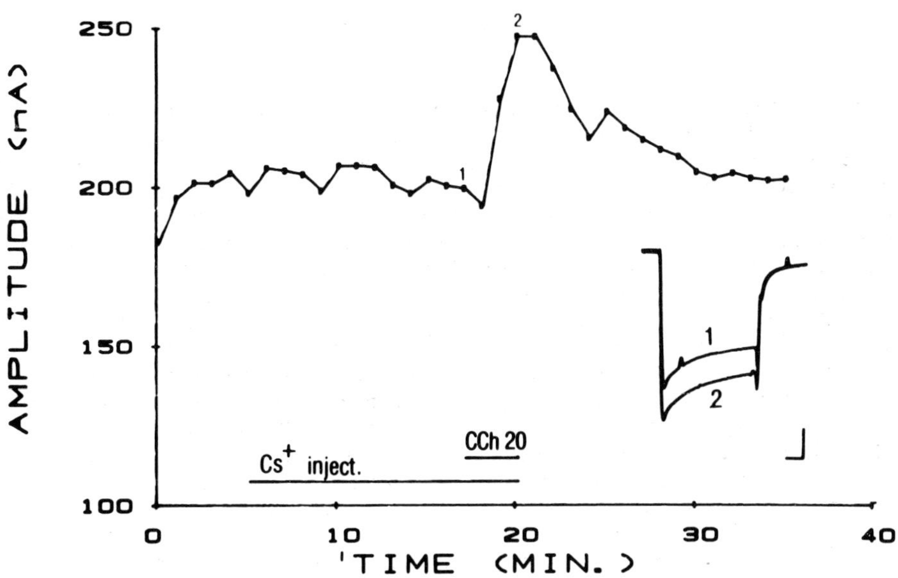

Fig. 2. Enhancement of the Ca current of a F1 neuron by carbachol (CCh). The amplitude of the Ca current was recorded as a function of time as explained in the legend of Fig. 1. The neuron was bathed in

a saline containing 1 mm 4-aminopyridine, 10 µM d-tubocurarine chloride and 10 µM hexamethonium bromide and in which Ca was replaced by Ba, and K by Cs. The cell was also impaled with a third micropipette filled with 1 M CsCl which was injected by pressure inside the cell to ensure a complete block of the outward K current components. The application of CCh (20 µM) after repetitive pressure injection of CsCl for 13 minutes evoked a marked increase in Ca current. The inset compares a recording of the control Ca current (1), with a recording of the Ca current obtained 2 minutes after the application of CCh (2).

Forskolin did not alter the Ca current of the F1 neuron or its enhancement by CCh. The extracellular application of either zaprinast or arachidonic acid had no effect on the Ca current or its modulation by CCh. In contrast, repetitive intracellular injections of EGTA prior to CCh application blocked the CCh-induced enhancement of the Ca current, suggesting that cytosolic Ca may be involved in the mechanism of the CCh-induced enhancement in Ca current.

It is known at least that the activation of two different kinds of protein-kinase involved in intracellular signalling, namely, PKC and Ca/calmodulin-dependent protein kinase (Ca/CaM-PK) requires an adequate cytosolic Ca concentration. PKC does not appear to be directly involved in the mechanism of the CCh-induced increase in Ca current because the extracellular application of diacylglycerol analogs such as dioleoylglycerol (DOG) or OAG induced a decrease in the Ca current amplitude and the blockade of the CCh-induced increase in Ca current. Therefore, the effect of PKC activation was opposite to that of CCh and moreover, it interfered in a yet undefined manner with the mechanism of CCh-induced response. In contrast, the calmodulin antagonist calmidazolium blocked the CCh-induced increase in Ca current. However, the specificity of the calmodulin antagonists is not high (it may be behaving, for instance, as an ACh antagonist). Indeed, we recently proceded to inject intracellularly Ca-CaM-PK of the Type II in the F1 neuron and observed that such injections did not affect the Ca current or its modulation by Ca.

The CCh-induced increase in Ca current involves an ACh receptor different from the three ACh receptors described in molluscan neurons (see above). The Ca current enhancement evoked by CCh and oxotremorine (10-25 µM) but not by pilocarpine (25 µM) or gallamine (25 µM). The effect of CCh is blocked by atropine (1-5 µM), pirenzepine (5-10 µM) and scopolamine (10-20 µM).

It can be concluded that the CCh-induced enhancement of the Ca current in snail neuron F1 results from the activation of an ACh receptor that resembles the type M1 muscarinic receptor of Vertebrates. Cytosolic Ca appears to play a role in the mechanism of this CCh response but the modalities by which it intervenes in the generation of the CCh-induced Ca current increase remains to be clarified.

II . NEUROTRANSMITTER-INDUCED DECREASES IN VOLTAGE-DEPENDENT CALCIUM CURRENTS IN SNAIL NEURONS

Cholecystokinin decreases irreversibly the voltage dependent Ca current of identified snail neurons. Role of PKC

Cholecystokinin is a naturally occurring peptide in identified neurons of the molluscs *Helix* (Osborne et al., 1982) and *Aplysia* (Ono, 1986). In the snail neurons D2 and F77, the 26-33 octapeptide of cholecystokinin (CCK 8, 5-20 nM) shortens the duration of the somatic Ca-dependent action potential. This effect had a latency of some minutes) and could not be reversed by prolonged wash-out.We also found that CCK 8 (5-20 nM) induced a marked decrease in the Ca current which took 7-9 minutes to reach a plateau and could not be reversed by prolonged wash out. Moreover, CCK 8 did not apparently alter any TEA- insensitive, Ca-independent, K^+ current in identified neurons (Hammond et al., 1988).

The long latency of the CCK 8-induced decrease in Ca current suggested the involvement of a second messenger mechanism. Intracellular injection of either cAMP or cGMP in the D2 and F77 neurons did not affect the amplitude of the Ca current or the CCK 8-induced decrease of this current. In contrast, the repetitive intracellular injection of EGTA for 10-15 minutes prior to the application of CCK 8, either depressed or blocked the effect of CCK 8. However, when a similar intracellular injection of EGTA was performed after the application of CCK 8, EGTA was unable to reverse the CCK 8-induced decrease in Ca current (Hammond et al., 1987).

These results suggest that cytosolic Ca plays a key role in the intracellular mechanism of the CCK 8-induced response, and accordingly, we explored whether the phospholipid intracellular messengers resulting from the activation of phospholipase C (see Berridge, 1986; Nishizuka, 1986), i.e. inositol trisphosphate (InsP3) and diacylglycerol (DAG), were involved in the CCK 8-induced modulation in Ca current. The intracellular injection of InsP3 in the neurons was found to elicit inconsistent effects on the Ca current and did not affect the CCK 8-induced response. In contrast, the application of OAG (250 nM-1 mM), decreased the Ca current in the D2 and F77 neurons and this effect of OAG was also depressed or blocked by prior intracellular injection of EGTA. When the concentration of OAG. Phorbol ester TPA, a PKC activator was also applied to the D2 and F77 neurons and found to mimic the CCK 8-induced decrease in Ca current at nanomolar concentrations. Such as in the case of CCK 8, the effect of either OAG or phorbol ester TPA could not be reversed by prolonged washing. These experiments strongly suggested that the CCK 8-induced reduction in Ca current in the D2 and F77 neurons involved PKC activation (Hammond et al., 1987).

To confirm this hypothesis, we analyzed the effect of the intracellular injection of PKC in the identified neurons. In collaboration with Paul Greengard and Angus Nairn (Hammond et al., 1987), we observed that the intracellular injection of PKC in the identified cells evoked a marked shortening of the duration of the somatic Ca-dependent action potential (Fig. 3, A). Moreover, PKC injection in the voltage-clamped neurons markedly reduced the amplitude of the Ca current (Fig. 3, B). The effect of PKC injections such as those of CCK 8, OAG and phorbol ester TPA, was irreversible. Moreover, it was abolished when PKC was inactivated by heating prior to its intracellular injection (Fig. 3, C).

The ensemble of these results suggest that the CCK 8-induced decrease in Ca current results from a chain of events in which the activation of CCK 8 receptors stimulate phospholipase C and the diacylglycerol formed, in the presence of an adequate cytosolic concentration of Ca, activates and translocates PKC which phosphorylates the Ca channels (Hammond et al., 1987). The irreversibility (or slow reversibility) of the CCK 8 effect remains to be explained. One possibility may be that a Ca-activated protease would fragment PKC, releasing the catalytic site from the control of both Ca and DAG allowing a long-lasting phosphorylation of the Ca channels (see Murray et al., 1987).

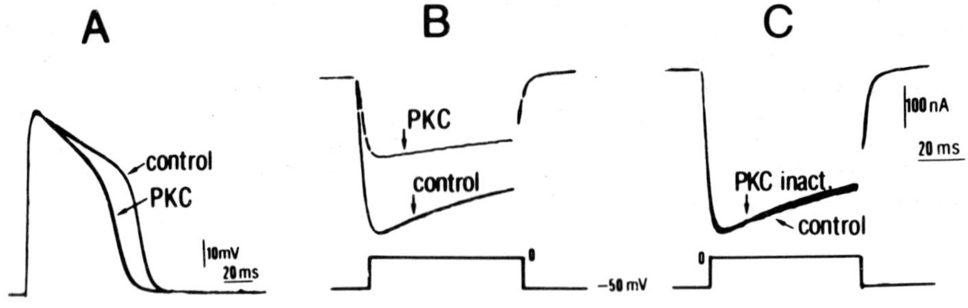

Fig. 3. Effect of the intracellular injection of PKC on the Ca-dependent action potential and on the Ca current of snail F77 neurons. **A**. In a F77 cell bathed in a TEA-containing saline, the control action potential shows a large Ca-dependent plateau phase. Intracellular pressure injection of PKC (2 pulses of 10 ms duration, pressure 2 bars) induces a decrease of the plateau phase and a shortening of the duration of the action potential. **B**. In another F77 neuron, bathed in a Ba/TEA saline, after recording the control Ca current, PKC was pressure injected inside the cells through a third micropipette (3 pulses of 10 ms, pressure 2 bars). After 7 minutes, a marked decrease of the Ca current was observed. **C**. Another F77 neuron bathed in Ba/TEA saline impaled with a third micropipette containing PKC inactivated by heating (60° for 12 minutes). The trace corresponds to two superimposed recordings of the Ca current, one in control conditions and another obtained after pressure injection (50 pulses of 20 ms duration, 2 bars) of inactivated PKC, which was totally ineffective. From Hammond et al. (1987).

Other neurotransmitter-induced regulations of the Ca channels may also involve PKC. We have already commented the probable involvement of PKC in the NA-induced decrease of Ca current in DRG neurons (Rane et al., 1989). Also in aortic muscle cells, vasopressin and somatostatin decrease the Ca influx through L-type channels and this effect is mimicked by phorbol esters (Galizzi et al., 1987). Moreover, phorbol esters and the intracellular injection of PKC increase the Ca current in other molluscan neurons, the bag-cells of Aplysia (DeRiemer et al., 1985) and phorbol esters seem to activate or unmask a new population of voltage-dependent Ca channels in these bag cells (Strong et al. 1987).

Dopamine reversibly decreases the voltage dependent calcium current in identified snail neurons. Role of a snail G protein related to mammalian Go.

In contrast to the irreversible effect of CCK 8 on the D2 and F77 snail neurons, the application of dopamine (DA, 1-5 µM) to these and other identified cells evokes a shortening of the duration of their somatic Ca-dependent action potential resulting from a decrease in the voltage-dependent Ca current (Fig. 4, A). The DA-induced responses are easily reversed by wash-out. The maximal effect of DA (1-5 µM), consists in a 30-35 % reduction of the initial Ca current (Paupardin-Tritsch et al., 1985).

The intracellular injection of either cAMP or cGMP, and the application of forskolin do not affect the DA-induced reduction of Ca current. Moreover, the intracellular injection of EGTA does not block the DA-induced decrease in Ca current indicating that cytosolic Ca is not involved in the generation of the DA-induced response. Extracellular application of arachidonic acid (50 µM) altered neither the Ca current nor its reduction by DA (Paupardin-Tritsch and Gerschenfeld, unpublished).

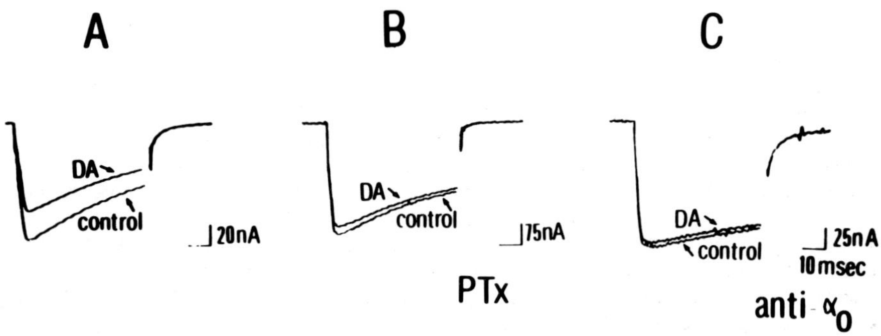

Fig. 4. **A.** DA-induced Ca current reduction in a snail D2 neuron bathed in a Ba/TEA saline. **B.** The intracellular pressure injection of PTX in another D2 neuron almost totally blocked the effect of DA on the Ca current. PTX was first activated by incubation with 25 mM dithithreitol at pH 7 for 30 minutes at 20°C and then diluted to a final concentration of 10 µM and injected in the cell by pressure for 30 minutes. The effect of DA was tested 60 minutes after the PTX injection to allow its intracellular diffusion. **C.** Intracellular injection of anti-α_O antibody blocks the DA-induced decrease in Ca current in a F77 neuron. After recording the control current the antibody was injected for 15 minutes and a 20 minutes period was allowed for the anti-α_O to diffuse inside the cell.

The intervention of a PTX-sensitive G protein having been postulated in other neurotransmitter-induced Ca current decreases (see Dunlap et al. 1987; Hescheler et al., 1987), we explored, in collaboration with J. Bockaert V. Homburger and B. Rouot (Centre CNRS-INSERM de Pharmacologie-Endocrinologie Montpellier), the possible involvement of a G protein in the DA-induced decrease in Ca current (see Harris-Warrick et al. 1988).

To confirm that a G protein intervened in the DA-induced decrease in Ca current, we injected intracellularly non-hydrolysable GTP analogs such as GTPγS and Gpp(NH)p in the identified neurons. These compounds mimicked the effect of DA and blocked the DA-induced reduction in Ca current probably by uncoupling of the DA receptors from the G proteins (Breitweiser and Szabo 1985). The maximal Ca current reduction induced by GTPγS was similar to that elicited by DA, i.e., 30-35%.

We examined next the effect of PTX on the DA-induced response. The intracellular injection of PTX (pre-activated by incubation with 25 nM dithiothreitol) blocked the DA-induced decrease in Ca current (Fig. 4, B). When PTX was inactivated by heating prior to its intracellular injection, it had no effect on the Ca current or on its modulation by DA.

PTX is known to ADP-ribosylate two different G-proteins present in bovine brain : Go and Gi (see Spiegel, 1987; Ross, 1989). However, in a membrane fraction of the nervous tissue of the snail *Helix aspersa*, PTX was found to ADP-ribosylate only one substrate (Homburger et al., 1987): the α subunit of a G protein of 40 KDa, a molecular mass between those of bovine brain α_o (39 KDa) and α_i (41 KDa). To investigate whether this snail 40 KDa α subunit was related to bovine brain α_o, we used an affinity purified polyclonal antibody raised against bovine brain α_o (anti-α_o, see Toutant et al., 1987). This anti-α_o antibody was found to recognize in immunoblots the 40 KDa snail α subunit, but did not recognize the α subunits of Gs, Gi and β of transducine and none of the α_{40} subunits found in bovine brain, C6 glioma cells or adrenal chromaffin granules (Toutant et al., 1987; Brabet et al., 1988). The intracellular injection of this anti-α_o antibody in the D2 and F77 neurons depressed or blocked of the DA-induced decrease of Ca-current (Fig. 4, C). This effect of the anti-α_o antibody disappeared when, prior to its intracellular injection the antibody was inactivated by heating.

In view of the immunological relationship between brain a_o and snail α_{40} subunit, we explored next whether the intracellular injection of α_o subunit purified from bovine brain had an effect on the Ca current of the identified neurons. Prior to its injection, the mammalian α_o was activated with GTPγS (10 μM), in the presence of 10 mM $MgCl_2$. The intracellular injection of the activated α_o subunit evoked a gradual and progressive decrease in Ca current, which was much larger than the 30-35% maximal reduction obtained with DA. Even though, further application of DA was still able to decrease the Ca as usual (Harris-Warrick et al., 1988). Therefore the action of injected α_o was not limited by the number of DA receptors or endogenous α_{40} subunits as was probably the case for DA and the irreversible GTP analogs and thus α_o could exert a modulatory effect on a larger number of Ca channels. Inspite of this effect, DA was still able to stimulate the endogenous protein because it was neither disconnected from the DA receptors, as in the case of the injections of GTPγS, nor inactivated, as in the case of the PTX or anti-α_o antibody injections (Harris-Warrick et al., 1988).

These results strongly suggest that the 40 KDa α subunit of a PTX-sensitive G protein of snail nervous tissue, immunologically and functionally related to mammalian brain α_o, mediates an essential step in the mechanism of the DA-induced decrease of Ca current in the D2 and F77 neurons of *Helix* . Having already ruled out an involvement of the major known second messengers in the generation of the DA-induced decrease in Ca current, the existence of a direct coupling of the DA receptors to the Ca channels by the α_{40} subunit remains to be proven.

CONCLUDING REMARKS

The classical idea that neurotransmitter receptors and ionic channels are part of the same protein macromolecule (Fatt and Katz, 1951) has been confirmed by modern studies (see Barnard et al., 1987) of the nicotinic cholinergic receptor of vertebrate neuromuscular junctions and fish electroplaques (Noda et al., 1983; see Changeux et al., 1987), the GABA-A receptor of brain synapses (Schofield et al., 1987) and the glycine receptor of spinal cord synapses (Grenningloh et al., 1987). However, many neurotransmitter receptor molecules have been shown to be independent from the ionic channel that they gate or regulate. In the latter cases, G-proteins, second messengers and protein kinases have been shown to couple the neurotransmitter receptors to the pre- or postsynaptic ionic channels.

As summarized above, from the work of other authors and from our own work it is clear that a great diversity of intracellular mechanisms underly the neurotransmitter-induced regulation of Ca channels in excitable cells. From the available exemples of neurotransmitter-induced enhancements of voltage-dependent Ca current it may be concluded at present that they generally involve phosphorylation of the channels by at least one of three protein kinases: the cAMP-dependent kinase (Osterrieder et al., 1982; Brum et al., 1983), the cGMP-dependent kinase (Paupardin-Tritsch et al., 1987) and protein kinase C (De Riemer et al., 1985).

Phosphorylation also appears to play a role in the mechanism of some neurotransmitter-induced decreases in voltage-dependent Ca current but, at present, only PKC has been shown to be involved in such kind of Ca current modulation (Hammond et al., 1987; Galizzi et al., 1987; Rane et al., 1989). An ACh-induced decrease in Ca current mediated by muscarinic receptors in cardiac muscle fibres has been found to be due to a decrease in cAMP-dependent phosphorylation resulting from an ACh-induced decrease in the intracellular cAMP concentration (Fischmeister and Harzell, 1986). For other known cases of neurotransmitter-induced decreases in Ca current, the most attractive explanation would be that they involve a direct coupling of the neurotransmitter receptor to the Ca channels via a G protein (see Dunlap et al., 1987) without any involvement of a second messenger system (see Yatani et al., 1987).

Acknowledgements

Our work was supported by the Centre National de la Recherche Scientifique, France (URA 295), the Institut National de la Santé et la Recherche Médicale, France, and the Université Pierre et Marie Curie, Paris France.

REFERENCES

Barnard E.A., Darlison M.G., and Seeburg, P. (1987) Molecular biology of the $GABA_A$ receptor: the receptor/channel superfamily. Trends Neurosci. **12**: 502-509

Bean, B.P. (1989) Classes of calcium channels in vertebrate cells. Ann. Rev. Physiol. **51**: 367-384

Bean B.P., Nowycky, M.C., Tsien R.W. (1984) β-adrenergic modulation of calcium channels in frog ventricular heart cells. Nature **307**: 371-375

Berridge M.J. (1986) Inositol phosphates as second messengers. In: J.W. Putney (ed.) Phosphoinositides and receptor mechanisms, pp. 25-39, New York : Alan Liss

Brabet, P., Dumuis, A., Sebben, M., Pantaloni, C., Bockaert, J., and Homburger, V. (1988) Immunocytochemical localization of the guanine nucleotide-binding protein Go in primary cultures of neuronal and glial cells. J. Neurosci. **8**: 701-708

Breitweiser, G.E., and Szabo, G. (1985) Uncoupling of cardiac muscarinic and B-adrenergic receptors from ion channels by a guanidine nucleotide analog. Nature **317**: 538-540
Brum, G., Flockerzi, V., Hofman, F., Osterrieder., W., and Trautwein W (1983) Injection of catalytic subunit of cAMP-dependent protein kinase into isolated myocytes. Pflügers Arch. **398**: 146-154
Brum., G., Osterrieder, W., and Trautwein, W. (1984) Beta-adrenergic increase in the calcium conductance of cardiac myocytes studied with the patch-clamp. Pflügers Arch. **401**: 111-118
Changeux J.P., Devilliers-Thiery, A., and Chemouilly, P. (1984) Acetylcholine receptor: an allosteric protein. Science **225**: 1335-1345
DeRiemer, S.A., Strong, J.A., Albert, K.A., Greengard, P., and Kaczmarek, L.K. (1985) Enhancement of calcium current in Aplysia neurones by phorbol-ester and protein kinase C. Nature **313**: 313-316
Dolphin, A.C., and Scott, R.H. (1987) Calcium channel currents and their inhibition by (-)-baclofen in rat sensory neurones: modulation by guanine nucleotides. J. Physiol. **386**: 1-17
Dunlap, K., and Fischbach, G.D. (1980) Neurotransmitters decrease the calcium conductance activated by depolarization of embryonic chick sensory neurones. J. Physiol.**317**: 519-535
Dunlap, K., Holz, G.G., and Rane, S.G. (1987) G proteins as regulators of ion channel function. Trends Neurosci. **10**: 241-244
Fatt, P., and Katz, B. (1951) An analysis of the end-plate potential recorded with an intra-cellular microelectrode. J. Physiol. **115**: 320-370
Fesenko, E.E., Kolesnikov, S.S., and Lyubarsky, A.L. (1985) Induction by cGMP of cationic conductance in plasma membrane of retinal rod outer segment. Nature **313**: 310-313
Fischmeister, R., and Harzell, H.C. (1986) Mechanism of action of acetylcholine on calcium current on single cells from frog ventricle. J. Physiol. **376**: 183-202
Galizzi, J.P., Qar, J., Fosset, M., Van Renterghem, C., and Lazdunski, M. (1987) Regulation of calcium channels in aortic cells by protein kinase activators (diacylglycerol et phorbol esters) and by peptides (vasopressin and bombesin) that stimulate phosphoinositide breakdown. J. Biol. Chem. **15**: 6947-6950
Galvan, M., and Adams P.R. (1982) Control of calcium current in rat sympathetic neurons by norepinephrine. Brain Res. **244**: 135-144
Gerschenfeld, H.M., and Paupardin-Tritsch, D. (1988) Acetylcholine enhances calcium current in a single identified snail neuron. Soc. Neurosci. Abstr. **14**: 754
Goldberg, N.D., and Haddox, M.K. (1977) Cyclic GMP metabolism and involvement in biological regulation. Ann. Rev. Biochem. **46**: 823-896
Greengard, P. (1978) Cyclic nucleotides, phosphorylated proteins and neuronal function, New York: Raven Press
Grenningloh, G., Rienitz, A., Schmitt, B., Methfessel, C., Gundelfinger, E.D. and Betz, H. (1987) The strychnine-binding subunit of the glycine receptor shows homology with nicotinic acetylcholine receptors. Nature **28**: 215-219
Hammond, C., Paupardin-Tritsch, D., Nairn, A.C., Greengard, P., and Gerschenfeld, H.M. (1987) Cholecystokinin induces a decrease in Ca current in snail neurons that appears to be mediated by protein kinase C. Nature **325**: 809-811
Harris-Warrick, R., Hammond, C., Paupardin-Tritsch, D., Homburger, V., Rouot B., Bockaert, J., and Gerschenfeld, H.M. (1988) An α_{40} subunit of a GTP-binding protein immunologically related to Go

mediates a dopamine-induced decrease of calcium current in snail neurones. Neuron **1**: 27-32

Hayne, L., and Yau K.W. (1985) Cyclic GMP-sensitive conductance in outer segment membrane of catfish cones. Nature **317**: 61-64

Hescheler, J., Rosenthal, W., Trautwein, W., and Schultz, G. (1987) The GTP-binding protein, Go, regulates neuronal calcium channels. Nature **325** 445-447

Hoffman F., Nastainczyk, W., Röhrkasten, A., Schneider, T., and Sieber, M. (1987) Regulation of L-type calcium channel. Trends Bioch. Sci. **8**: 393-398

Holz, G.G., Rane, S.G., and Dunlap, K. (1986) GTP-binding proteins mediate transmitter inhibition of voltage-dependent calcium channels. Nature **319**: 670-672

Homburger, V., Brabet, O., Audigier, Y., Pantaloni, C., Bockaert, J, and Rouot, B. (1987) Immunological localization of the GTP-binding protein Go in different tissues of vertebrates and invertebrates. Mol. Pharmac. **31**: 313-319

Horn, J.P., and McAffee, D.A. (1980) Alpha adrenergic inhibition of calcium-dependent potentials in rat sympathetic neurones. J. Physiol. **301**: 109-204

Hosey, M.M., and Lazdunski, M. (1988) Calcium channels: molecular pharmacology, structure and regulation. Membr. Biol. **104**: 81-105

Kehoe, J.S. (1972) Three acetylcholine receptors inAplysia neurones. J. Physiol. **225**: 115-146

Levitan, I (1988) Modulation of ion channels in neurons and other cells. Ann. Rev. Neurosci. **11**: 119-136

Murray, A.W., Fournier, A., and Hardy, S.J. (1987) Proteolytic activation of protein kinase C: a physiological reaction ? Trends Bioch. Sci. **12**: 53-54

Nishizuka, N. (1986) Studies and perspectives of protein kinase C. Science **233**: 305-312

Noda, M., Takahashi, H., Tanabe, T., Toyosato, S., Kikyotani, S., Furutani Y., Takashima, H., Inayama, S., Miyata, T., Numa, S. (1983) Structural homology of Torpedo californica acetylcholine receptors subunits. Nature **305**: 818-223

Ono, J. (1986) Localization and identification of neurons with cholecystokinin and gastrin-like immunoreactivity in wholemounts of Aplysia ganglia. Neurosci. **18**: 957-974

Osborne, N.N., Cuello, .A.C., and Dockeray, G.J. (1982) Substance P cholecystokinin and serotonin in a giant neuron. Science **216**: 409-411

Osterrieder, W., Brum, G., Hescheler, J., Trautwein, W., Flockerzi, V., and Hofman, F. (1982) Injection of subunits of cyclic AMP-dependent protein kinase into cardiac myocytes modulates Ca current. Nature **298**: 576-57838

Paupardin-Tritsch, D., Colombaioni, L., Deterre, P., and Gerschenfeld, H.M. (1985) Two different mechanisms of calcium spike modulation by dopamine. J. Neurosci. **5**: 2522-2532

Paupardin-Tritsch, D., Hammond, C., and Gerschenfeld, H.M. (1986) Serotonin and cyclic GMP both induce an increase of the calcium current in the same identified molluscan neurones. J. Neurosci. **6**: 2715-2723

Paupardin-Tritsch, D., Hammond, C., Gerschenfeld, H.M., Nairn, A.C. and Greengard, P. (1986) cGMP-dependent protein kinase enhances Ca current and and potentiates the serotonin-induced increase of Ca current in identified snail neurones. Nature **323**: 812-814

Rane, S.G. and Dunlap, K. (1986) Kinase activator 1,2 oleylacetylglycerol attenuates voltage-dependent calcium current in sensory neurones. Proc. Natl. Acad. Sci. USA **83**:184-188

Rane, S.G., Walsh, M.P., McDonald, J.R., and Dunlap, K. (1989) Specific inhibitors of protein kinase C block transmitter-induced modulation of sensory neuron calcium current. Neuron **3**: 239-245

Reuter, H., Cachelin, A.B., De Peyer, J.E., and Kobuku, S. (1983) Modulation of calcium channels in cultured cardiac cells by isoproterenol et 8-bromo-cAMP. Cold Spring Harb. Symp. Quant. Biol. **48**: 193-200

Ross, E.M. (1989) Signal sorting and amplification through G-coupled receptors. Neuron **3**: 141-152

Schofield P.R., Darlison, M.G., Fujita, N., Burt, D.R., Stephenson, F.A. Rodriguez, H., Rhee, L., Ramachandran, J., Reale, V., Glencorse, T.A. Seeburg, P., and Barnard, E. (1987) Sequence and functional expression of the $GABA_A$ receptor shows a ligand-gated receptor super-family. Nature **328**: 221-227

Spiegel, A.M. (1987) Signal transduction by guanine nucleotide binding proteins. Mol. Cell Endocrinol. **49**: 1-16

Strong, J.A., Fox, A.P., Tsien, R.W., and Kaczmarek, L.K. (1987) Stimulation of protein kinase C recruits covert calcium channels in Aplysia cells. Nature **325**: 714-717

Tauc, L., and Gerschenfeld, H.M. (1961) Cholinergic transmission mechanism for both excitation and inhibition in molluscan central synapses. Nature **192**: 366-367

Tillotson, D. (1979) Inactivation of Ca-conductance on entry of Ca ions in molluscan neurones. Proc. Natl. Acad. Sci. USA **76**: 1497-1500

Toutant, M., Aunis, D., Bockaert, J., Homburger, V., and Rouot, B. (1987) Presence of three Pertussis toxin substrates and Go immunoreactivity in both plasma and granule membranes of chromaffin cells. FEBS Lett. **215**: 339-344

Tsien, R.W., Lipscombe, D., Madison, D.V., Bley, K.R., and Fox A.P. (1988) Multiple types of calcium channels and their selective modulation. Trends Neurosci. **11**: 431-438

Waldman, S.A., and Murad, F. (1987) Cyclic GMP synthesis and function. Pharmacol. Rev. **39**: 163-193

Winquist, R.J., Faison, E.P., Waldman, S.A., Schwartz, K., Murad, F., and Rapoport, R.M. (1984) Atrial natriuretic factor elicits a endothelium-independent relaxation and activates particulate guanylate cyclase in vascular smooth muscle. Proc. Natl. Acad. Sci. USA **81**: 7661-7664

Yatani, A., Codina, J., Brown, A.M., and Birnbaumer, L. (1987) Direct activation of mammalian atrial muscarinic potassium channels by GTP regulatory protein Gk. Science **235**: 207-211

Action of Ca^{2+} agonists/antagonists in mammalian peripheral neurons

E. Carbone[*,$] , F. Clementi[o], A. Formenti[x], A. Pollo[*] and E. Sher[o]

[*] Dept. Anatomy and Human Physiology, I-10125 Torino
[o] Dept. Medical Pharmacology, Ctr. Cytopharmacology C.N.R., I-20129 Milano
[x] II Inst. Human Physiology, I-20152 Milano (Italy)
[$] To whom reprint requests should be addressed

Abstract

The action of several ligands on the low- (LVA,T) and high-threshold (HVA,L and N) Ca channels of adult rat sensory neurons and human neuroblastoma IMR32 cells has been investigated. In both cell types, 40 μM Cd^{2+} and 6.4 μM ω-Conotoxin (ω-CgTx) selectively blocked the HVA channels, sparing the majority of LVA channels that were antagonized by amiloride and Ni^{2+}. In 50% of the cells, however, ω-CgTx spared also a 15% of HVA channels that proved to be sensitive to BAY K 8644. The agonistic action of BAY K 8644 on ω-CgTx-resistant HVA channels caused a large Ba current increase, prolonged current deactivation and acceleration of HVA channels inactivation that was particularly evident in adult rat DRG.

Introduction

Pharmacological identification of neuronal Ca channels is conditional for understanding the complexity of neuronal functioning. At present, a number of Ca channel ligands have been proved effective in distinguishing low-threshold from high-threshold Ca channels (Carbone and Lux, 1984; Nowycky et al., 1985a). In a variety of neurons, micromolar concentrations of Cd^{2+} and ω-CgTx are sufficient to depress HVA Ca currents, sparing most of the LVA currents (see Tsien et al., 1988). In contrast, the K^+ sparing diuretic amiloride (500 μM) selectively blocks the LVA Ca currents in mouse neuroblastoma, chick DRG and rat sensory neurons (Tang et al., 1988; Carbone et al., 1989). Also Ni^{2+} blocks efficiently LVA channels but its action appears species-specific. It is prominent in avian sensory neurons (Fox et al., 1987; Carbone et al.,1987) but weak and unselective in adult rat DRG (Ferroni et al., 1989; Formenti et al., 1989) and human neuroblastoma cells (Carbone et al., 1989).

Still controversial, however, remains the classical identification of high threshold Ca channels into L- and N-subtypes (Nowycky et al., 1985a). Recent reports find inconsistencies with common classifications and provide a more reasonable way to distinguish HVA channels by their sensitivity to ω-CgTx and dihydropyridines (DHP) (Sher et al., 1988, Aosaki and Kasai, 1989; Plummer et al., 1989; Carbone et al., 1989).

Here we report that, based on sensitivity to Ca-antagonists/agonists, we could distinguish different Ca current components in mammalian peripheral neurons: a low-threshold and two high-threshold (one ω-CgTx-sensitive and one DHP-sensitive). The two HVA components were otherwise poorly resolved in terms of their inactivation kinetics, range of activation and sensitivity to holding potentials (see Carbone and Lux, 1987; Swandulla and Armstrong, 1988). The low-threshold current is shown to persist in the presence of ω-CgTx and Cd^{2+} but revealed a weaker sensitivity to Ni^{2+} and amiloride than in other neurons (Fox et al., 1987; Carbone et al., 1987; Tang et al., 1988). Our findings suggest that currently used criteria for identifying multiple types of neuronal Ca channels (T, L, N), based on activation-inactivation kinetics, Ca/Ba permeability and sensitivity to holding potentials can be misleading if not supported by pharmacological assays.

Materials and Methods

Cell Culture

In vitro differentiated human neuroblastoma IMR32 cells were grown in culture as already described (Clementi et al., 1986). Thoracic and lumbar dorsal root ganglia were isolated from rats older than 7 weeks as described by Scott (1982). The anesthetized animals were decapitated and ganglia collected after dorsal laminectomy and removal of the spinal cord. The ganglia were then minced with fine iridectomy scissors in a cold Ca-free Tyrode solution. Cell dissociation was achieved by sequential incubation (37°C) of the tissue in a Ca-free Tyrode solution containing first 1.2 mg/ml collagenase (45 min) and then 0.4 mg/ml Trypsin (20 min) , followed by gentle trituration with a fine tip pasteur pipette. After centrifugation the cells (30 to 50 µm in diameter) were plated on collagene-coated petri dishes and maintained in normal Tyrode at 37°C in a air humidified incubator.

Patch-clamp recordings and solutions

Whole-cell membrane currents were measured according to the method of Hamill et al.,1981. Details on patch-pipette fabrication, I-V converter, stimulation and data acquisition are given elsewhere (Carbone and Lux, 1984; 1987). The external bath contained Ca or Ba and choline while the pipette filling solution contained Cs and TEA (see Carbone and Lux, 1987).

Results

LVA and HVA Ca currents in adult rat DRG and IMR32 neuroblastoma cells

Adult rat DRG and IMR32 cells were found to possess low- and high-threshold Ca currents with properties close to those described in other neurons (Carbone and Lux, 1984). LVA currents activated positive to -50 mV (in 20 mM Ca_o). Their inactivation was fast, complete in 200 ms and sharply voltage dependent (Fig.1a, left). HVA currents activated positive to -10 mV and had slow and incomplete inactivation (Fig.1a, right). As in chick and rat embryonic DRG (Carbone and Lux, 1987), their rate of inactivation decreased with increasing membrane depolarization.

Other features provided evidence for two classes of

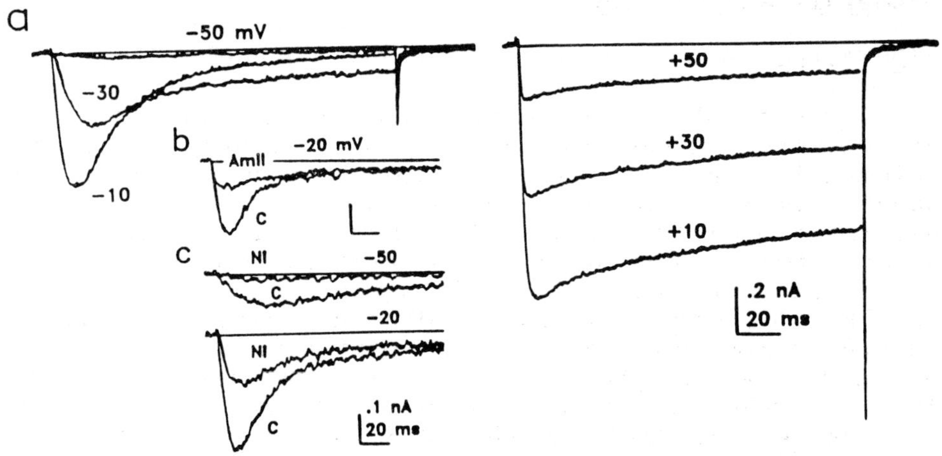

Fig.1- a) Family of Ca currents recorded from an adult rat DRG neuron bathed in 20 mM Ca_o at the potential indicated. Vh -90 mV. b) Blocking action of Amiloride on LVA Ca currents in 5 mM Ca_o. Current traces were obtained before (C) and after application of 500 μM amiloride to the bath. Vh -90 mV. c) Action of 100 μM Ni^{2+} on LVA Ca currents in 5 mM Ca_o at the potentials indicated.

Ca channels in adult rat DRG and IMR32 cells: i) Replacing Ca_o with Ba_o decreased by 10 to 20% the size of LVA currents and doubled that of HVA currents. ii) LVA currents where fully inactivated at holding potentials positive to -60 mV and iii) LVA currents survived longer than HVA currents during prolonged cell dialysis (Fenwick et al., 1982).

LVA channels blockers

As in mouse neuroblastoma cells (Tang et al., 1988), bath application of 500 μM amiloride caused a selective depression of fast inactivating LVA currents in adult rat DRGs (Fig.1b). The action of amiloride was complete in few seconds, fully reversible and independent of membrane potential. We could never observe full block of LVA currents, even at higher amiloride concentrations (1 mM). This suggests either the presence of two distinct LVA channels in our cells or a partial modulatory action of the drug on a LVA-channel type.

The blocking action of Ni^{2+} on LVA currents showed interesting features (Fig.1c). In preliminary experiments with 100 μM Ni^{2+} LVA currents were strongly depressed at potential below -40 mV but only weakly reduced above -20 mV. Thus, like Mg^{2+} and Cd^{2+} (Fukushima and Hagiwara, 1985; Lansmann et al., 1986; Lux et al.,1989; Swandulla and Armstrong,1989) Ni^{2+} may block Ca^{2+} passage through open LVA channels by binding to a site inside the channel sensing the intramembrane electric field. Increasing negative membrane voltages would enhance the block by Ni^{2+}, while positive potentials would facilitate the clearing of Ni^{2+} from occluded channels.

HVA channels blockers

As in other neurons, HVA Ca channels can be selectively blocked by micromolar amounts of Cd^{2+} and ω-CgTx. In half of the IMR32 cells and adult rat DRGs tested, ω-CgTx (6.4 μM) caused a nearly complete block of HVA Ca currents sparing a small transient LVA component (see Fig.2a). Also Cd^{2+} was very effective in selectively blocking HVA currents. At concentrations around 40 μM, Cd^{2+} fully blocked the HVA channels with little effects on LVA channels (Fig.2b).

The antagonistic action of 1 μM nitrendipine (NTP) was more puzzling. NTP was uneffective when applied at very negative holding potentials (-90 mV; Fig.2c top), but caused a nearly 50% depression of HVA currents when the cell was held at -50 mV holding potential (Fig. 2c bottom). NTP action, however, showed little sign of recovery upon washing, thus complicating the separation of NTP blockade from the fast "run down" of HVA channels at this holding potential (Fig.2c bottom).

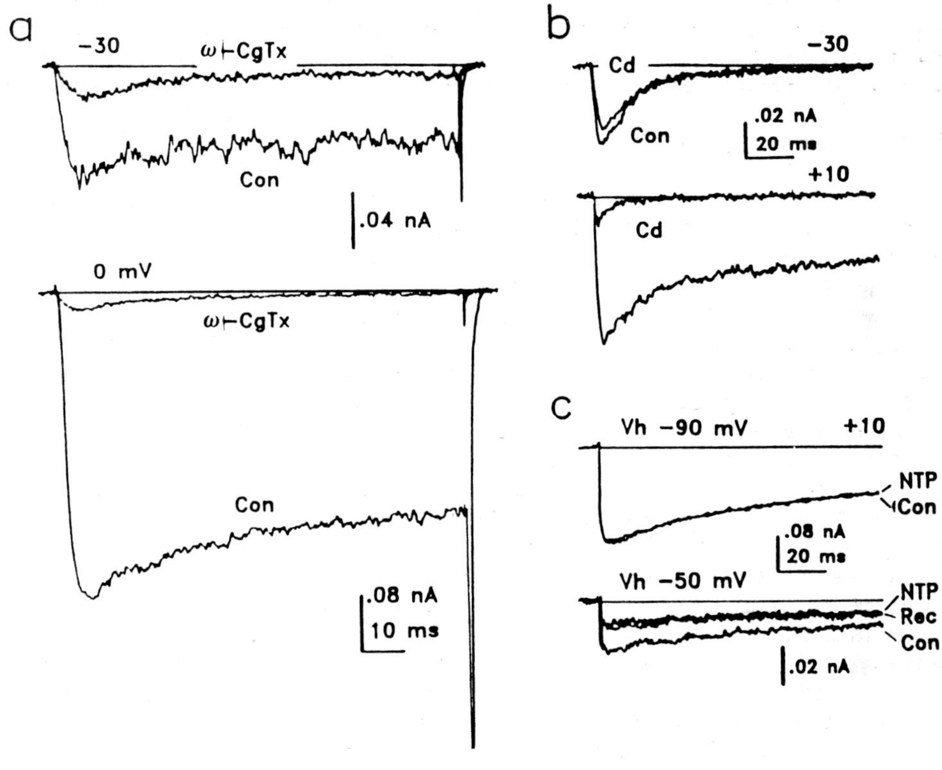

Fig 2- Antagonistic actions of 6.4 µM ω⊢CgTx (a), 40 µM Cd^{2+} (b) and 1 µM NTP (c) on HVA Ba currents in a human neuroblastoma IMR32 cell. The records were obtained before (Con) and after addition of the antagonist to the bath. Vh -90 mV.

ω⊢CgTx and BAY K 8644 distinguish two classes of HVA Ca channels

Contrary to previous reports in chick DRG, about 50% of human neuroblastoma and DRG neurons preincubated in saturating concentrations of ω⊢CgTx (6.4 µM for 30 min) exhibited residual HVA currents. The average size of ω⊢CgTx-resistant currents was 15 to 20% that of Ca currents in untreated cells (n=32), suggesting a predominance of ω⊢CgTx-sensitive Ca channels in mammalian peripheral neurons. Fig.3a shows the kinetic features of ω⊢CgTx-sensitive and ω⊢CgTx-resistant Ba currents in a human IMR32 cell acutely treated with 6.4 μM ω-CgTx. The toxin blocked about 85% of the control current with little changes to the activation-inactivation kinetics and voltage-dependence of spared HVA channels (fig. 2b).

Residual ω-CgTx-insensitive HVA channels showed an extraordinary sensitivity to BAY K 8644. Addition of 1 μM BAY K 8644 after ω-CgTx application caused a 20 mV hyperpolarizing shift of the peak I/V relationship (open circles in Fig.3b), a nearly 3-fold increase of peak Ba currents, and a prolongation of the deactivation time course at -50 mV.

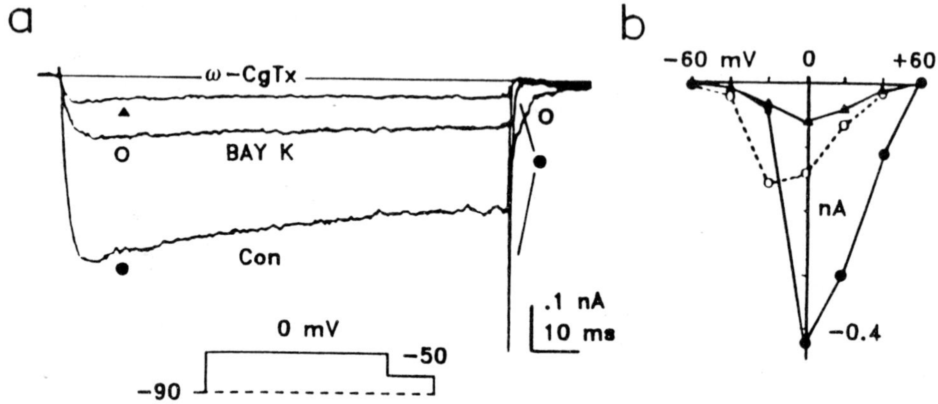

Fig.3- a) Time course of ω-CgTx- and DHP-sensitive HVA Ba currents. The records were obtained from a human neuroblastoma IMR32 cell before (filled circles), 2 min after application of 6.4 μM ω-CgTx (filled triangles) and in the presence of 1 μM BAY K 8644 (open circles) in 10 mM Ba. b) Current-voltage relationships determined at the peak of Ba currents of panel a.

The agonistic action of BAY K 8644

In IMR32 cells and adult rat DRG poisoned with ω-CgTx, the agonistic action of BAY K 8644 was maximal at very negative holding potentials (Vh -90 mV). BAY K 8644 action was fully reversible and caused always HVA Ba current increase and prolongations of HVA channel deactivation (about one order of magnitude on return to -50 mV; Fig. 4). There was, however, a different modulatory action of BAY K 8644 on the HVA channel inactivation of the two types of neurons (Fig.4). In rat DRG, BAY K 8644 caused a sharp acceleration of HVA channel inactivation which was virtually absent in human IMR32 cells. This is reminescent of the BAY K-induced Ca channel inactivation observed in cardiac L-type channel (Hess et al., 1984; Brown et al., 1984; Sanguinetti et al., 1986), suggesting pharmacological similarities among neuronal and cardiac DHP-sensitive Ca channels. Indeed, the weak sensitivity of neuronal Ca channels to other DHP-derivatives (nitrendipine, nifedipine etc...) and the variable action of BAY K 8644 on different types of neurons (see Fig. 4), suggest differences among DHP-receptors and/or different interactions between DHP-receptors and Ca channels gating.

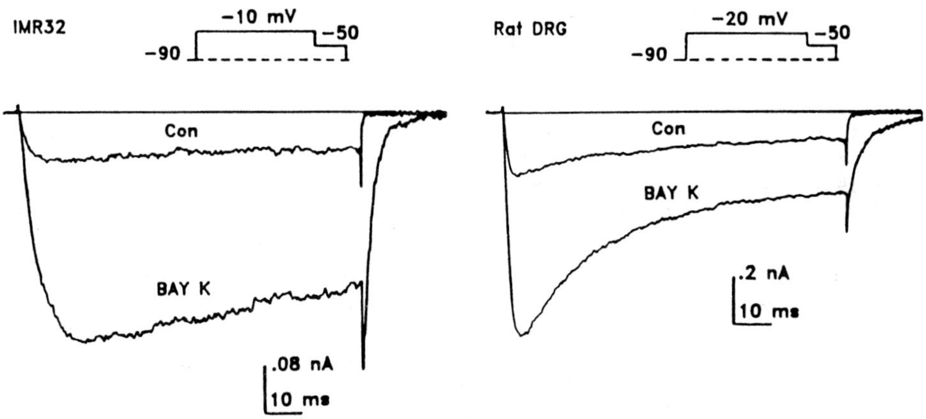

Fig.4- Action of BAY K 8644 on |ω-CgTx-resistant Ba currents in a human neuroblastoma IMR32 cell (left) and an adult rat DRG (right). Current traces were recorded before (Con) and during addition of 1 μM BAY K 8644. Pulse protocols as indicated. Vh -90 mV.

Discussion

Our data show that adult rat DRGs and IMR32 human neuroblastoma cells possess both low- and high-threshold Ca channels with distinct kinetics and sensitivity to drugs. LVA channels possess similar voltage-dependent kinetics and resistance to Cd^{2+} and |ω-CgTx but a weaker sensitivity to Ni^{2+} and amiloride than in other neurons (Fox et al., 1987; Carbone et al., 1987; Tang et al, 1988). Ni^{2+} and amiloride were, on the other hand, rather effective to block the LVA channels of two clonal lines of mouse neuroblastoma (NB-N18 and NB-41A3; Augusti-Tocco and Carbone,unpublished observations). We conclude therefore that either functionally similar LVA channels display some variability to Ca-antagonists depending on the cell type, or that multiple types of LVA channels coexist in neurons.

Based on the activation-inactivation kinetics and sensitivity to Cd^{2+}, the HVA currents of IMR32 cells and adult rat DRG are nearly indistinguishable from those of other neurons (Carbone and Lux, 1987; Swandulla and Armstrong, 1988; Plummer et al., 1989). They would hardly suggest the existence of multiple HVA components in these neurons (see also Ferroni et al., 1989). In contrast to this, HVA currents in human IMR32 cells and adult rat DRGs displayed clear differential sensitivity to BAY K 8644 and ω-CgTx. Saturating concentrations of ω-CgTx, which proved to exert full block in avian DRG (McCleskey et al., 1987; Carbone and Lux, 1989), only partly depress the HVA currents in our cells (85%). BAY K 8644 action, on the other hand, appeared maximal on ω-CgTx-treated neurons but smaller and variable in untreated cells. Although kinetically unresolved, HVA channels can be distinguished in two classes one more sensitive to ω-CgTx and the other to DHP.

Identification of ω-CgTx -sensitive channels with N-types Ca channels and DHP-sensitive with L-types (Plummer et al., 1989; Aosaki and Kasai, 1989) would imply a substantial redefiniton of the N channel concept. In this case the N channel would contribute to most of the HVA current, including transient and long lasting components, and not only to fast HVA current decays as proposed by Nowycky et al., 1985a. Indeed, this redefinition of neuronal N channels fits rather closely that of the HVA channel given by Carbone and Lux (1984; 1987).

Among DHP-compounds we found the action of BAY K 8644 the most suitable for HVA currents separation. BAY K 8644 acts reversibly and independently of holding potential (-90 to -50 mV) producing unequivocal Ba current increases and marked tail current prolongations. In this respect our data fit well previous observations on BAY K 8644-treated neurons (Nowycky et al., 1985b; Plummer et al., 1989) and cardiac cells (Hess et al., 1984; Brown et al., 1984), showing prolongations of the mean open time of L-type Ca channels. Our data, however, underly differences between neuronal and cardiac DHP-sensitive channels. In neurons, BAY K 8644 action varies depending on the cell type (see Fig.4) and nitrendipine is a weak HVA channel antagonist. A possibility is that neuronal and cardiac DHP-receptors differ in their affinity for various DHP-compounds, and that given a high affinity binding (as for BAY K 8644 in our cells) the DHP-modulatory action on Ca channels may not be stereotyped.

References

Aosaki, T. and Kasai, H. (1989) Characterization of two kinds of high-voltage-activated Ca channel currents in chick sensory neurons. Differential sensitivity to

dihydropyridines and ω-conotoxin GVIA. Pflügers Arch. **414**:150-156.
Bean, B. (1989) Classes of calcium channels in vertebrate cells. Ann. Rev. Physiol **51**:367-384.
Brown, A.M., Kunze, D.L. and Yatani, A. (1984) The agonistic effect of dihydropyridines on Ca channels. Nature **311**:570-572.
Carbone, E. and Lux, H.D. (1984) A low voltage-activated, fully inactivating Ca channel in vertebrate sensory neurones. Nature **310**:501-502.
Carbone, E. and Lux, H.D. (1987) Kinetics and selectivity of a low-voltage-activated calcium current in chick and rat sensory neurones. J. Physiol. **386**:547-570.
Carbone, E. and Lux, H.D. (1989) ω-Conotoxin blockade distinguishes Ca from Na permeable states in neuronal calcium channels. Pflügers Arch. **413**:14-22.
Carbone, E., Morad, M. and Lux H.D. (1987) External Ni^{2+}selectively blocks the low-threshold Ca^{2+} current of chick sensory neurons. Pflügers Arch **408**:R60.
Carbone, E., Sher, E. and Clementi, F. (1989) Pharmacological identification of Ca channels in a human neuroblastoma cell line. Europ. J. Neurosci. Suppl. **2**:157.
Clementi, F., Cabrini, D., Gotti, C. and Sher, E. (1986) Pharmacological characterization of cholinergic receptors in a human neuroblastoma cell line. J. Neurochem. **47**:291-297.
Fenwick, E.M., Marty, A., Neher, E. (1982) Sodium and calcium channels in bovine chromaffine cells. J. Physiol. **331**:599-635.
Ferroni, A., Mancinelli, E., Camagni, S. and Wanke, E.(1989) Two high voltage-activated calcium currents are present in isolation in adult rat sensory neurons. Biochem. Biophys. Res. Comm. **168**:379-384.
Formenti, A., Pollo, A., Taglialatela, M. and Carbone,E. (1989) Low and high threshold Ca currents in adult rat sensory neurons. Europ. J. Neurosci.Suppl.2:156.
Fox, A.P., Nowycky, M.C., Tsien, R.W. (1987) Kinetic and pharmacological properties distinguishes three types of calcium currents in chick sensory neurones. J. Physiol. **394**:149-172.
Fukushima, Y. and Hagiwara, S. (1985). Currents carried by monovalent cations through calcium channels in mouse neoplastic B lymphocytes. J. Physiol. **358**:255-284.
Hamill, O.P., Marty, A., Neher, E., Sakmann, B. and Sigworth, F.J. (1981) Improved patch-clamp techniques for high-resolution current recording from cells and cell-free membrane patches. Pflügers Arch. **391**:85-100.
Hess., P., Lansman, J.B. and Tsien, R.W. (1984)

Different modes of Ca^{2+} channel gating behavior favored by dihydropyridine Ca^{2+} agonists and antagonists. Nature **311**:538-544.

Lansman, J.B., Hess, P. and Tsien R.W. (1986). Blockade of Ca current through single calcium channels by Cd^{2+}, Mg^{2+} and Ca^{2+}: Voltage and concentration dependence of calcium entry into the pore. J. Gen Physiol. **88**:321-347.

Lux, H.D.,Carbone, E. and Zucker, H. (1989) Block of Na^{+} ion permeation and selectivity of Ca channels. Ann. N.Y. Acad. Sci. **560**:94-102.

McCleskey, E.W., Fox, A.P., Feldman, D.H., Cruz, L.J. Olivera, B.M., Tsien, R.M. and Yoshikami, D. (1987) ω-Conotoxin: Direct and persistent blockade of specific types of calcium channels in neurons but not in muscle. Proc. Natl. Acad. Sci. USA **84**:4327-4331.

Nowycky, M.C., Fox, A.P. and Tsien, R.W. (1985a) Three types of neuronal calcium channels with different calcium agonist sensitivity. Nature **316**:440-443.

Nowycky, M.C., Fox, A.P. and Tsien, R.W. (1985b) Long-opening mode of gating of neuronal calcium channels and its promotion by the dihydropyridine calcium agonist Bay K 8644. Proc. Natl. Acad. Sci. (USA) **82**:2178-2182.

Plummer, M.R., Logothetis, D.E.and Hess, P. (1989) Elementary properties and pharmacological sensitivities of calcium channels in mammalian peripheral neurons. Neuron **2**:1453-1463.

Sanguinetti, M.C., Krafte, D.S., Kass, R.S. (1986) Voltage-dependent modulation of Ca channel current in heart cells by Bay K 8644. J. Gen Physiol. **88**:369-392.

Scott, B.S. (1982) Adult neurons in cell culture: electrophysiological characterization and use in neurological research. Progr. Neurobiol. **19**:187-211.

Sher, E., Pandiella, A. and Clementi, F. (1988). w-Conotoxin binding and effects on calcium channel function in human neuroblastoma and rat pheochromocytoma cell lines. FEBS Lett **235**:178-182.

Swandulla, D. and Armstrong, C.M. (1988) Fast deactivating calcium channels in chick sensory neurons. J. Gen. Physiol. **92**:197-218.

Swandulla,D. and Armstrong C.M. (1989) Calcium channel block by cadmium in chicken sensory neurons. Proc. Natl. Acad. Sci. USA **86**:1736-1740.

Tang, C., Presser, F. and Morad, M. (1988). Amiloride selectively blocks the low threshold (T) calcium channel. Science **240**:213-215.

Tsien, R.W., Lipscombe, D.V., Madison, K.R., Bley, K.R. and Fox, A.P. (1988) Multiple types of neuronal calcium channels and their selective modulation. Trends in Neurosci. **11**:431-438.

CROSS-TALK BETWEEN RECEPTORS COUPLED TO CALCIUM CURRENTS IN ADULT BUT NOT NEONATAL RAT SENSORY NEURONS

E. WANKE, A. BECCHETTI, L. BERTOLLINI AND A. FERRONI

Dept. General Physiology and Biochemistry, University of Milan, 20133 MILANO, Italy.

ABSTRACT.

In adult rat sensory neurons Ca^{2+} currents were studied with the whole-cell patch-clamp technique. Two categories of neuromodulators, known to activate different 2nd messenger systems: 1) angiotensin II (AII), bovine serum albumin (BSA), Acetylcholine (ACh) and 2) GABA, stimulated the low-voltage activated (LVA) and inhibited the high voltage activated (HVA) currents, respectively. The simultaneous application of the two types of drugs failed to inhibit the HVA current via a putative cross-talk between the two 2nd messengers.

INTRODUCTION

In many neurons, the voltage-dependent Ca^{2+} current is depressed or enhanced by neurotransmitters or hormones. Is is known that calcium entry is essential for neurotransmitter release. Thus, the modulation of $[Ca^{2+}]_i$ through the inward Ca^{2+} current is a possible mechanism for the control of presynaptic release. There is evidence that, for some neurotransmitters, the release is predominantly evoked by the selective activation of Ca^{2+} currents in different physiological ranges (Rane et al., 1987; Hirning et al, 1988). The discovery of: i) kinetically different macroscopic currents and ii) different single channels conductances (although in unphysiological conditions) was sufficient to propose various types of Ca^{2+} channels, namely a low voltage activated (LVA) or T-channel , two high voltage activated channels (HVA): the N-channel and the L-channel (Carbone & Lux, 1984; Fedulova et al., 1985; Bossu et al., 1985; Nowycky et al., 1985). Initially, the selective blockage of these currents by drugs and toxins was considered as a strong proof of the existence of different channel-proteins. Recently, however, it has been shown that the peculiar sensitivity to these drugs (dihydropyridines, omega-conotoxin) for some channels is not general but cell-dependent (Plummer et al., 1989; Akaike et al., 1989; Toselli and Lux, 1989).

We here report an interesting and peculiar difference between adult and neonatal rat sensory neurons. It consists of a cross-talk between two different types of receptors which, as a rule, modulate voltage-dependent Ca^{2+} currents. It is known from the work of Fischbach and Dunlap (1981) that GABA has inhibitory action on the Ca^{2+} current. We have detected an inhibitory action on the high voltage activated (HVA) currents. On the contrary, Angiotensin II (see Kass and Blair, 1981; Cohen et al., 1988; Herscheler et al., 1988.), and other peptides (as shown here) are stimulatory for the T-channel in these neurons. We find that the simultaneous application of the two types of neuromodulators is additive in neonatal neurons, as if the two modulatory mechanisms were acting independently, but that this is not true in adult neurons, where the action of GABA is suppressed. We think that this effect could be explained by a possible interaction of two diverse second messenger systems in the cell.

Methods

Ca^{2+} currents were studied, at 24°C, on freshly disperded sensory neurons (Ferroni et al., 1989) with the whole-cell patch-clamp technique (Hamill et al., 1981).

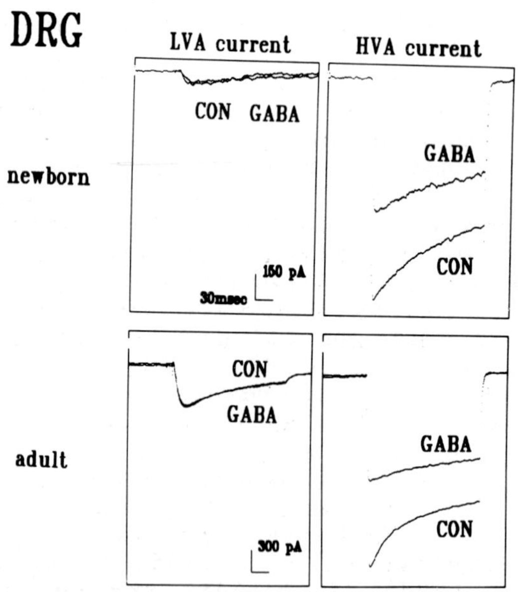

Fig.1 HVA (right) but not LVA (left) Ca2+ currents are inhibited by GABA in a similar fashion in newborn (upper) and in adult (lower) dorsal root ganglion neurons. Neurons: newborn D9511, adult C9503.

The composition of the external medium during the experiments was (in mM): 86 ChoCl, 50 TEACl, 2 KCl, 2 $CaCl_2$, 1 4-AP, 1 $MgCl_2$, 10 HEPES, 15 glucose, pH 7.3. Composition of the internal solution was (in mM): 100 CsAspartate, 20 TEACl, 2 BAPTA, 10 HEPES, 2 MgATP, 0.5 GTP, 20 creatine phosphate, 50 Uml^{-1} creatine phosphokinase, pH 7.3. The neuron under study was continuously perfused with the standard solution and, when necessary, with the various drugs, via a multi-barreled metal pipette positioned about 0.3 mm from the soma. Patch pipettes had resistances of 0.5-2 MOhm. Analog and digital (P/4 technique, Armstrong & Bezanilla, 1974) subtraction was used for correction of the traces; Cd^{2+} was used several times during each experiment to correct for the Cd-insensitive current. The pClamp (Axon Instrum., USA) software and hardware was used during experiments and analysis. The drug concentration was 50 µM for GABA and ACh, 0.5 µM for AII and 20 µM for the compound called here BSA which was obtained from commercial bovine serum Albumine (SIGMA A0281, A4378 or MILES V-81-003-3) after fractionation by heat shock and selective microconcentration (<10000 MW cutoff, Centricon). The response (a transient increase of an inward chloride current) of the $GABA_A$ receptor was seen in about 75% of the neurons.

Results

In neonatal and in adult sensory neurons the low-threshold activated current (much smaller in the neonatal rats) is completely inactivated at -30 mV and the long-lasting current is not yet activated at this membrane potential. We took advantage of this property of the cells to develop two protocols, one to test the T-channel and the other to test the L-channel in such a way that the recorded currents are pure LVA or HVA currents. To activate the T-channel the neuron was preconditioned at -90 mV for 0.5 sec and tested at -30 mV; to activate the L-channel the preconditioning voltage was set at -30 mV and the test-command was +10 mV. The effect of applying GABA is shown in Fig. 1. As already mentioned in the introduction the inhibitory action is selective for the HVA current. On the other hand, as shown in Fig. 2 and 3, the application of either AII (fig.2) or a contaminant present in bovine serum albumin (here called BSA, fig.3) produced always a stimulatory action on the T-current and a negligible effect on the HVA. In the same neurons shown in Fig. 1, we tested (two min later) also the simultaneous application of GABA and BSA. The result is shown in Fig. 4. It can be seen that the inhibitory action of GABA, for the HVA channel, was no longer present in the adult neuron while the stimulatory action of BSA for the T-channel was still present in both types

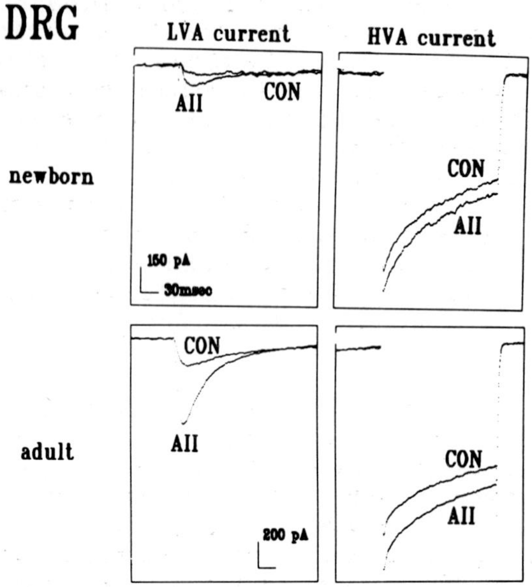

Fig.2 In the two types of neurons (upper: newborn, lower: adult) LVA (left) currents are increased (about 300%) while HVA (right) currents are poorly affected by AII. Neurons: newborn C9519, adult B9526.

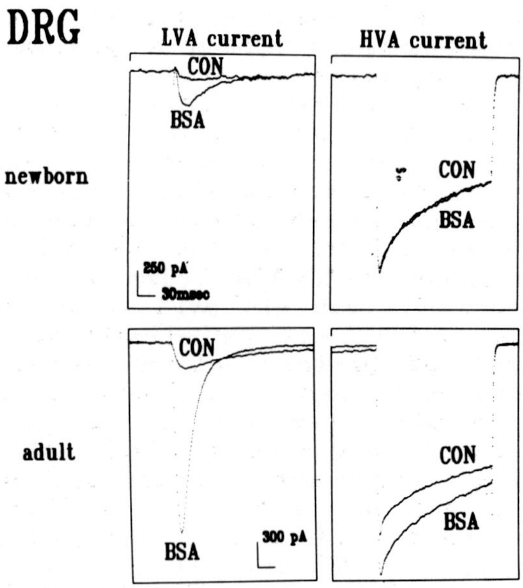

Fig.3 In the two types of neurons (upper: newborn, lower: adult) LVA (left) currents are greatly enhanced (about 700%) while HVA currents (right) are poorly affected by BSA (see methods). Neurons: newborn C9519, adult B9526.

of neurons. The removal of the GABA action could be seen also with Ach (see Fig.5) and AII (not shown).

It is well known that two possible second messenger systems characterize the muscarinic response (Peralta et al., 1988). We thus decided to apply also ACh in order to compare its modulatory action with that reported before (Wanke et al., 1987; Plummer et al., 1989; Toselli & Lux, 1989). The result is shown in Fig.5. It can be seen that the LVA current was enhanced while the HVA current was inhibited only in the newborn neuron. In the two neurons used in fig.5 the effects of the other drugs were identical to those presented in figs.1, 2, 3 (not shown).

Discussion

In order to explain the competitive action of two drugs (when applied simultaneously) on the modulation of the long-lasting Ca^{2+} channel in the adult neuron, it is useful to summarize the results previously recorded on the three Ca^{2+} currents (T, N, L) in different laboratories. These results were obtained in neurons (DRG or others) of different sources (*e*mbryonic, *n*eonatal, *a*dult) and animals (*c*hick, *r*at, *m*ouse) using various drugs addressed to different receptors such as ALFA for α-adrenergic, M_1-M_2 for muscarinic, ADEN for adenosine and OPIO for opiod. In the following table the modulatory effects are classified, in two groups according to the mechanisms supposed to be involved : those where PI turnover and protein kinase C are supposed (or demonstrated) to be activated (first box) and those where this mechanism is excluded and/or G-proteins-Ca^{2+}-channel coupling is evident (second box).

Although we have no proof that the positive modulation of the T-current seen in all the experiments mentioned in the present work depends on PI hydrolysis (as suggested by Rasmussen et al., 1985, for AII), we may assume that in our case this is the mechanism. For neurotransmitters listed in the second box, there is conclusive evidence that GABA is acting via a G-protein, but probably not via cAMP (Dolphin et al., 1986). For the α-adrenergic receptor there are conflicting results and the involvement of protein kinase C, as suggested by Dunlap and coworkers, has to be reconsidered in view of more recent results (Hockberger et al., 1989). The muscarinic effects described by Wanke et al., 1989 and Mancinelli et al., 1989 are similar to those described in the sympathetic neuron (Wanke et al., 1987) where it was shown that neither cAMP neither protein kinase C are involved.

During our combined experiments (GABA+BSA) it is reasonable to suppose that we were stimulating both the PI hydrolysis (first box) and G-protein coupling (second box). It may be worth-noticing that according to the

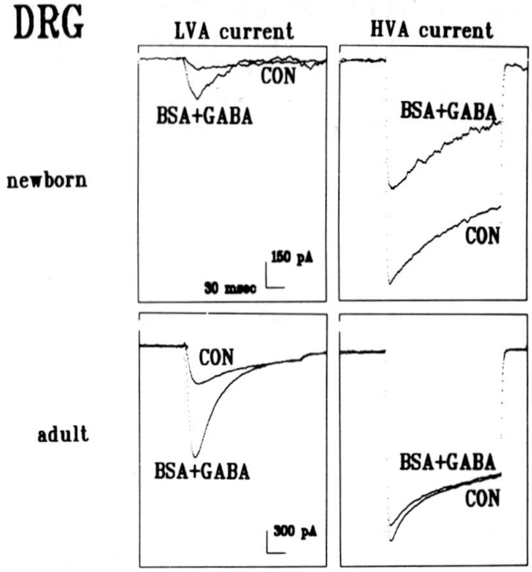

Fig.4 In the same neurons of fig.1 (tested also for the stimulatory action of BSA, not shown) the action of GABA+BSA corresponds to the independent effects of the two drugs only in the newborn neuron (upper). In the adult neuron (lower) the action of GABA was inhibited.

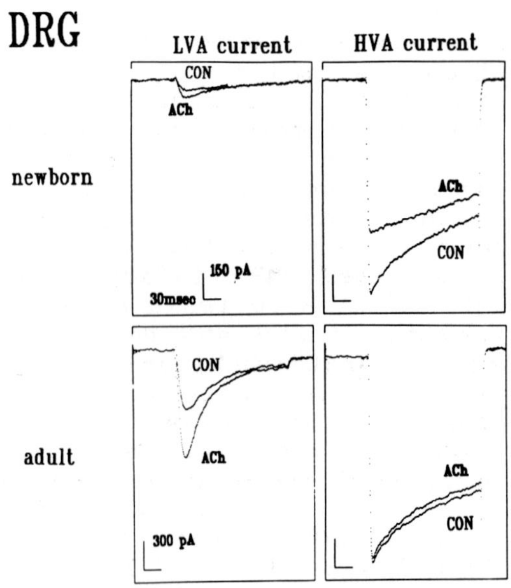

Fig.5 The action of ACh is stimulatory for the LVA current (about 165%) while for the HVA current it is without effect in the adult neuron and inhibitory in the neonatal neuron. Neurons: newborn D9511, adult B9504.

Modulatory effects on calcium currents reported from various laboratories (indicated) and obtained after application of various drugs (see text).

TABLE I

RECEPTORS	LABORATORY	SECOND MESSENGERS	NEURON	Ca^{2+} CHANNEL T	Ca^{2+} CHANNEL N	Ca^{2+} CHANNEL L
AII	Rasmussen et al.	PI-PKC	Adren	+T		
AII	Herscheler et al.	?	Y1		+N	+L
AII	This work	?	nDRGr	+T		
AII	This work	?	aDRGr	+T		
BSA	This work	?	nDRGr	+T		
BSA	This work	?	aDRGr	+T		
M_1	Mancinelli et al.	?	nDRGr	+T		
M_1	Mancinelli et al.	?	aDRG	+T		
$GABA_B$	Holz IV et al.	G (no cAMP)	eDRGc			-L
$GABA_B$	Dolphin et al.	G (no cAMP)	nDRGr		-N	
$GABA_B$	This work	?	nDRGr		-N	-L
$GABA_B$	This work	?	aDRGr		-N	-L
ALFA	Marchetti et al	?	eDRGc	-T		-L
ALFA	Holz IV et al.	G (no cAMP)	eDRGc			-L
ALFA	Gray et al.	Gs cAMP	aHIPgp			+L
M_2	Mancinelli et al.	?	aDRGr			-L
M_2	Wanke et al.	G (no cAMP)	nDRGr		-N	-L
ADEN	Dolphin et al.	?	nDRGr		-N	
OPIO	MacDonald et al.	?	eDRGm		-N	

Caron group (Yoshimasa et al., 1987) various second messenger systems (once activated) could talk to each other producing various effects. In our case, the particularly high concentration of the drugs could produce enough protein kinase C to inhibit the still unknown coupling mechanism between GABA receptors and L-type channels. A similar effect was already mentioned by Worley et al., 1987, when they showed that the overproduction of protein kinase C could block the inhibitory action of GABA and Adenosine in hippocampal neurons. According to our opinion, the fact that in new-born rats the cross-talk is not present, is extremely interesting from the point of view of the postnatal ontogenetic development.

It is worth mentioning that, according to the Peralta group (Peralta et al., 1988) the family of muscarinic receptors can be subdivided into two groups: the M_1 (with M_3 and M_5) and the M_2 (with M_4) groups. The former group acts through PI turnover, while the latter acts through the inhibition of Adenylate cyclase (in their cells). More precisely the first group (at high drug concentration) could *stimulate* Adenylate cyclase. This consideration suggests that the results of Fig.5 can be interpreted as follows: in the newborn rat, where we suppose the cross-talk is not functioning (see fig.4), the action of ACh is double (1) excitatory for the LVA channel through the M1 receptor and (2) inhibitory for the HVA channel through the M2 receptor. In the adult rat, where the cross-talk is active (Fig.4), the stimulatory effect for the LVA channel is still present while the inhibitory effect is blocked.

Obviously, the mechanisms of all these actions have to be further demonstrated by the extensive use of both selective muscarinic agonists and antagonists and blockers of the PI and G-protein dependent processes.

We thank Jacopo Meldolesi and Dario DiFrancesco for useful comments, Drs. E. Mancinelli and S. Camagni and Mr. G. Mostacciuolo for expert assistance. This work was supported in part by grants from Ministero Pubblica Istruzione, Membrane Physiology Program (to A.F. and E.W.) and from the Consiglio Nazionale delle Ricerche, International Joint Project Italia/USA (to E.W.).

References

Akaike N., Kostyuk P.G., Osipchuk Y.V. (1989) Dihydropyridine-sensitive low-threshold calcium channels in isolated rat hypothalamic neurons. J. Physiol., (Lond.) 412:181-196

Armstrong C.M. and Bezanilla F. (1974) Charge movement associated with the opening and closing of the activation gates of Na channels. J. Gen. Physiol. 63:533-552.

Bossu J.L., Feltz A. and Thomann J.M. (1985) Depolarization elicits two distinct calcium currents in vertebrate sensory neurons. Pfluegers Arch. 403:360-368.

Carbone E. and Lux H.D. (1984) A low voltage-activated calcium conductance in embryonic sensory neurons. Biophys. J., 46:413-418.

Cohen C.J., McCarthy R.T., Barrett P.Q., Rasmussen H. (1988) Ca channels in adrenal glomerulosa cells: K and angiotensin II increase T-type Ca channel current. Proc. Natn. Acad. Sci. U.S.A 85:2412-2416.

Dolphin A.C., Scott R.H. (1987) Calcium channel currents and their inhibition by (-) Baclofen in rat sensory neurons: modulation by guanine nucleotides. J. Physiol., (Lond.) 386:1-17

Dunlap K., Fischbach G.D. (1981) Neurotransmitters decrease the calcium conductance activated by depolarization of embryonic chick sensory neurons. J. Physiol., (Lond.) 317:519-535.

Fedulova S.A., Kostyuk P.G. and Veselovsky N.S. (1985) Two types of calcium channels in the somatic membrane of new-born rat dorsal root ganglion neurons. J. Physiol., (Lond.) 359:431-446.

Ferroni A., Mancinelli E., Camagni S., Wanke E. (1989) Two high voltage-activated calcium currents are present in isolation in adult rat spinal neurons. Biochem. Biophys. Res. Commun. 159:379-384.

Fox A.P., Nowycky M.C. and Tsien, R. (1987) Single channel recordings of three types of calcium channels in chick sensory neurons. J. Physiol., (Lond.) 394:173-200.

Gray R., Johnston D. (1987) Noradrenalin and adrenoceptor agonists increase activity of voltage-dependent calcium channels in hippocampal neurons. Nature 327:620-622.

Hamill O.P., Marty A., Neher E., Sakmann B. and Sigworth F.J. (1981) Improved patch clamp techniques for high resolution current recording from cells and cell-free membrane patches. Pfluegers Arch. 391:85-100.

Herschler J., Rosenthal., Hinsch K.D., Wulfern M., Trautwein W., Schultz G. (1988) Angiotensin II induced stimulation of voltage-dependent Ca currents in an adrenal cortical cell line. EMBO J. 7:619-624

Hirning L.D., Fox A.A., McCleskey E.W., Olivera B.M., Thayer S.A., Miller R.J., Tsien R.W. (1988) Dominant role of N-type Ca channels in evoked release of Norepinephrine from sympathetic neurons. Science 239:57-60.

Hockberger P., Toselli M., Swandulla D., Lux H.D. (1989) A diacylglycerol analogue reduces neuronal calcium currents independently of protein kinase C activation. Nature 338:340-342.

Holz IV G.G., Rane S.G., Dunlap K. (1986) GTP-binding proteins mediate transmitter inhibition of voltage-dependent calcium channels. Nature 319:670-672.

Mancinelli E., Becchetti A., Camagni S., Wanke E., Ferroni A. (1989) Adult rat sensory neurons: muscarinic modulation of Ca^{2+} currents. 12th Ann.Meet.ENA, Torino, 3-7 Sept., 1989, 152.

Marchetti C., Carbone E., Lux H.D. (1986) Effects of Dopamine and Noradrenaline on Ca channels of cultured sensory and sympathetic neurons of chick. Pfluegers Arch. 406:104-111.

McDonald R.L., Werz M.A. (1986) Dynorphin A decreases voltage-dependent calcium conductance of mouse dorsal root ganglion neurons. J. Physiol., (Lond.) 377:237-249.

Nowycky M.C., Fox A.P. and Tsien R. (1985) Three types of neuronal calcium channel with different calcium agonist sensitivity. Nature 316:440-443.

Peralta E.G., Ashkenazi A., Wislow J.W., Ramachandran J., Capon D.J. (1988) Differential regulation of PI hydrolysis and adenylyl cyclase by muscarinic receptor subtypes. Nature 334:434-438.

Plummer M.R., Logothetis D.E., Hess P. (1989) Elementary properties and pharmacological sensitivities of calcium channels in mammalian peripheral neurons. Neuron 2:1453-1463.

Rane S.G., Holz IV G.G., Dunlap K. (1987) Dihydropyridine inhibition of neuronal calcium current and substance P release. Pfluegers Arch. 409:361-366.

Toselli M., Lux, H.D. (1989) GTP-binding proteins mediate acetylcholine inhibition of voltage dependent calcium channels in hippocampal neurons. Pfluegers Arch. 413:319-321.

Tsien, R.W., Lipscombe, D., Madison, D.V., Bley, K,R, and Fox, A.P. (1988) Multiples types of neuronal calcium channels and their selective modulation. Trends Neurosci. 11:431-438.

Wanke E., Ferroni A. (1988) Modulation of neuronal excitability by Acetylcholine. In neurotransmitters & Cortical Functions. (Avoli et al., eds.) Plenum Press., 227-286.

Wanke E., Ferroni A., Malgaroli A., Ambrosini A., Pozzan T., Meldolesi J. (1987) Activation of a muscarinic receptor selectively inhibits a rapidly inactivated Ca^{2+} current in rat sympathetic neurons. Proc. Natn. Acad. Sci. U.S.A 84:4313-4317.

Wanke E., Ferroni A., Sardini A. (1989) L and N Ca^{2+} channels coupled to muscarinic receptors in rat sensory neurons. Ann. N.Y. Acad. Sci. 560:398-400.

Worley T., Baraban J.M., McCarren M., Snyder S.H., Alger B.E. (1987) Cholinergic phosphatidylinositol modulation of inhibitory, G protein-linked, neurotransmitter actions: electrophysiological studies in rat hippocampus. Proc. Natl. Acad. Sci. U.S.A 84:3467-3471.

Yoshimasa T., Sibley D.R., Bouvier M., Lefkowitz R.J., Caron M.G. (1987) Cross-talk between cellular signalling pathways suggested by phorbol ester induced adenylate cyclase phosphorylation. Nature 327:67-70.

CROSS-TALK BETWEEN DIFFERENT INTRACELLULAR SIGNALLING PATHWAYS IN THE RAT HIPPOCAMPUS

M. Parenti[1], G. Ceresoli, S. Consolo* and A. Groppetti

"E. Trabucchi" Department of Pharmacology, University of Milano and * "Mario Negri" Institute, Milano, Italy.

ABSTRACT

The activation of α1-adrenergic receptors in rat hippocampal slices enhances polyphosphoinositide (PPI) breakdown and cyclicAMP (cAMP) accumulation. The latter effect is antagonized by different protein kinase C (PKC) inhibitors and mimicked by a diacylglycerol (DAG) analogue, 1,2-diolein, which activates PKC, suggesting that cAMP synthesis is indirectly affected by α1-adrenoceptors through the stimulated generation of DAG upon PPI hydrolysis. Furthermore the elevation of hippocampal cAMP decreases the ability of α1-receptor agonists to enhance PPI breakdown. It is proposed that the observed effects are part of a complex cross-talk between PPI and AC signalling pathways operating in hippocampal neurons.

INTRODUCTION

Hydrophilic hormones, growth factors and neurotransmitters bind to specific receptors on the external surface of the cell. Their message is thus transmitted across the plasma membrane and transduced into stimulation of second messenger-generating systems which synthesize the signal molecules responsible for the activation of the intracellular pathways, ultimately leading to the biological response. Due to the multiplicity of the extracellular signals continuously perceived by a cell, the proper integration of second messenger-activated pathways is an absolute requirement for the proper coordination of cellular responses. This may be achieved by cross-talk among second messenger-generating systems. By regulating the synthesis of second messengers, these systems exchange informations related to their functional status, so to coordinate their activity. Second messengers appear therefore to perform a dual function: as signals, to intracellularly convey the message generated by receptor activation, and as communication carriers among different intracellular signalling pathways.

A vast repertoire of second messengers is available for cellular signalling. However, despite the number, their generation so far appear to be linked to a relatively limited variety of systems. Of these, the best characterized is the receptor-coupled adenylate cyclase (AC; Levitzki, 1986). Stimulation of the AC enzyme enhances the conversion of adenosine trisphosphate (ATP) to 3′:5′-cyclic adenosine monophosphate (cAMP), while the inhibition decreases cAMP production.

[1]To whom all correspondence should be addressed

The cyclic nucleotide then acts as a second messenger by activating cAMP-dependent protein kinases (PKA) that phosphorylate selected proteins. Another important receptor-coupled enzyme effector is phospholipase C (PLC), that cleaves phosphatidylinositol 4,5-bisphosphate [PtdIns(4,5)P_2], a minor membrane phospholipid present in all eukaryotic cells (Berridge, 1987). The products of this rection are 1,2-diacylglycerol (DAG) and inositol(1,4,5)trisphosphate [Ins(1,4,5)P_3], two established second messengers, that together form a bifurcating signal pathway: one limb, controlled through DAG, activates protein kinase/s C (PKC), whereas the other limb is triggered by Ins(1,4,5)P_3, whose primary function is to mobilize calcium from intracellular non-mitochondrial store/s. Calcium itself acts as a messenger through activation of Ca^{2+}/calmodulin-dependent protein kinases (Kennedy and Greengard, 1981) and, synergistically with DAG, of PKC.

Recently a direct coupling of membrane receptors to phospholipase A_2 (PLA_2) has been shown (Burch et al., 1986): stimulation of this enzyme triggers a reaction cascade with generation of arachidonic acid (AA) and a number of active metabolites, the eicosanoids (Smith, 1989), some of which may serve as intracellular messengers (Piomelli et al., 1987).

All second messenger-generating systems so far mentioned show a remarkable similarity in their molecular organization: the signal generated by receptor activation is transmitted to the enzyme effector (AC, PLC, PLA_2) through a GTP-binding regulatory protein (G protein; Gilman, 1987). The structural analogy may imply a similar mode of functioning, as recently suggested for AC- and PLC-coupled systems by Downes (1989) and perhaps provides a "common language" for intracellular signal cross-talk.

α1-ADRENERGIC RECEPTORS EVOKE PLEIOTYPIC CELL RESPONSES

The majority of extracellular signals evoke multiple receptor-mediated responses on their target cells. Figure 1 shows that accumulation of both inositol phosphate (IP; panel A) and cAMP (panel B) is increased in a rat brain region, the hippocampus, after activation of α1-adrenergic receptors by the selective, partial agonist, phenylephrine (Phe). The cAMP response seems to be a peculiarity of the brain tissue (Johnson and Minneman, 1987) whereas the coupling of α1-adrenergic receptors to polyphosphoinositide (PPI) breakdown has been observed in all examined tissues (see Minneman, 1988 for review). PLC is therefore considered the cellular effector for these receptors. However, additional responses have also been reported following activation of α1-adrenoceptors, such as an increased release of AA (Burch et al., 1986) and the opening of dihydropyridine-sensitive voltage-gated Ca^{2+} channels (Han et al., 1987). Multiple responses upon α1-adrenergic receptor stimulation are observed not only in tissues which include heterogeneous cell populations (like the hippocampus), but also in homogeneous cell lines, such as the FRTL 5 rat thyroid and MDCK-D1 canine kidney epithelial cells, where α1-agonists increase both IP accumulation and AA release (Burch et al., 1986; Terman et al.,

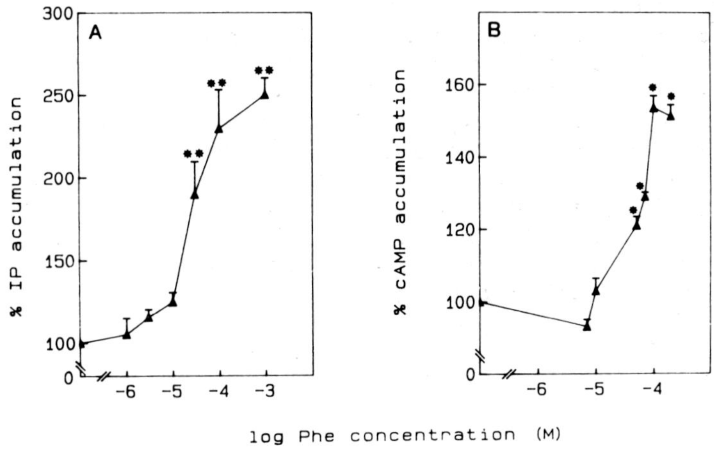

Figure 1. Effect of α1-adrenergic receptor stimulation by phenylephrine (Phe) on inositol phosphate (IP; panel A) and cAMP (panel B) accumulations in rat hippocampal slices. IP and cAMP were assayed as described by Consolo et al. (1988). Incubation of the slices was carried out at 37°C for 20 (IP) and 15 (cAMP) min. * $P < 0.005$ and ** $p < 0.001$ vs basal values by Student 't' test.

1987). These observations can be simply explained by assuming the existence of distinct α1-adrenoceptor subtypes, each one linked to a specific transduction mechanism. For some receptor families this assumption has received a clear-cut experimental support from biochemical and molecular biological studies. It is well known that human muscarinic acetylcholine receptors represent a family of at least five gene products which have distinct primary sequences, ligand-binding selectivities and tissue-specific patterns of expression (Bonner et al., 1988). However, for many other receptors, like α1-adrenergic receptors, for which such evidences are still lacking, the possibility of alternative interpretations still exists to explain the multiplicity of evoked cellular responses. A pharmacologically homogeneous class of receptors may thus be coupled (1) to distinct transduction mechanisms according to different tissue and cellular localization, modulation by the extracellular environment and/or the surrounding components of the plasma membrane or (2) to a unique transduction mechanism whose activation may in turn affect other mechanisms (cell signalling pathway cross-talk). Evidence obtained with the rat hippocampus may favour the latter hypothesis, suggesting that α1-agonist-mediated cAMP accumulation could be an indirect effect. Figure 2 compares the time course of the cAMP increases induced by isoproterenol (Iso), a selective ß-receptor agonist, and by Phe. When the ß-adrenergic stimulant is used, elevation of the cyclic nucleotide content is a rapid event, being already significant after 1 min incubation, whereas a considerable lag time (about 10 min) is needed before Phe can alter the cAMP levels. This slow kinetics may underlie an indirect control of AC activity since fast responding β-receptors are known to be directly coupled to this enzyme. Moreover Iso and Phe, when simultaneously present at maximally effective concentrations,

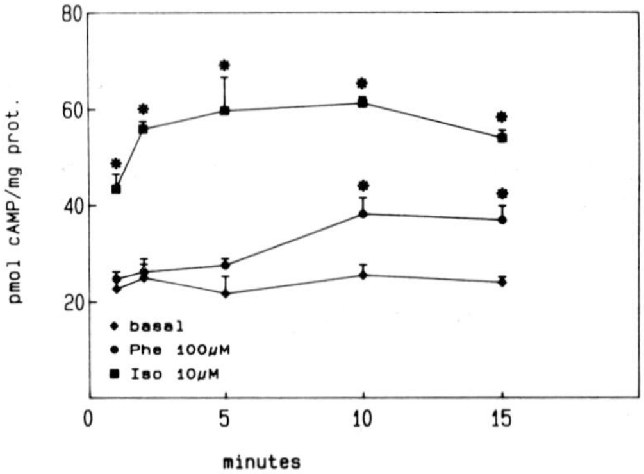

Figure 2. Time courses of ß- and α1-adrenergic stimulation by isoproterenol (Iso) and phenylephrine (Phe) of hippocampal cAMP accumulation. * P< 0.001 vs basal values by Dunnet 't' test.

elicit additive increments of cAMP (data not shown), a result which strengthen the idea that AC is stimulated through independent pathways by ß- and α1-adrenergic receptors.

PROTEIN KINASE C IS INVOLVED IN CELL SIGNALLING PATHWAY CROSS-TALK

It is possible that hippocampal cAMP could be secondarily increased as a result of α1-adrenoceptor activation of PLC, thus involving the second messengers generated at either one or both limbs of the reaction cascade triggered by the phosphodiesteratic cleavage of PtdIns(4,5)P_2. The results reported in Table I and Figure 3 suggest an involvement of PKC in the cAMP response. Table I shows that different compounds (H-7, staurosporine, palmitoylcarnitine and polymyxin B), known to block PKC with various degrees of selectivity (Hidaka and Hagiwara, 1987), all inhibited Phe-induced accumulation of cAMP. Moreover the direct activation of PKC by the cell permeant synthetic DAG analogue, 1,2-diolein, causes an increase of cAMP, already significant at 2 min and maximal at 5 min following diolein addition (Fig. 3, panel A). Surprisingly, the phorbol ester PMA (phorbol 12-myristate, 13-acetate), a potent activator of PKC, is completely ineffective by itself, even at the highest concentration tested, 10^{-5} M (shown in Fig. 3, panel A), whereas it potentiates the accumulation of cAMP elicited by ß-receptor stimulation with Iso (Fig. 3, panel B). We can conclude that stimulation of PKC by DAG and phorbol esters affects AC activity albeit involving different mechanisms. Therefore it is possible to hypothesize that cAMP elevation induced by α1-agonists might occur through PKC activation by DAG generated from PPI breakdown. The synthesis of cAMP could then be accelerated by PKC-induced phosphorylation of either a G protein (Katada et al., 1985) and/or the catalytic subunit of AC (Yoshimasa et al., 1987). Some experimental evidence obtained in the rat pineal gland supports such an hypothesis. The activation of pineal α1-adrenoceptors, shown to be coupled to PLC, has no effect on cAMP accumulation by itself, but enhances the

Table 1. Effect of protein kinase C inhibitors on cAMP accumulation in rat hippocampal slices.

Additions[a]	pmol cAMP/mg prot.	% cAMP accumulation
None	16.1 + 0.3	100
Phe 100 μM	23.6 + 0.8 **	147
H-7 15 μM	16.3 + 0.5	101
H-7 + Phe	20.5 + 1.6	127
Sta 30 nM	16.5 + 0.2	102
Sta + Phe	19.2 + 1.2	119
Pac 30 μM	21.0 + 2.1 **	130
Pac + Phe	20.0 + 0.8 *	124
Pmx 10 μM	13.2 + 1.2	82
Pmx + Phe	15.3 + 0.8	95

[a] 1-(5-Isoquinolinesulfonyl)-2-methylpiperazine (H-7), staurosporine (Sta), palmitoylcarnitine (Pal) and polymyxin B (Pmx) were added 15 min before Phe. * $P< 0.005$ and ** $p> 0.001$ vs "no addition" by Dunnet 't' test.

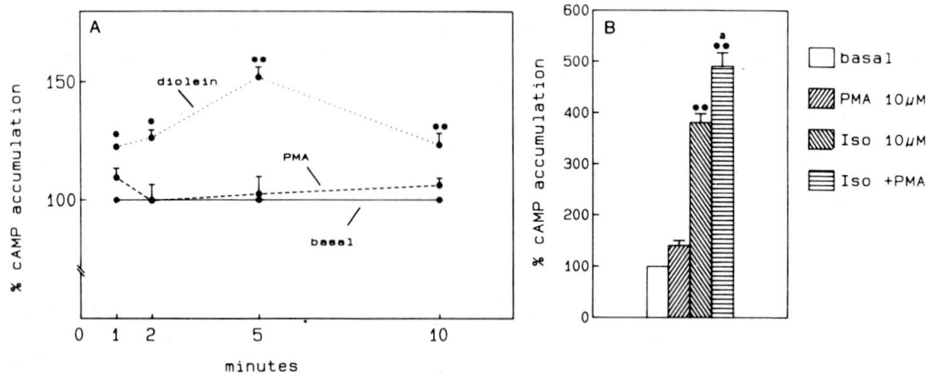

Figure 3. Panel A: time courses of 1,2-diolein (5 μg) and phorbol 12-myristate 13-acetate (PMA; 10 μM) effects on hippocampal cAMP accumulation. * P< 0.005 and ** p< 0.001 vs basal values by Dunnet 't' test. **Panel B:** potentiation of isoproterenol (Iso)-induced cAMP accumulation by PMA. PMA was added 15 min before Iso and incubation was continued for 15 min. ** P< 0.001 vs basal values; [a] p< 0.005 vs Iso alone by Dunnet 't' test.

ß-adrenergic response, resulting in 100- to 300-fold increase in the cyclic nucleotide content. Such an effect is mimicked by phorbol esters and synthetic DAG and blocked by H-7 (Ho et al., 1988). Our results however differ from the data obtained in the pineal gland because of the different effect of DAG and phorbol esters on hippocampal cAMP. This may involve distinct patterns of protein phosphorylation in response to activation of PKC by the two agents, as shown to occur in liver membranes (Kiss and Luo, 1986). The recent discovery that multiple isoforms of PKC exist may explain such different substrate specificity (Nishizuka, 1988). Indeed, all the seven subspecies of PKC identified in the rat brain by molecular cloning appear to be alike in their phorbol ester-binding activities and requirements for Ca^{2+} and phospholipids, but show some differences with respect to their effector-mediated stimulation (Huang et al., 1988). One of these, the γ-subspecies, apparently expressed only in the central nervous system, is selectively activated by both AA and a lipoxygenase metabolite, lipoxin A (Shearman et al., 1989). Finally the different kinetics of activation of PKC by DAG and phorbol esters, and DAG metabolism may be also taken into account to temptatively explain the discrepancy observed in their effects on AC. While DAG is very rapidly degraded, so to assure only a transient activation of PKC, phorbol esters are stable compounds which cause a very long-lasting stimulation of the enzyme. Moreover, the metabolism of DAG can give rise to active molecules. In particular phosphorylation to phosphatidic acid, a compound shown to promote Ca^{2+} influx in some cellular systems (Ohsako and Deguchi, 1981), might ultimately activate Ca^{2+}-binding proteins, such as calmodulin, which is known to stimulate brain AC activity (Brostrom et al., 1977). Alternatively, DAG is metabolized by lipase enzyme. The released AA and its metabolites, among which some prostaglandins (PG), may then stimulate AC activity. While at present we can not rule out an involvement of phosphatidic acid in mediating hippocampal cAMP accumulation by α1-agonists, a possible action of PG is excluded by the observation that blockade of PG synthesis with indomethacin, a cycloxygenase inhibitor, does not prevent Phe action (data not shown). Also the PLA_2 blocker quinacrine is ineffective (data not shown), ruling out that α1-adrenergic receptors could alter hippocampal AC activity through an involvement of the PLA_2 reaction cascade.

CYCLIC AMP AFFECTS POLYPHOSPHOINOSITIDE BREAKDOWN

In the preceding paragraph we have hypothesized a potential role of PKC in mediating the regulation of hippocampal AC-linked receptors by α1-adrenergic receptors coupled to PPI breakdown. Additionally PKC could act as a negative feedback regulator of hippocampal α1-adrenergic receptor function, similarly to many other PPI-coupled receptors. Figure 4 shows that the activation of PKC by PMA significantly reduces Phe-stimulation of IP accumulation. This might occur as a consequence of the direct phosphorylation of α1-adrenoceptors by PKC, leading to their functional uncoupling from PLC, as demonstrated by Leeb-Lundberg et al. (1985). Similarly to PMA, also cAMP negatively affects the accumulation of IP that follows α1-adrenergic receptor activation. The elevation of the cyclic nucleotide levels by forskolin, a diterpene which directly interacts with the AC enzyme, decreases the extent of Phe stimulation (Fig.4). Although the effect has been observed in a number of cellular systems, the mechanism by which cAMP inhibits agonist-stimulated PPI breakdown is still unknown, even if an involvement of PKA has been postulated (Takai et al., 1982). While it is possible that inhibition of receptor-dependent PLC activity could be directly caused by PKA-catalyzed phosphorylation of the enzyme

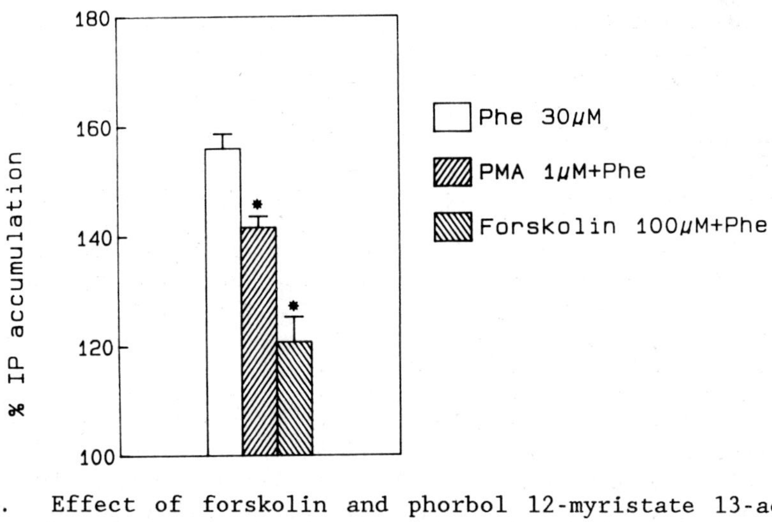

Figure 4. Effect of forskolin and phorbol 12-myristate 13-acetate (PMA) on phenylephrine (Phe)-stimulated inositol phosphate (IP) accumulation in rat hippocampal slices. Incubations were carried out for 20 min with all compounds added simultaneously. * $P < 0.05$ vs Phe alone by Dunnet 't' test.

molecule, evidence, obtained in platelets, suggests that this inhibition reflects a decreased availability of the PPI substrate for agonist-induced breakdown (Lapetina, 1986). Recently, an action of cAMP on the cellular targets of PPI-generated second messengers has also been reported. Supattapone and coll. (1988) demonstrated a cAMP-dependent phosphorylation of the intracellular receptors for Ins(1,4,5)P_3 purified from rat cerebellum, leading to a 10-fold decrease in the ability of Ins(1,4,5)P_3 to release Ca^{2+}. The activation of PKA may also affect the DAG limb of the PPI cascade since it causes a diminished PKC activity, presumably due to an indirect action via a substrate that regulates the PKC enzyme (Narindrasorasak et al., 1987).

CONCLUSION

We have shown that α1-adrenergic receptors in the rat hippocampus activate PPI and AC second messenger-generating pathways. While a direct α1-receptor coupling to PLC can be assumed in brain as demonstrated in a number of tissues and cell lines, AC activity seems to be indirectly affected as a consequence of the DAG activation of PKC that follows α1-agonist-induced PPI breakdown. The recent demonstration that different molecular components of the AC complex may serve as substrates for PKC-induced phosphorylation supports such an hypothesis. Therefore the function of receptors coupled to AC can be enhanced by the parallel activation of α1-adrenergic receptors linked to PLC and present on the same cell population/s. Since a negative regulation of α1-adrenergic receptor function can be exerted by co-localized AC-coupled receptors, the existence of a cross-talk between different cell signalling systems can be hypothesized. Moreover the indirect cAMP elevation by α1-receptor agonists could be part of a negative feedback autoregulatory control of PLC-coupled α1-receptor function, operated through PKC interaction with AC. This would provide a further, "longer", pathway working synergistically with the "short" negative feedback regulation, also involving PKC.

REFERENCES

Berridge, M. J. (1987) Inositol trisphosphate and diacylglycerol: two interacting second messengers. Ann. Rev. Biochem. 56: 159-193.

Bonner, T.J., Young, A.C., Brann, M.R. and Buckley, N.J. (1988). Cloning and expression of the human and rat m5 muscarinic acetylcholine receptor genes. Neuron 1: 403-410.

Brostrom, C. O., Brostrom, M. A. and Wolff, D. J. (1977) Calcium-dependent adenylate cyclase from rat cerebral cortex. J. Biol. Chem. 252: 5677-5685.

Burch, R. M., Luini, A. and Axelrod, J. (1986) Phospholipase A_2 and phospholipase C are activated by distinct GTP-binding proteins in response to α1-adrenergic stimulation in FRTL 5 thyroid cells. Proc. Natl. Acad. Sci. USA 83: 7201-7205.

Consolo, S., Cicioni, P., Ladinsky, H., Rusconi, L., Parenti, M. and Vinci, R. (1988) Serotonergic control of phenylephrine-induced cyclic 3',5'-adenosine monophosphate and inositol phosphate formation in rat hippocampus. J. Pharm. Exp. Ther. 247: 1187-1192.

Downes, C. P. (1989) The cellular function of myo-inositol. Biochem. Soc. Trans. 17: 259-268.

Gilman, A. G. (1987) G-proteins: transducers of receptor-generated signals. Ann. Rev. Biochem. 56: 615-649.

Han, C., Abel, P. W. and Minneman, K. P. (1987) α1-Adrenoceptor subtypes linked to different mechanisms for increasing intracellular Ca^{2+} in the smooth muscle. Nature 329: 333-335.

Hidaka, H. and Hagiwara, M. (1987) Pharmacology of the isoquinoline sulfonamide protein kinase C inhibitors. Trends Pharm. Sci. 8: 162-164.

Ho, A. K., Chik, C. L. and Klein, D. C. (1988) Effects of protein kinase inhibitor (1-(5-isoquinolinesulfonyl)-2-methylpiperazine (H7) on protein kinase C activity and adrenergic stimulation of cAMP and cGMP in rat pinealocytes. Biochem. Pharm. 37: 1015-1020.

Huang, K.-P., Huang, F. L., Nakabayashi, H. and Yoshida, Y. (1988) Biochemical characterization of rat protein kinase C isozymes. J. Biol. Chem. 263: 14839-14845.

Johnson, R. D., and Minneman, K. P. (1987) Differentiation of α1-adrenergic receptors linked to phosphatidylinositol turnover and cyclicAMP accumulation in rat brain. Mol. Pharm. 31: 239-246.

Katada, T., Gilman, A. G., Watanabe, Y., Bauer, S. and Jakobs, K. H. (1985) Protein kinase C phosphorylates the inhibitory guanine nucleotide-binding regulatory component and apparently suppresses its function in hormonal inhibition of adenylate cyclase. Eur. J. Biochem. 151: 431-437.

Kennedy, M. B. and Greengard, P. (1981) Two calcium/calmodulin-dependent protein kinases, which are highly concentrated in brain, phosphorylate protein I. Proc. Natl. Acad. Sci. USA 78: 1293-1297.

Kiss, Z. and Luo, Y. (1986) Phorbol ester and 1,2-diolein are not fully equivalent activators of protein kinase C in respect to phosphorylation of membrane proteins in vitro. FEBS Lett. 198: 203-207.

Lapetina, E. G. (1986) Incorporation of synthetic 1,2-diacylglycerol into platelet phosphatidylinositol is increased by cAMP. FEBS Lett. 195: 111-114.

Leeb-Lundberg, L. M. F., Cotecchia, S., Lomasney, J. W., De Bernardis, J. F., Lefkowitz, R. J. and Caron, M. G. (1985) Phorbol esters promote α1-adrenergic receptor phosphorylation and receptor uncoupling from inositol phospholipid metabolism. Proc. Natl. Acad. Sci. USA 82: 5651-5655.

Levitzki, A. (1986) β-Adrenergic receptors and their mode of coupling to adenylate cyclase. Physiol. Rev. 66: 819-854.

Minneman, K. P. (1988) α1-Adrenergic receptor subtypes, inositol phosphates and sources of cell Ca^{2+}. Pharmacol. Rev. 40: 87-119.

Narindrasorasak, S., Brickenden, A., Ball, E. and Sanwal, B. D. (1987) Regulation of protein kinase C by cyclic adenosine 3':5'-monophosphate and a tumor promoter in skeletal myoblasts. J. Biol. Chem. 262: 10497-10501.

Nishizuka, Y. (1988) The molecular heterogeneity of protein kinase C and its implications for cellular regulation. Nature 334: 661-665.

Ohsako, S. and Deguchi, T. (1981) Stimulation by phosphatidic acid of calcium influx and cyclicGMP synthesis in neuroblastoma cells. J. Biol. Chem. 256: 10945-10948.

Piomelli, D., Volterra, A., Dale, N., Siegelbaum, S. A., Kandel, E. R., Schwartz, J. H. and Belardetti, F. (1987) Lipoxygenase metabolites of arachidonic acid as second messengers for presynaptic inhibition of Aplysia sensory cells. Nature 328: 38-43.

Shearman, M. S., Naor, Z., Sekiguchi, K., Kishimoto, A. and Nishizuka, Y. (1989) Selective activation of the γ-subspecies of protein kinase C from bovine cerebellum by arachidonic acid and its lipoxygenase metabolites. FEBS Lett. 243: 177-182.

Smith, W. L. (1989) The eicosanoids and their biochemical mechanism of action. Biochem. J. 259: 315-324.

Supattapone, S., Danoff, S.K., Theibert, A., Joseph, S. K., Steiner, J. and Snyder, S. H. (1988) Cyclic AMP-dependent phosphorylation of a brain inositol trisphosphate receptor decreases its release of calcium. Proc. Natl. Acad. Sci. USA 85:8747-8750.

Takai, Y., Kaibuchi, K., Sano, K. and Nishizuka, Y. (1982) Counteraction of calcium-activated, phospholipid-dependent protein kinase activation by adenosine 3',5'-monophosphate and guanosine 3',5'-monophosphate in platelets. J. Biochem. 91: 403-406.

Terman, B. I., Slivka, S. R., Hughes, R. J. and Insel, P. A. (1987) α1-Adrenergic receptor-linked guanine nucleotide-binding protein in muscle and kidney epithelial cells. Mol. Pharm. 31: 12-20.

Yoshimasa, T., Sibley, D. R., Bouvier, M., Lefkowitz, R. J. and Caron, M. G. (1987) Cross-talk between cellular signalling pathways suggested by phorbol-ester-induced adenylate cyclase phosphorylation. Nature 327: 67-70.

ARACHIDONIC ACID METABOLITES AS MEDIATORS OF SYNAPTIC MODULATION

Andrea Volterra

Department of Pharmacology, Center for Neurobiology and Behavior, Howard Hughes Medical Institute, Columbia University, New York N.Y. 10032, U.S.A.

Present address: Center of Neuropharmacology and Institute of Pharmacological Sciences, University of Milan, Via Balzaretti 9, 20133 Milan, Italy.

ABSTRACT

The neurotransmitters histamine, dopamine and the peptide Phe-Met-Arg-Phe-NH2 (FMRFa) cause presynaptic inhibition in the nervous system of the marine mollusk Aplysia Californica by combined down-modulation of a Ca^{++} conductance and up-modulation of a K^{+} conductance. The action of FMRFa on the S-type K^{+} channels of Aplysia sensory neurons is mediated by a metabolite of the 12-lipoxygenase pathway of arachidonic acid, possibly 12-HPETE. A Pertussis toxin-sensitive GTP binding protein couples FMRFa receptor to the activation of the arachidonic cascade. Once produced, 12-HPETE does not require ATP- or GTP-dependent processes to act on the K^{+} channels, but it may directly modulate the channel via an external membrane receptor. Based on this observation, a role for eicosanoids as possible intercellular messengers in the C.N.S. is discussed.

INTRODUCTION: the action of inhibitory transmitters is mediated by a diffusable second messenger in Aplysia nervous system.

At least three different neurotransmitters - histamine, dopamine and the tetrapeptide Phe-Met-Arg-Phe-NH2 (FMRFa) - have been shown to cause presynaptic inhibition with similar ionic mechanisms in the nervous system of the marine mollusk Aplysia Californica (Abrams et al., 1984; Kretz et al., 1986; Brezina et al., 1987). The effects of FMRFa and dopamine have been studied at the level of the mechanoreceptor sensory neurons which represent the presynaptic pole of the excitatory sensory-motor connection mediating the defensive gill- and siphon-withdrawal reflex in Aplysia. When applied to a sensory neuron, the peptide FMRFamide (as well as dopamine) induces a slow hyperpolarization of the membrane potential accompanied by an increase in membrane conductance, a decrease in action potential duration, and a decrease in the transmitter release from the sensory neuron terminals (Fig. 1). Combined activation of a K^+ current and decrease of a Ca^{++} current by FMRFamide is thought to account for the presynaptic inhibitory action of the peptide. In particular, FMRFamide causes up-modulation of a specific class of K^+ channels named S-type K^+ channels (S channels) since they were first described to be closed by serotonin. These channels show outward rectification and relative voltage independence. They are at least partially open at most membrane potentials and contribute to the resting value as well as to the repolarization phase of the action potential (Siegelbaum et al., 1982). Recently, FMRFa has been shown to decrease also a transient, dihydropiridine-insensitive Ca^{++} conductance in Aplysia sensory neurons (Edmonds et al., 1988).

With the patch-clamp technique it has been possible to study the action of FMRFa at the molecular level of single S channel function. Application of FMRFa consistently induces a several-fold increase in S channel activity in cell-attached patches. This increase in activity is due to an increased probability of opening of the channels caused by the peptide (Belardetti et al., 1987).

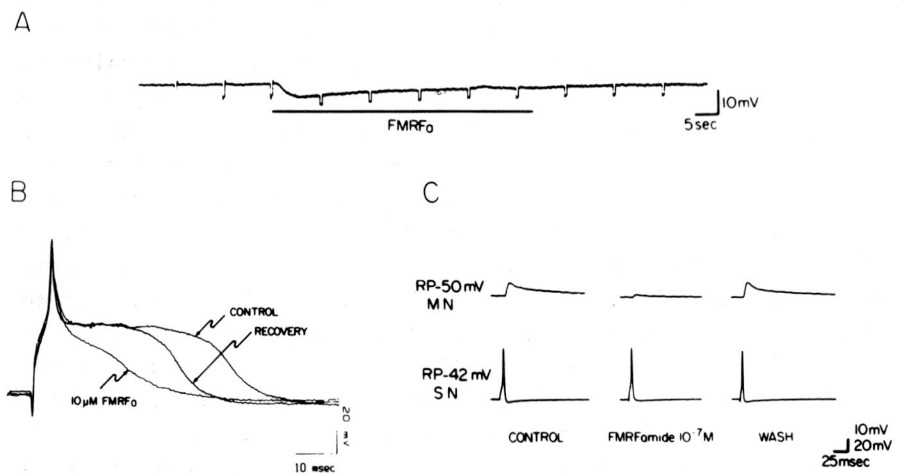

Fig. 1 - FMRFa produces a slow hyperpolarization of the sensory neuron resting potential, accompanied by an increase in membrane conductance (A), a reversible decrease in action potential duration (B), and a reduction in the fast EPSP in follower motor neuron (C:upper traces) in response to firing an action potential in sensory neuron (C:lower traces).

The above experiment provides another important piece of information: FMRFa must act on the S channels through an internal second messenger. Thus, the patch pipette in the cell-attached mode forms a very stable, high resistance seal with the cell membrane that is thought to prevent diffusion of transmitters applied externally to the area under the patch pipette where channel activity is recorded. This observation implies that internal second messengers must exist that diffuse within the cell to couple the FMRFa receptors to the K^+ channels under the pipette.

Lipoxygenase metabolites of arachidonic acid mediate the action of the inhibitory transmitters.

What is the identity of the second messenger system activated by FMRFa? None of the major known diffusable second messengers proved to be a good candidate in mediating FMRFamide action. Thus, FMRFa does induce neither increase nor decrease in cAMP accumulation in intact sensory neurons. Moreover, neither IP_3, nor phorbol esters (protein kinase C activators) nor cGMP, when applied to sensory neurons, simulate FMRFa effects. Many transmitter receptors are thought to be directly coupled to ion channels via a GTP-binding protein (G protein) (Dunlap et al., 1987). Many lines of evidence argue against this mechanism in FMRFa action (see also next paragraph): in particular, application of GTP-gamma-S, an irreversible G protein activator, to cell-free inside-out patches proved ineffective in increasing S channel activity (Buttner, Siegelbaum & Volterra, unpublished results). The first clue as to the nature of the second messenger utilized by FMRFa action came from a biochemical study of arachidonic acid metabolism in Aplysia (Piomelli et al., 1987a). This study showed that arachidonic acid is a prominent component of membrane phospholipids in Aplysia nervous tissue and is metabolized by two major kinds of enzymatic pathways, a ciclooxygenase pathway and two (5- and 12-) lipoxygenase pathways. Moreover, release of arachidonic acid and formation of lipoxygenase metabolites is a receptor-mediated process, induced by the modulatory transmitter histamine and blocked by the histamine receptor antagonist cimetidine. When applied to isolated sensory neuron clusters preincubated with ^3H-arachidonic acid, FMRFa caused a marked release of radioactive material, which, following reverse-phase HPLC chromatography, was identified as a mixture of products of the 5- and 12-lipoxygenase metabolism (Piomelli et al., 1987b). In order to assess whether this effect of the peptide is related to its action in channel modulation, experiments utilizing inhibitors of arachidonic acid metabolism were carried out. Both bromophenacylbromide - a phospholipase inhibitor that blocks release of arachidonic acid from membranes - and nordihydroguaiaretic acid - which preferentially blocks lipoxygenases - but not indomethacin - a cicloxygenase inhibitor - were able to block the hyperpolarizing response of the sensory neurons to FMRFa. These results confirm that the effects of FMRFa are mediated by arachidonic acid metabolites and suggest that lipoxygenase, rather than cyclooxigenase metabolites are involved in the response. Recently, it has been shown that the same inhibitors block also dopamine action on the sensory neurons (Yaari, 1988). One prediction from the above observations is that either arachidonic acid or its active lipoxygenase products should mimic the effects of FMRFa and dopamine on sensory cell ionic conductances. When tested, both arachidonic acid and 12-hydroperoxyeicosatetraenoic acid (12-HPETE), the first unstable product of the 12-lipoxygenase pathway, proved very effective in simulating the effects of the inhibitory transmitters on the sensory neuron resting potential and on the action potential duration. 12-HPETE was the most potent compound, being markedly more effective than the 5-lipoxygenase derivative, 5-HPETE, and than the two reduction products, 12-hydroxyeicosatetrenoic acid (12-HETE) and 5-HETE, which proved almost ineffective (Piomelli et al., 1987b). Therefore, 12-HPETE is a good candidate for the active second messenger in FMRFa's and dopamine's action. However, it has been recently shown that 12-HPETE in Aplysia can be further processed to other compounds, some of which are active on ionic conductances (Piomelli et al. 1989).

A Pertussis toxin-sensitive GTP-binding protein is involved in the receptor-mediated activation of the arachidonic acid cascade.

At this point, studies were carried out to assess how the arachidonic acid cascade is activated by the receptors for inhibitory transmitters. Several mechanisms have been described in vertebrate cells for receptor-induced release of arachidonic acid from membrane phospholipids, including indirect activation of phospholipase A_2 following an increase in intracellular Ca^{++}, intracellular alkalinization due to Na^+/H^+ exchange or direct phospholipase activation via GTP-binding proteins. In Aplysia sensory neurons FMRFa receptor activation seems to require an increase neither in intracellular Ca^{++} nor in pH (Blumenfeld et al., 1988), whereas a role for a G protein at a stage before arachidonic acid release has been clearly demonstrated (Volterra and Siegelbaum, 1988). The intracellular Ca^{++} levels were measured using the fluorescent Ca^{++} indicator dye Fura-2. No appreciable changes in resting intracellular Ca^{++} levels were detected in response to FMRFa concentrations that induced marked effects on the sensory cell S current. Moreover, when the internal pH was measured with the pH-sensitive dye BCECF, no changes were seen in response to FMRFa application. The peptide also did not speed the recovery from acidification following exposure to NH_3, arguing against a marked stimulation of the Na^+/H^+ exchange. Next, a possible role for G proteins in the response to FMRFa was investigated. As a first step, GTP-gamma-S was iontophoretically injected into sensory neurons. The nucleotide produced a slow, irreversible hyperpolarization of the membrane potential associated with an increase in conductance, due to activation of an outward current with the characteristics of the S current. Moreover, GTP-gamma-S altered the kinetics of the normally transient hyperpolarization in response to FMRFa into an irreversible response. On the contrary, the hyperpolarization following arachidonic acid application was not affected by the presence of GTP-gamma-S. Evidence for an obligatory role of G proteins in the response to FMRFa came when the bacterial toxin Pertussis toxin, which blocks the activation of several distinct G proteins through covalent ADP-rybosilation, was pressure injected into the sensory neurons. Pertussis toxin almost completely abolished the FMRFa-induced hyperpolarization in a long-lasting manner. In the same experiment, the arachidonic acid response was not affected. However, preincubation of the sensory neurons with either p-bromophenacylbromide or nordihydroguaiaretic acid - two blockers of the arachidonic acid cascade - prevented the GTP-gamma-S-induced hyperpolarization. Taking together these data, they suggest that a Pertussis toxin-sensitive G protein mediating FMRFa action is involved at an early stage in the intracellular cascade, before arachidonic acid release, probably coupling FMRFa receptor to phospholipase activation. No other G proteins seem to be involved in the cascade. In particular, no G protein seems to mediate S channel modulation by the lipoxygenase metabolites.

Lipoxygenase metabolites directly modulate S-K^+ channel activity in cell-free patches

Among the possible molecular mechanisms leading to ion channel modulation by second messengers, phosphorylation (e.g. cAMP-dependent phosphorylation of L-type Ca^{++} channels following beta-adrenergic receptor activation in the heart) or direct interaction (e.g. cGMP binding to the cationic channels in the rod outer segments) have been described. The experiments illustrated in the previous section rule out activation of a GTP-binding protein as a possible mechanism to couple the lipoxygenase metabolites to the S channel. Another likely possibility is that the arachidonic acid cascade activates a phosphoprotein phosphatase. Thus, FMRFa has been shown to induce protein dephosphorylation in Aplysia sensory neurons (Volterra et al., 1988). A reversible modulatory action through a phosphorylation/ dephosphorylation process involves an enzyme-driven transfer of a phosphate group to or from a substrate protein. In order to distinguish between this possibility and a direct action, cell-free patch-clamp experiments - where a small patch of membrane containing the active channels is excised from the remaining of the cell - have been undertaken, where S channel modulation by lipoxygenase metabolites has been evaluated after replacing the internal cell medium with an artificial one lacking the high energy nucleotide ATP, the phosphate group donor (Buttner, Siegelbaum & Volterra, submitted). In experiments utilizing cell-free inside-out patches, where the cytoplasmic side of the membrane is exposed to the bathing solution, application of 12-HPETE induced a clear, reversible increase in S channel activity. The reduced derivative 12-HETE proved only slightly effective, and arachidonic acid was totally devoid of activity. This data suggests that arachidonic acid, which is very potent in increasing S channel activity in cell-attached patches, in order to act requires some internal factor (probably the 12-lipoxygenase enzyme) which is washed away in the cell-free patches. On the contrary, 12-HPETE is still effective when applied to the isolated patches of membrane, even in absence of ATP (and GTP). This observation makes phosphorylation an unlikely mechanism of 12-HPETE action. Similarly, dephosphorylation is unlikely because it cannot explain the reversible nature of the increase in S channel opening with 12-HPETE. Therefore, 12-HPETE may act directly on the S channel or a protein coupled to the S channel in the cell-free patches.

However, 12-HPETE, when applied to inside-out patches seems in some way less effective and slower in its action than when applied to intact sensory neurons, as seen with intracellular recording. One possible explanation for this fact is that the 12-HPETE site of action on the S channel is on the outer side of the membrane and, for this reason, it is not easily accessible to the metabolite in the inside-out configuration. To test this idea,

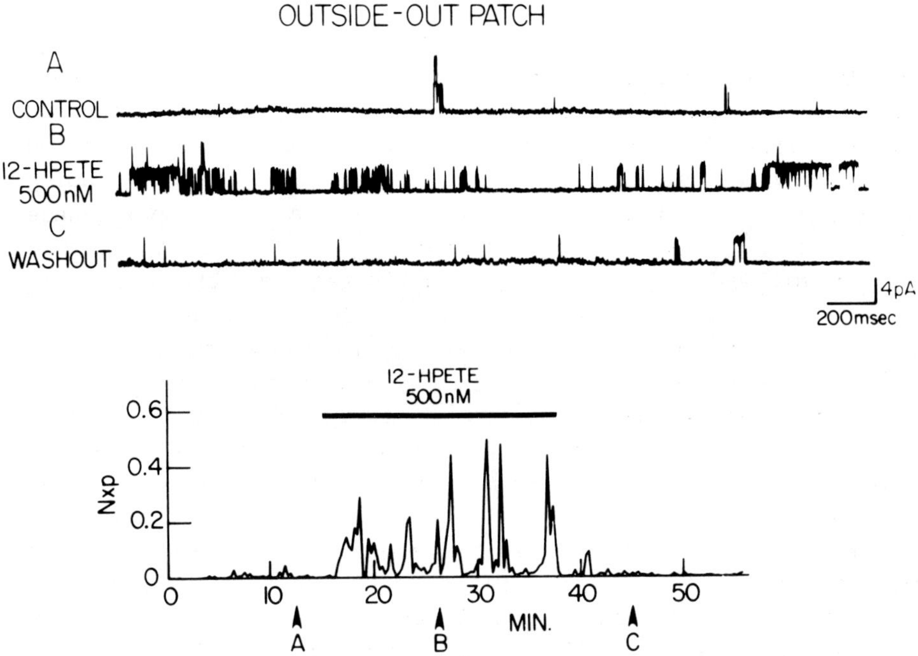

Fig. 2 - 12-HPETE increases S-K^+ channel activity in cell-free outside-out patches of membrane. Upper part: records of single S channel currents before (A), during (B) and after washout (C) of 500 nM 12-HPETE. Lower part: Analysis of channel activity measured as Np (number of channels x open probability) during entire experiment shown in the upper part.

experiments in the cell-free outside-out configuration were carried out, where the outer side of the membrane was exposed to the metabolites. Again, arachidonic acid and 12-HETE proved almost ineffective, in parallel to what seen in the inside-out experiments. On the contrary, 12-HPETE was markedly more effective and faster in increasing S channel activity (Fig. 2). In particular, the threshold concentration of 12-HPETE for an appreciable effect on S channel activity was at least two orders of magnitude lower in outside-out vs. inside-out experiments, ranging approximately around 50 nM (Buttner et al., 1989). Interestingly, it has been recently reported that a metabolite of 12-HPETE, 8-hydroxy-11, 12-epoxyeicosatrienoic acid (8-HEpETE or Hepoxilin A) has a similar potency in modulating S channels in inside-out patches (Belardetti et al., 1988). Therefore, the possibility exists that 12-HPETE and its metabolites may act at two sites on S channel function: an external site that responds to 12-HPETE at concentrations above 50 nM, and an internal site, that is preferentially activated by 12-HPETE metabolites, possibly involving 8-HEpETE (Fig. 3).

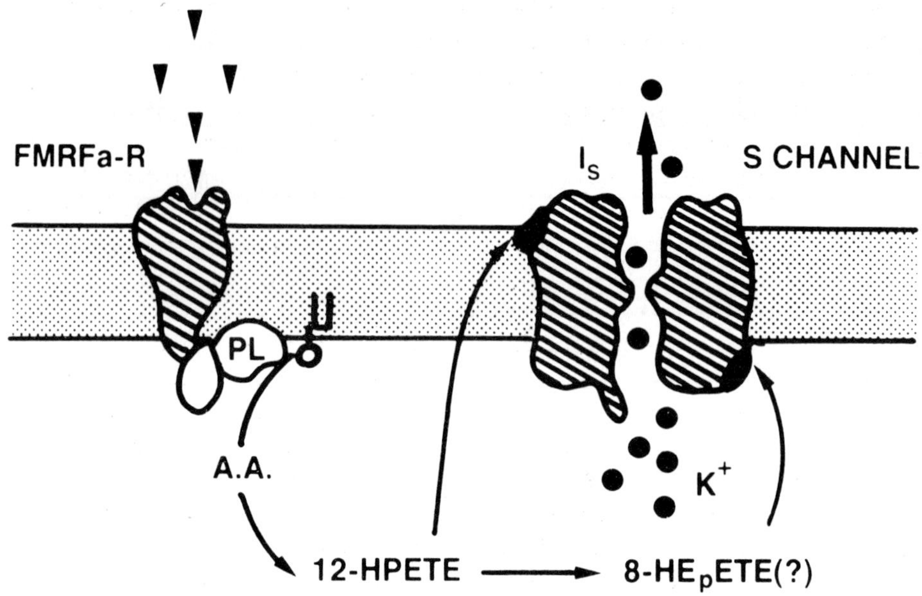

Fig. 3 - Model for S channel modulation by 12-HPETE and downstream metabolites. Binding of FMRFa to receptor (R) activates a pertussis-toxin sensitive G protein which then activates phospholipase (PL) leading to release of arachidonic acid. 12-HPETE produced through action of 12-lipoxygenase may directly interact with site near outer surface of membrane. In addition, further metabolism of 12-HPETE, perhaps to 8-HEpETE (see text), produces compounds that may act at inner surface of membrane.

CONCLUDING REMARKS: Lipoxygenase metabolites of arachidonic acid may be relevant to cell-to-cell communication in the C.N.S.

In this review we have seen that lipoxygenase metabolites of arachidonic acid mediate the presynaptic inhibitory action of FMRFa in Aplysia sensory neurons. This role for arachidonic acid metabolites in ion channel modulation is not unique to FMRFa action or to Aplysia sensory neurons. Thus, dopamine, acting through a D-2-like receptor, is also able to induce an increase in the sensory neuron S current that is inhibited by nordihydroguaiaretic acid (but not indomethacin). Presynaptic inhibition of the L10 neuron in the abdominal ganglion of Aplysia is induced by histamine which activates the 12-lipoxygenase pathway. In the neuroinhibitory action of FMRFa and dopamine it has been clearly shown that lipoxygenase metabolites increase a K^+

channel activity, probably via a direct action. A similar effect for lipoxygenase metabolites has been recently described in heart atrial miocytes: here, 5-lipoxygenase products activate (even in cell-free patches) a class of K^+ channels that are modulated by acethylcholine (Kurachi et al., 1989; Kim et al., 1989).

Arachidonic acid metabolites differ from other intracellular second messengers in one important way: they can cross the cell membrane and leave the cell in which they are generated to act on neighbouring cells due to their amphiphylic nature. This phenomenon has been clearly demonstrated in the cross-talk between platelets and vascular endothelium. The present data suggests that arachidonic acid metabolites may have a similar role in the C.N.S. Thus, 12-HPETE seems to bind to surface receptors and thereby directly modulate ion channel activity. Based on this evidence, it is conceivable that 12-HPETE may exert its action not only on the cell where it has been produced, but also on a neighbouring one, possibly the opposite side of a synaptic connection. The existance of a trans-synaptic messenger able to bring a signal from a postsynaptic cell to a presynaptic one, could explain the operation of Hebbian synapses, of the kind postulated to be important for long-term potentiation (LTP) of pyramidal cells in the CA_1 region of the hippocampus. In this region, a glutamate-induced depolarization of the postsynaptic pyramidal neurons in response to repetitive stimulation of afferent inputs leads to enhanced release of glutamate from the presynaptic region. Indeed, recent evidence suggests a role for the arachidonic acid cascade in this phenomenon. Thus, stimulation of the NMDA-type of glutamate receptors, which is central to LTP induction, leads to release of arachidonic acid and some lipoxygenase metabolites (Dumuis et al., 1988; Wolfe and Pellerin, 1988). Moreover, induction of LTP in the hippocampal dentate gyrus as well as in the CA_1 region can be prevented by the lipoxygenase blocker nordihydroguaiaretic acid (Williams and Bliss, 1988).

REFERENCES

1. Abrams T.W., Castellucci V.F., Camardo J.S., Kandel E.R. and Lloyd P.E., (1984) Two endogenous neuropeptides modulate the gill and siphon withdrawl reflex in Aplysia by presynaptic facilitation involving cAMP-dependent closure of a serotonin-sensitive potassium channel. Proc.Natl.Acad.Sci.USA, **81**, 7956-7960
2. Belardetti F., Kandel E.R. and Siegelbaum S.A., (1987) Neuronal inhibition by the peptide FMRFamide involves opening

of S K^+ channels. Nature, **325**, 153-156

3. Belardetti F., Campbell W., Charbert P., Falck J.R., Mioskowsky C. and Rosolowsky M., (1988) A novel molecular mechanism for presynaptic inhibition: the arachidonic derivative hepoxilin - A directly acts on the serotonin-sensitive "S" K^+ channel to increase its opening in Aplysia sensory neurons. Soc.Neurosci.Abstr., **14**, 1207
4. Blumenfeld H., Bug B., Buttner N., Sweatt J.D. and Siegelbaum S.A., (1988) Does FMRFamide-stimulated release of arachidonic acid depend on Na/H exchange or internal calcium?. Soc. Neurosci.Abstr., **14**, 1206
5. Brezina V., Eckert R. and Erxleben C., (1987) Suppression of calcium current by an endogenous neuropeptide in neurones of Aplysia californica. J.Physiol., **388**, 565-596
6. Buttner N., Siegelbaum S.A. and Volterra A., (1989) 12-Lipoxygenase metabolites of arachidonic acid open single S-K^+ channels: role for an external membrane receptor?. Soc. Neurosci. Abstr., **15**, in press.
7. Dumuis A., Sebben M., Haynes M., Pin J.P. and Bockaert J., (1988) NMDA receptors activate the arachidonic acid cascade system in striatal neurons. Nature, **336**, 68-70
8. Dunlap K., Holtz G.G. and Rane S.G., (1987) G proteins as regulators of ion channel function. Trends Neurosci., **10**, 241-244
9. Edmonds B., Kandel E.R. and Klein M., (1988) Different functional roles for two components of calcium current in Aplysia sensory neurons. Soc. Neurosci.Abstr., **14**, 1206
10. Kim D., Lewis D.L., Graziadei L., Neer E.J., Bar-Sagi D. and Clapham D.E., (1989) G-protein betagamma-subunits activate the cardiac muscarinic K^+ channel via phospholipase A2. Nature, **337**, 557-560
11. Kretz R., Shapiro E. and Kandel E.R., (1986) Presynaptic inhibition produced by an identified presynaptic inhibitory neuron. I. Physiological mechanisms. J.Neurophysiol., **55**, 131-146
12. Kurachi Y., Ito H., Sugimoto T., Shimuzu T., Miki I. and Ui M., (1989) Arachidonic acid metabolites as intracellular modulators of the G protein-gated cardiac K^+ channel. Nature, **337**, 555-557
13. Piomelli D., Shapiro E., Feinmark S.J. and Schwartz J.H., (1987a) Metabolites of arachidonic acid in the nervous system of Aplysia: possible mediators of synaptic modulation. J. Neurosci., **7**, 3675-3686
14. Piomelli D., Volterra A., Dale N., Siegelbaum S.A., Kandel

E.R., Schwartz J.H. and Belardetti F., (1987b) Lipoxygenase metabolites of arachidonic acid as second messengers for presynaptic inhibition of Aplysia sensory cells. Nature, **328**, 38-43

15. Piomelli D., Shapiro E., Zipkin R., Schwartz J.H. and Feinmark S.J., (1989) Formation and action of 8-hydroxy-11, 12-epoxy-5, 9, 14-icosa trienoic acid in Aplysia: a possible second messenger in neurons. Proc.Natl.Acad.Sci.USA, **86**, 1721-1725
16. Siegelbaum S.A., Camardo J.S. and Kandel E.R., (1982) Serotonin and cyclic AMP close single K^+ channels in Aplysia sensory neurones. Nature, **299**, 413-417
17. Volterra A. and Siegelbaum S.A., (1988) Role of two different guanine nucleotide-binding proteins in the antagonistic modulation of the S-type K^+ channel by cAMP and arachidonic acid metabolites in Aplysia sensory neurons. Proc.Natl.Acad. Sci.USA, **85**, 7810-7814
18. Volterra A., Siegelbaum S.A., Kandel E.R. and Sweatt J.D., (1988) FMRFamide antagonizes S current modulation and protein phosphorylation produced by 5-HT and cAMP. Soc.Neurosci. Abstr., **14**, 152
19. Williams J.H. and Bliss T.V.P., (1988) Induction but not maintenance of calcium-induced long-term potentiation in dentate gyrus and area CA1 of the hippocampal slice is blocked by nordihydroguaiaretic acid. Neurosci.Lett., **88**, 81-85
20. Wolfe L.S. and Pellerin L., (1988) Glutamate induces 12-HETE synthesis through NMDA receptor activation in rat cerebral cortex. Soc. Neurosci. Abstr., **14**, 131
21. Yaari Y. (1988) Evidence that lipoxygenase metabolites link dopamine D_2 receptors to potassium S-channels in Aplysia sensory neurons. Soc.Neurosci.Abstr., **14**, 1205

DESTABILIZATION OF IONIZED Ca^{2+} HOMEOSTASIS IN EXCITATORY AMINO ACID NEUROTOXICITY: ANTAGONISM BY GLYCOSPHINGOLIPIDS

Manev, H., Favaron, M., De Erausquin, G., Guidotti, A., Brooker, G.* and Costa, E.

FIDIA-Georgetown Institute for the Neurosciences
and *Department of Biochemistry
3900 Reservoir Road, N.W.
Washington, D.C. 20007
U.S.A.

Introduction

An insignificant proportion of the Ca^{2+} present in tissues of higher organisms is ionized in extra and intracellular fluids while most of the body's Ca^{2+} is immobilized in a dynamic steady state in bone and teeth. Most of the intracellular ionized Ca^{2+} is compartmentalized in endoplasmic reticulum (ER) and mitochondria, and the ionized cytosolic Ca^{2+} is less than 0.1μM (Carafoli, 1987). However, the ionized Ca^{2+} pool in ER and plasma, though small in size, plays a major physiological role as a reservoir to mediate the increase in the ionized cytosolic Ca^{2+} that may occur during neuron to neuron signalling at metabolotropic and ionotropic receptors. The metabolotropic signalling device can transduce extracellular chemical signals (transmitters and neuromodulators) into precise intracellular messages by releasing Ca^{2+} from ER through the action of a second messenger (Nahorski, 1988; Meldolesi et al., 1988). When the ionized cytosolic Ca^{2+} concentrations increase, specific Ca^{2+}-dependent intracellular enzymes are activated to catalyze covalent structural modifications of neuronal proteins, including metabolotropic and ionotropic membrane receptors for neurotransmitters. When neuron to neuron signalling involves cationic channels, ionized cytosolic Ca^{2+} transiently increases (Murphy et al., 1987; Connor et al., 1988). In CNS, even minor changes in the transmembrane Ca^{2+} fluxes brought about by the transduction of transmitters at cationic receptors may produce significant changes in ionized Ca^{2+} without the participation of a second messenger response (Wroblewski and Danysz, 1989). Similar changes can also be induced, as mentioned earlier, by mobilizing Ca^{2+} from ER stores through the activation of phospholipase C and the formation of inositol 1,4,5, phosphate ($InsP_3$). Many studies have suggested that ER membranes are the site of $InsP_3$ action; others have suggested that the $InsP_3$ acts on receptors located in membranes of a newly described smooth surfaced intracellular structure termed calciosome (Meldolesi et al., 1988; Volpe et al., 1988). These $InsP_3$ receptors, located in distinct intracellular organelles, may have diverse functions: some may mediate a rapid release of Ca^{2+} from stores while those located in rough ER near the nucleus might be related to a process whereby transmitters, through $InsP_3$, transfer information from the cell membranes to the nucleus to regulate the transcriptional activation of specific genes (Ross et al., 1988).

In order to facilitate the exposition of our hypothesis that a destabilization of the delicately balanced homeostasis of ionized Ca^{2+} mediates the neurotoxic action of excitatory amino acids (EAA), we should distinguish the main mechanisms regulating the ionized intracellular Ca^{2+}. These are 1) the Ca^{2+} transporting systems of plasma membranes which include a) the transmitter modulated cationic channels that can carry Ca^{2+}, b) the voltage dependent Ca^{2+} channels, c) the $Na^{\pm}$ Ca^{2+} exchange, d) the Ca^{2+} ATPase; 2) the Ca^{2+} transporting systems across intracellular membranes which include a) the smooth ER, b) the rough ER, c) the mitochondrial transport of Ca^{2+} (for review see Carafoli, 1977; Nahorski, 1988).

An analysis of the balance between Ca^{2+} influx and efflux regulatory mechanisms indicates that homeostasis can be destabilized when cationic channels carrying Ca^{2+} are activated persistently and continuously. Such a persistent stimulation occurs during cerebral edema when EAA are released in the extracellular space. Thus, high levels of EAA become available and the unregulated stimulation of the ubiquitous cationic (Ca^{2+}) channels responsive to these transmitters ensues (Benveniste et al., 1984, 1988).

Homeostasis of cytosolic ionized Ca^{2+} during physiologically intermittent or experimentally induced persistent activation of EAA amino acid receptors

In neurons, the physiological intermittent and transient activation of ionotropic and metabolotropic EAA receptors (Wroblewski and Danysz, 1989) induces fleeting oscillations of cytosolic ionized Ca^{2+} (Connor et al., 1988) which function as a second messenger, transiently activating a number of enzymes, including Ca^{2+} and lipid dependent protein kinases (Nishizuka, 1988; Vaccarino et al., 1987). These physiological spikes of cytosolic ionized Ca^{2+} are very short lasting because of the channel kinetic properties and because of the participation of appropriate compensatory mechanisms which almost instantaneously revert Ca^{2+} levels to homeostatic conditions. Thus, as soon as the ionized cytosolic Ca^{2+} returns to its low steady state level, this signalling device is ready to function again in the transduction of new information. Furthermore, the Ca^{2+} activated enzymes, synchronously with the Ca^{2+} spikes, promptly revert to their steady state catalytic activity. Such a sequence of events follows the physiological release of EAA from axon terminal mediated by intermittent depolarization. However, in a number of pathological processes, including the paroxysmal stimulation of EAA receptors caused by continuous unrelenting EAA amino acids release during cerebral edema, the content of cytosolic ionized Ca^{2+} tends to accumulate because the specific ionized Ca^{2+} homeostasis processes become overwhelmed (Ogura et al., 1988; Manev et al., 1989a; Connor et al., 1988). We do not understand the molecular mechanisms involved but we know that in neuronal model of excitotoxicity, characterized by paroxysmal stimulation of EAA receptors, the abrupt termination of such receptor activation by receptor antagonists or EAA withdrawal is followed by a persistent increase of Ca^{2+} (Ogura, et al. 1988; Manev et al., 1989a). In figure 1 we have contrasted the duration of the increase of ionized cytosolic Ca^{2+} after termination of the EAA receptor activation elicited by an excitotoxic dose of glutamate and by a high dose of glutamate that fails to cause neuronal death. After ionized cytosolic Ca^{2+} is

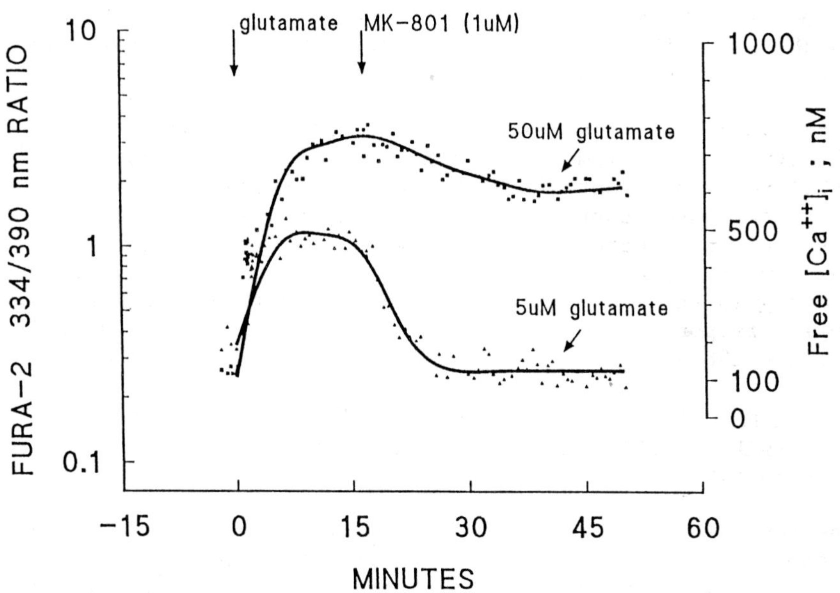

Figure 1: Neurotoxic pulse of glutamate (50μM) induces protracted elevation of free cytosolic Ca^{2+}.
Primary cultures of cerebellar granule neurons were incubated with 5μM fura-2 AM for 30 min. Thereafter, cultures were washed with Mg^{2+}-free buffer and exposed to 5 or 50μM glutamate. Glutamate exposure was terminated by perfusion (5 min at a rate of 1ml/min) with glutamate-free buffer containing 1mM $MgCl_2$ and 1μM MK-801. Background-corrected fluorescence intensity recordings from excitation at 334 and 390 nm were converted to ratios and the $[Ca^{2+}]_i$ values were calculated (Attofluor system). Presented are results of a typical experiment in which representative neurons were selected.

increased for 1 hour or longer, neuronal death within 24 hours is the inevitable consequence (Manev et al., 1989a). In this condition of abusive stimulation of EAA receptors, Ca^{2+} dependent enzymes remain activated persistently after agonist withdrawal. Consequently, these enzymes (i.e. protein kinase C) may translocate from their physiologic cytosolic domain to a domain associated with neuronal membranes and change the tertiary structure of important proteins located proximally to their site of translocation. Among various molecular forms of protein kinase C (PKC) (Nishizuka, 1988) that are translocated from cytosol to the plasma membrane domain during the pathological state elicited by continuous EAA receptor stimulation are those including in their structure lipophylic domains, facilitating a specific binding of the enzyme to phosphatidylserine and diacylglycerol molecules associated with the neuronal membrane (Huang et al., 1989). In fact, the sustained increase in extent and duration of ionized cytosolic Ca^{2+} shifts the steady state of PKC from an equilibrium in which the molecular form of PKC_S (soluble PKC) prevails over the PKC_{MB} (membrane bound PKC) to a new equilibrium where PKC_{MB} becomes the prevailing molecular form of the enzyme. Probably, the sustained increase of ionized Ca^{2+} has an additional action on phosphoprotein phosphatases, maintaining a high level of phosphorylation in proteins functioning in Ca^{2+} homeostasis. This modification may contribute to a destabilization of ionized Ca^{2+} regulatory mechanisms.

The data of figure 1 show that in primary cultures of cerebellar granule cells the duration of the transient increase of free Ca^{2+} becomes a function of the concentration of glutamate added to the cultures. In the presence of a prolongation of the increase in ionized cytosolic Ca^{2+}, the duration of the shift in the molecular transition of PKC from PKC_S to PKC_{MB} is also greatly prolonged (Fig. 2).

Since the duration of the change in the equilibrium among the two molecular forms of PKC occurs as a function of glutamate concentration and the consequent persistence of the increase in ionized cytosolic Ca^{2+} content, one might infer that, in vivo, the neurons close to the source of unrelenting release of glutamate exhibit a protracted increase in PKC_{MB}. One might surmise that the increase in the number of PKC molecules associated with the membrane is a triggering point for the long-term destabilization of the of cytosolic ionized Ca^{2+} homeostasis. If this were the case, then prevention of this shift in the steady state equilibrium of PKC favoring PKC_{MB} might become an important target to be used in the study of drugs that limit glutamate neurotoxicity. However, it appears to be difficult to dissociate increase of ionized Ca^{2+} from shifts of PKC_S/PKC_{MB} in favor of PKC_{MB}. The only instance in which this dissociation is possible, is when primary cultures are treated for a short time (20 min) with phorbol 12-myristate, 13-acetate (TPA), a PKC activator (Castagna et al., 1982). This causes a prolonged destabilization of the equilibrium

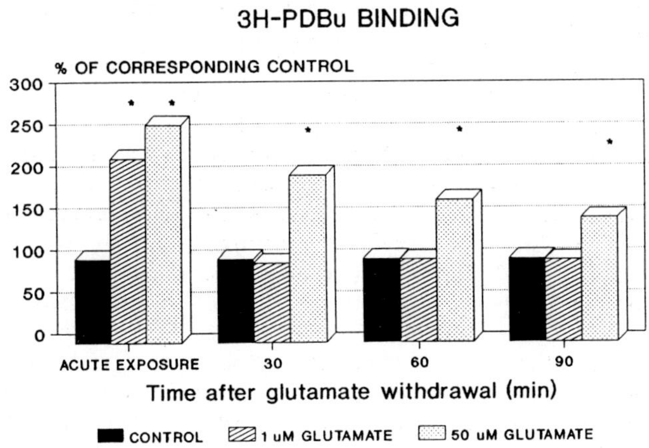

Figure 2: Dose-dependent glutamate-induced protracted increase of PKC_{MB} in cerebellar granule neurons. Protracted enhancement of ^{3}H-PDBu binding (an index of PKC_{MB}) was observed after application of higher, toxic (50μM) but not lower, nontoxic (1μM) doses of glutamate (Manev et al., 1989). Results (% of corresponding control) are means of at least three experiments. SEM did not exceed 15%. $*p<0.05$ when compared with the corresponding control.

between PKC_S/PKC_{MB} in favor of the latter without increasing ionized cytosolic Ca^{2+}. It is important to note that acute TPA treatment fails to cause neuronal death. Thus, a persistent increase of PKC_{MB}, per se, may be a process necessary, but not sufficient, to cause neurotoxicity.

<u>Role of extracellular Ca^{2+} in the destabilization of cytosolic ionized Ca^{2+} homeostasis</u>

Since PKC translocation is not sufficient to elicit glutamate neurotoxicity, one must consider whether the persistent destabilization of Ca^{2+} homeostasis is "per se" sufficient to elicit excitotoxicity. Moreover, it is important to evaluate whether this destabilization results from abnormalities in the communication between the extracellular and intracellular pools of ionized Ca^{2+} that persists after termination of EAA receptor stimulation.

The data shown in table 1 clearly indicates that a reduction of extracellular Ca^{2+} content during glutamate application dramatically reduces the excitotoxicity of this EAA. Thus, within the limits of the glutamate concentrations operative in the experiments of table 1, Ca^{2+} influx appears to be the determinant of glutamate neurotoxicity. Indeed, in absence of Ca^{2+}, the glutamate causes neuronal swelling and other signs of abnormality that persist for about 30 min following glutamate withdrawal but

TABLE 1: ION DEPENDENCY OF GLUTAMATE-INDUCED NEUROTOXICITY

Ions in Incubation Buffer			Time after 50μM Glutamate	
Mg^{++} (1 mM)	Ca^{++} (2.3 mM)	Na^{+} (154 mM)	30 min (viability: % cells alive)	24 hours
+	+	+	95	95
-	+	+	93	20
-	-	-	0	0
-	-	-[a]	95	95
-	+	-[a]	94	40

[a]154 mM NaCl was substituted by equimolar amount of choline chloride.
Cerebellar granule neurons in primary culture were exposed for 15 min to 50 uM glutamate in Locke's buffer containing the indicated concentrations of Mg^{++}, Ca^{++}, and Na^{+}. After washing, neurons were returned to the culture conditioned medium and viability was estimated by intravital staining with fluorescein diacetate\propidium iodide (Favaron et al., 1988). Results are means of a typical experiment repeated at least three times. SEM did not exceed 10%.

these changes are brief and reversible. Therefore, one might surmise that the influx of other ions secondary to the persistent activation of cationic channels by glutamate is not a cause of neurotoxicity in absence of a Ca^{2+} influx. Thus, glutamate neurotoxicity in vivo might be prevented by blocking Ca^{2+} entry through glutamate regulated channels by using specific allosteric and isosteric glutamate receptor antagonists. The validity of such inference is supported by published reports (Choi, 1988; Favaron et al., 1988). In granule cells and other CNS neurons, glutamate ionotropic receptors include two structural types of cationic channels which have a different activation specificity (Vicini et al., 1989). One (40-60 pS) is sensitive to glutamate and NMDA but not to quisqualate and kainate; the other (10-15pS) is sensitive to kainate and quisqualate but fails to respond to NMDA. The pharmacology of the high conductance channel differs from that of the low conductance channel (Wroblewski and Danysz, 1989). Thus, in neuronal cultures used as models to study glutamate neurotoxicity, blockers of the high conductance NMDA-sensitive glutamate receptors prevent neuronal death elicited by NMDA but not by kainate; conversely, blockers of kainate receptors fail to prevent NMDA-induced neuronal death (Favaron et al., 1988; Manev et al., 1989a). However, such a protective mechanisms cannot be safely used <u>in vivo</u> to antagonize the neurotoxicity elicited by glutamate released during brain edema and ischemia. In fact, glutamatergic synapses represent about 30% of CNS synapses which function in the regulation of several vital processes. Hence, one cannot block persistently NMDA receptors without causing an important reduction in the ability of brain to compensate for those mechanisms that are affected by the primary source of glutamate damage. Thus, blockers of NMDA receptors cannot be used to limit glutamate neurotoxicity in patients with brain ischemia because they cause severe untoward effects and also impair compensatory processes. Moreover, these drugs, in the high doses required to protect from glutamate neurotoxicity, are "per se" neurotoxic (Abrahams et al., 1988; Olney et al., 1989).

That glutamate receptors play a role in the regulation of essential physiological processes is vastly supported in the literature. Moreover, the evidence that treatment of healthy animals with allosteric antagonists of EAA receptors causes neuronal degeneration (Olney et al., 1989) suggests that glutamate receptors may function in some unknown manner in the neurotrophic processes that we must preserve to assure compensatory repair of ongoing ischemic brain damage.

These considerations have suggested to us that in order to protect from glutamate neurotoxicity operative in cerebral edema and ischemias, one should devise a strategy directed to inhibit those processes that are specifically elicited by the persistent pathological stimulation of glutamate receptors. Not only must these drugs specifically inhibit those processes triggered by unrelenting, continuous and abusive stimulation of EAA receptors, but they must also act down stream from the transmitter recognition site in order to limit drug action to the area affected by the pathological process.

A departure point for the application of such research strategy to drug discovery was a report in the literature that sphingosine could inhibit the progressive accumulation of cytosolic Ca^{2+} caused by repeated prolonged application of NMDA to isolated hippocampal neurons (Connor et al., 1988). Since sphingosine was "per se" neurotoxic, we decided to test whether gangliosides which are not neurotoxic (Favaron et al., 1988) and contain sphingosine in their structure could reduce persistent accumulation of ionized cytosolic Ca^{2+} elicited by prolonged glutamate application. We believe that drug-induced limitation of glutamate-induced accumulation of ionized cytosolic Ca^{2+} may be a sign indicating an inhibition of the destabilization of ionized Ca^{2+} homeostasis induced by glutamate.

PKC translocation and ionized cytosolic Ca^{2+} homeostasis

Since the extracellular ionized Ca^{2+} functions as the reservoir subserving steady state changes of ionized cytosolic Ca^{2+}, we tested whether the PKC translocation that persists following withdrawal of neurotoxic glutamate concentrations and is associated with an increase of cytosolic ionized Ca^{2+} provided the molecular mechanism responsible for a sustained influx of extracellular Ca^{2+} that destabilizes the homeostasis of ionized cytosolic Ca^{2+}. The data of table 2 show that radioactive Ca^{2+} flows more abundantly in cultured granule cells after withdrawal of neurotoxic doses of glutamate (50μM) than in untreated granule cell cultures. Moreover, it should be noted that in this neuronal model the neurotoxic doses of glutamate are not causing immediate neuronal death but begin to cause neuronal death 2 hours after glutamate withdrawal and express their maximal cytotoxic action within 16 to 24 hours after glutamate withdrawal. Hence, the

TABLE 2: GANGLIOSIDE (GT1b) AND TPA PRETREATMENT PREVENT THE INCREASED NEURONAL 45 Ca UPTAKE IN THE POSTGLUTAMATE PERIOD

GLUTAMATE (uM)	^{45}Ca Uptake 30 min after Glutamate Removal
0	11 $\pm$ 0.6
1	12 $\pm$ 1.6
50	22 $\pm$ 1.6*
50 + GT1B	11 $\pm$ 1.4
50 + TPA	12 $\pm$ 1.3

Cerebellar granule neurons were exposed for 15 min at room temperature (22 C) to glutamate in the absence of Mg^{++}. Ganglioside pretreatment was performed by incubating the culture with 60 uM GT1b for 2 hours and removing the free ganglioside from the incubation medium prior to glutamate exposure. TPA (100 nM) pretreatment was carried out for 24 hours in order to down regulate PKC (Manev et al., 1989b) prior to glutamate exposure. After glutamate exposure, cultures were washed three times and incubated at 37 C for the next 30 min. At the end of this period, ^{45}Ca uptake was measured for 1 min (Manev et al., 1989). Results are mean $\pm$ SEM of five to six experiments. *p<0.01 in comparison with untreated control.

increased Ca^{2+} influx shown to occur in the immediate postglutamate period (Table 2) cannot be attributed to the permeability change associated with neuronal death. Thus, the persistent PKC translocation which occurs after application of neurotoxic doses of glutamate (Fig. 2) is not the only residual effect persisting after the withdrawal of neurotoxic doses of glutamate because Ca^{2+} content is also sharply elevated.

In order to decide on the causal value of PKC translocation on glutamate neurotoxicity, we treated the granule cell cultures with doses of a phorbol ester (TPA) which were known to reduce by 80% or more PKC immunoreactivity and catalytic activity. As shown in table 3, in cells with reduced PKC content and catalytic activity, the standard neurotoxic doses of glutamate used in our experiments fail to cause neurotoxicity. Moreover, in TPA treated cultures, the influx of radioactive Ca^{2+} fails to increase following the withdrawal of the doses of glutamate that are neurotoxic in normal neuronal cultures (Table 2).

TABLE 3: TPA PRETREATMENT DOWN REGULATES PKC AND PROTECTS NEURONS FROM GLUTAMATE-INDUCED DEATH

TREATMENT	PKC ACTIVITY (% control)		PKC IMMUNOREACTIVITY (% control)		VIABILITY (% cells alive) 24 h after glut.
	supernatant	pellet	supernatant	pellet	
CONTROL	100	100	100	100	20
TPA 24 h	12	8	0	29	95

Cerebellar granule neurons were exposed to 100 nM TPA or vehicle for 24 hours. PKC activity (phosphorylation of histone-III S), and PKC immunoreactivity (Western immunoblot followed by densitometric analysis) (Roth et al., 1989), were measured in the 100,000 x g supernatant and pellet fraction. In parallel, experiment cultures were exposed for 15 min to 50 uM glutamate in Mg^{++}-free medium, and viability was assayed 24 hours later (Favaron et al., 1988). Results are means of a typical experiment expressed as % of the corresponding control. SEM did not exceed 10%.

These experiments suggest that PKC translocation might have two roles: 1) It is a necessary, albeit insufficient step in mediating the neurotoxic action of the doses of glutamate used in our experiments. 2) It is a necessary and sufficient step to cause the persistent influx of Ca^{2+} during the postglutamate period if associated with persistent influx of Ca^{2+} in the period of abusive stimulation of NMDA-sensitive glutamate receptors. It is possible that when PKC translocation occurs in association with high levels of cytosolic ionized Ca^{2+} it destabilizes the regulation of the homeostasis of ionized cytosolic Ca^{2+}. As a corollary of these suggestions, we propose that the phosphorylation of one of the membrane components regulating Ca^{2+} homeostasis may reduce its function and facilitate persistence of high levels of ionized cytosolic Ca^{2+}. Perhaps, this phosphorylation by impairing Ca^{2+} ATPase may also facilitate Ca^{2+} fluxes from the extracellular space to the cytosol.

Inhibitors of glutamate neurotoxicity acting downstream of the glutamate regulated cationic channels

As mentioned above, because of the consideration given to Ca^{2+} in the genesis of the neurotoxicity elicited by glutamate, and the knowledge that sphingosine-inhibited Ca^{2+} accumulation elicited in neurons by NMDA, this molecule became a natural prototype for the design of drugs to be studied as antagonists of EAA induced neurotoxicity. In fact, sphingosine inhibits Ca^{2+} and lipid dependent kinases (Hannun and Bell, 1989; Vaccarino, 1987). However, we found that sphingosine could not be used as an antagonist of glutamate neurotoxicity due to its strong direct cytolytic action. Since natural gangliosides are sphingosine-related molecules and are devoid of intrinsic neurotoxicity, we tested whether gangliosides act on glutamate-regulated cationic channels. We found that GM_1 and GT_{1B} (see fig. 3 for structure) do not change the glutamate regulation of high and low conductance cationic channels sensitive to NMDA and kainic acid, respectively. Then we tested whether these compounds could protect from glutamate neurotoxicity and our results showed that glutamate neurotoxicity was markedly reduced in granule cells incubated with GM_1 or GT_{1B} for two hours and then thoroughly washed before application of neurotoxic doses of glutamate (Fig. 4). Gangliosides not only inhibit the neurotoxicity but also block

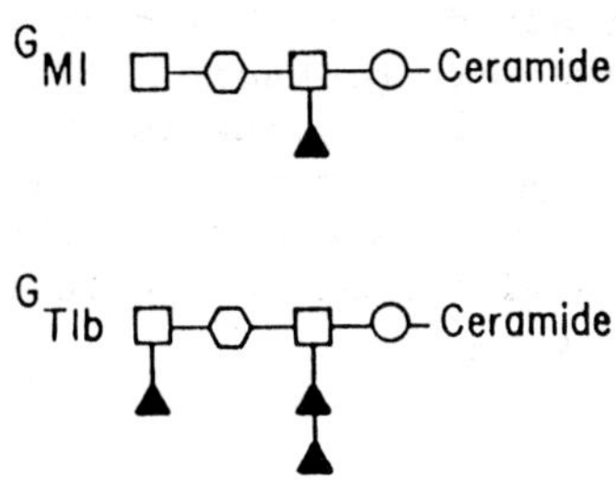

Figure 3: Chemical structure of gangliosides GM1 and GT1b. Symbols: circle, glucose; square, galactose; hexagon, N-acetylgalactosamine, filled triangle, neraminic acid.

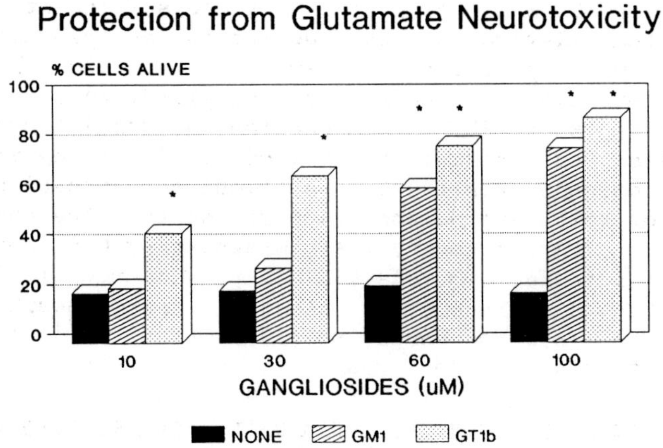

Figure 4: Gangliosides prevent glutamate-induced neuronal death.
Cerebellar granule neurons in primary culture were incubated with the indicated concentrations of gangliosides (GM1, GT1b) for 2 hours. Thereafter, cultures were washed three times and exposed to 50 μM glutamate, 15 min in absence of Mg^{++}. Following the removal of glutamate, cultures were returned to the culture-containing medium, and viability was estimated 24 hours later (Favaron et al., 1988). Results are means of at least five experiments. SEM did not exceed 15%. *$p<0.05$ in comparison with glutamate treated control.

the persistent high levels of ionized Ca^{2+} (Table 2) and the sustained translocation of PKC (Manev et al., 1989a) elicited by the neurotoxic doses of glutamate which persist even after EAA has been withdrawn from the culture media. Thus, GM_1 and GT_{1B} are the prototypes of a new class of drugs that reduce neurotoxicity without blocking the physiological transient increase of ionized cytosolic Ca^{2+} elicited by EAA applied either in low doses or intermittently to mimic the physiological action of glutamate. In contrast, gangliosides block the glutamate neurotoxicity that depends on the protracted destabilization of ionized cytosolic Ca^{2+} homeostasis which is probably mediated by the prolonged translocation of PKC. To distinguish this new type of glutamate neurotoxicity antagonism, we propose the term of "receptor abuse dependent antagonism". Consequently, the drugs acting in a mode similar to that of gangliosides can be termed RADA (Receptor Abuse Dependent Antagonists) drugs.

REFERENCES

1. Abrahams, T.P., Gillis, R.A., Hamosh, P. and Taveria Da Silva, A.M. (1988) Soc. Neurosci. Abstr., 14, 937.

2. Benveniste, H., Drejer, J., Schousboe, A. and Diemer, N.H. (1984) J. Neurochem., 43, 1369-1374.
3. Benveniste, H., Jorgesen, M.B., Diemer, N.H. and Hansen, J.A. (1988) Acta Neurol. Scand., 78, 529-536.
4. Carafoli, E. (1987) Ann. Rev. Biochem., 56, 395-433.
5. Castagna, M., Takai, Y., Kaibuchi, K., Sano K., Kikkawa, U. and Nishizuka, Y. (1982) J. Biol. Chem., 257, 7847-7851.
6. Choi, D.W. (1988) Neuron, 1, 623-634.
7. Connor, J.A., Wadman, W.J., Hockberger, P.E. and Wong, R.K.S. (1988) Science, 240, 649-656.
8. Favaron, M., Manev, H., Alho, H., Bertolino, M., Ferret, B., Guidotti, A. and Costa, E. (1988) Proc. Natl. Acad. Sci. USA, 85, 7351-7355.
9. Hannun, Y.A. and Bell, R.M. (1989) Science, 243, 500-507.
10. Huang, F.L., Yoshida, Y., Cunha-Melo, J.R., Beaven, M.A. and Huang, K.P. (1989) J. Biol. Chem. 264, 4238-4243.
11. Manev, H., Favaron, M., Guidotti, A. and Costa, E. (1989a) Molec. Pharmacol., 36, 106-112.
12. Manev, H., Favaron, M., Brooker, G., Guidotti, A. and Costa, E. (1989b) Soc. Neurosci. Abstr., 15, 479.
13. Meldolesi, J., Volpe P. and Pozzan, T. (1988) TINS, 11,449-452.
14. Murphy, S.N., Thayer, S.A. and Miller, R.J. (1987) J. Neurosc., 7(12), 4145-4158.
15. Nahorski, S.R. (1988) TINS, 11, 444-448.
16. Nishizuka, Y. (1988) Nature, 334, 661-665.
17. Olney, J.W., Labruyere, J. and Price, M.T. (1989) Science, 244, 1360-1362.
18. Ogura, A., Miyamoto, M. and Kudo, Y. (1988) Exp. Brain. Res., 73, 447-458.
19. Ross, C.A., Meldolesi, J., Milner, T.A., Satoh, T., Supattapone, S. and Snyder S.H. (1989) Nature, 339, 468-470.
20. Roth, B.L., Mehagan, J.P., Jacobowitz, D.M., Robey, F. and Iadarola, M.J. (1989) J. Neurochem., 52, 215-221.
21. Vaccarino, F., Guidotti, A. and Costa, E. (1987) Proc. Natl. Acad. Sci. USA, 84, 8707-8711.
22. Vicini, S., Bertolino, M. and Costa, E. (1989) Allosteric Modulation of Amino Acid Receptors: Therapeutic Implications, Raven Press, New York, pp. 249-257.
23. Volpe, P., Krausen, K.H., Hashimoto, S., Zorzato, F., Pozzan, T., Meldolesi, J. and Lew, D.P. (1988) Proc. Natl. Acad. Sci. USA, 85, 1091-1095.
24. Wroblewski, J.T. and Danysz, W. (1989) Ann. Rev. Pharmacol. Toxicol., 29, 441-474.